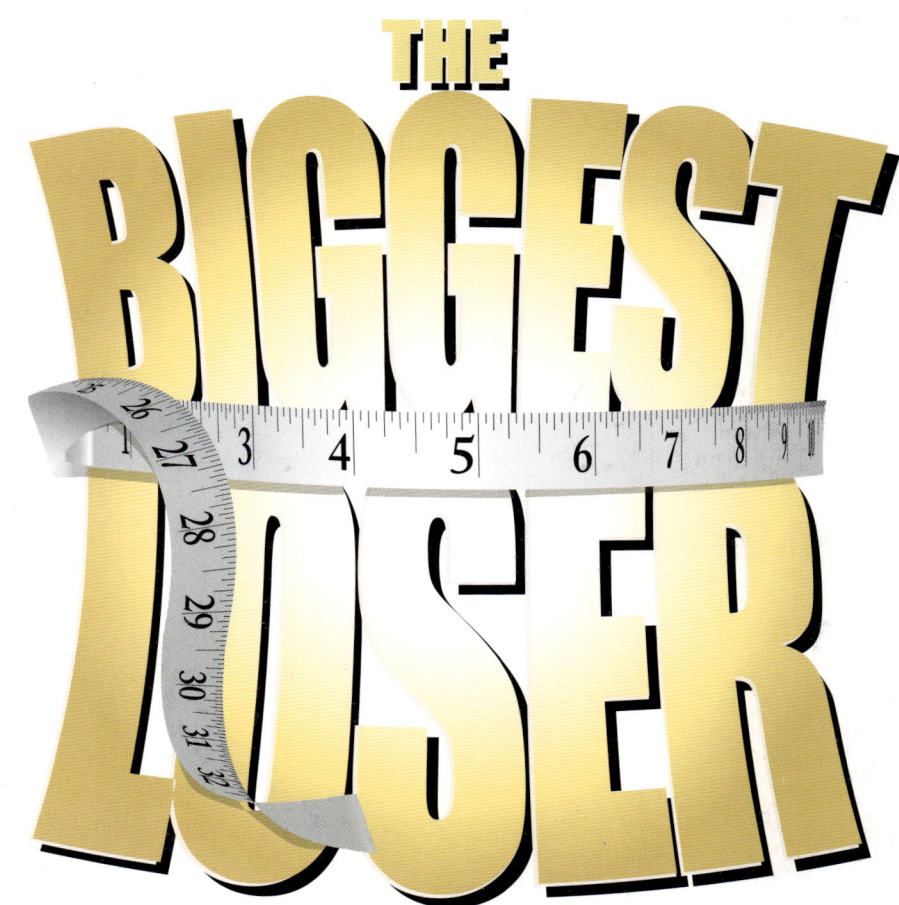

THE BIGGEST LOSER

Change Your Life

The diet and fitness program to help you lose weight and keep it off

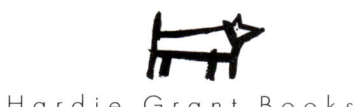

Hardie Grant Books

Published in 2007 by
Hardie Grant Books
85 High Street
Prahran, Victoria 3181, Australia
www.hardiegrant.com.au

All rights reserved. No part of this publication may be reproduced, stored in a retrieval system or transmitted in any form by any means, electronic, mechanincal, photocopying or otherwise, without the prior written permission of the publisher, copyright holders and trademark owners.

The moral right of the authors has been asserted.

Copyright text © Hardie Grant Books 2007
Copyright photography (food) © Ian Hofstetter 2007

Photography on pages 3, 14, 46, 63, 78, 92: istockphoto.com

Cataloguing-in-Publication Data is available from the National Library of Australia.

ISBN 13: 978 1 74066 500 1
ISBN 10: 1 74066 500 7

Printed in China by SNP Leefung

10 9 8 7 6 5 4 3 2

Disclaimer
The information provided in this book is for general reference only. It is not a substitute for professional medical advice or an individualised health program. See a doctor before you begin any diet and exercise program. The publisher has taken care in researching and preparing this book, but accepts no responsibility for any claims arising from the material within this book.

The Biggest Loser is a trademark of Reveille LLC and operated under licence by FremantleMedia Australia Pty Limited.
The Biggest Loser is produced by FremantleMedia Australia Pty Limited in association with Reveille LLC.
www.fremantlemedia.com

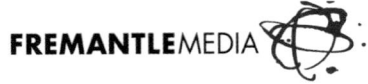

Project editor
Alexandra Payne

Authors
Carolyn Bell
Alexandra Payne
Sophie Russell

The Biggest Loser consultants
Dr Clare Collins,
PhD, BSc, Dip Nutr&Diet,
Dip Clin Epi, AdvAPD
Shannan Ponton,
Cert IV Personal Training, NSCA Level II
Strength & Conditioning Coach,
SMA Level I Sports Trainer

Cover and text design
Ellie Exarchos

Food and exercise photography
Ian Hofstetter

Food styling
Katy Holder

Food preparation
Wendy Quisumbing

Food props
MUD Australia
David Edmonds

Text layout
Pauline Haas, bluerinse setting

Contents

Foreword vii

Part 1: READY?

Why are you reading this book?	2
Why lose weight?	4
Are you overweight?	6
Why are you overweight?	8
How do you lose weight?	12
Setting lifestyle and health goals	18
Dealing with bad days	23

Part 2: SET

THE BIGGEST LOSER EATING PLAN — 27

How much food do you need?	28
What to eat	31
What to drink	34
10 Biggest Loser steps to weight-loss success	37
The KickStart Plan	48
The LifeStyle Plan	50
What is healthy eating?	53

THE BIGGEST LOSER EXERCISE PLAN — 61

Why exercise?	62
The Biggest Loser programs	64
Where do you start?	66
7 Biggest Loser steps to fitness success	72
What else do you need to know?	76

Part 3: GO!

THE KICKSTART PLAN — 83

Eating	84
Exercise	92

THE LIFESTYLE PLAN — 97

Eating	98
Exercise – Program 1	108
Exercise – Program 2	119

THE EXERCISES — 129

RECIPES FOR LIFE — 147

Breakfasts	148
Soups, salads and light meals	166
Dinners	194
Desserts and sweet treats	231

Index 243

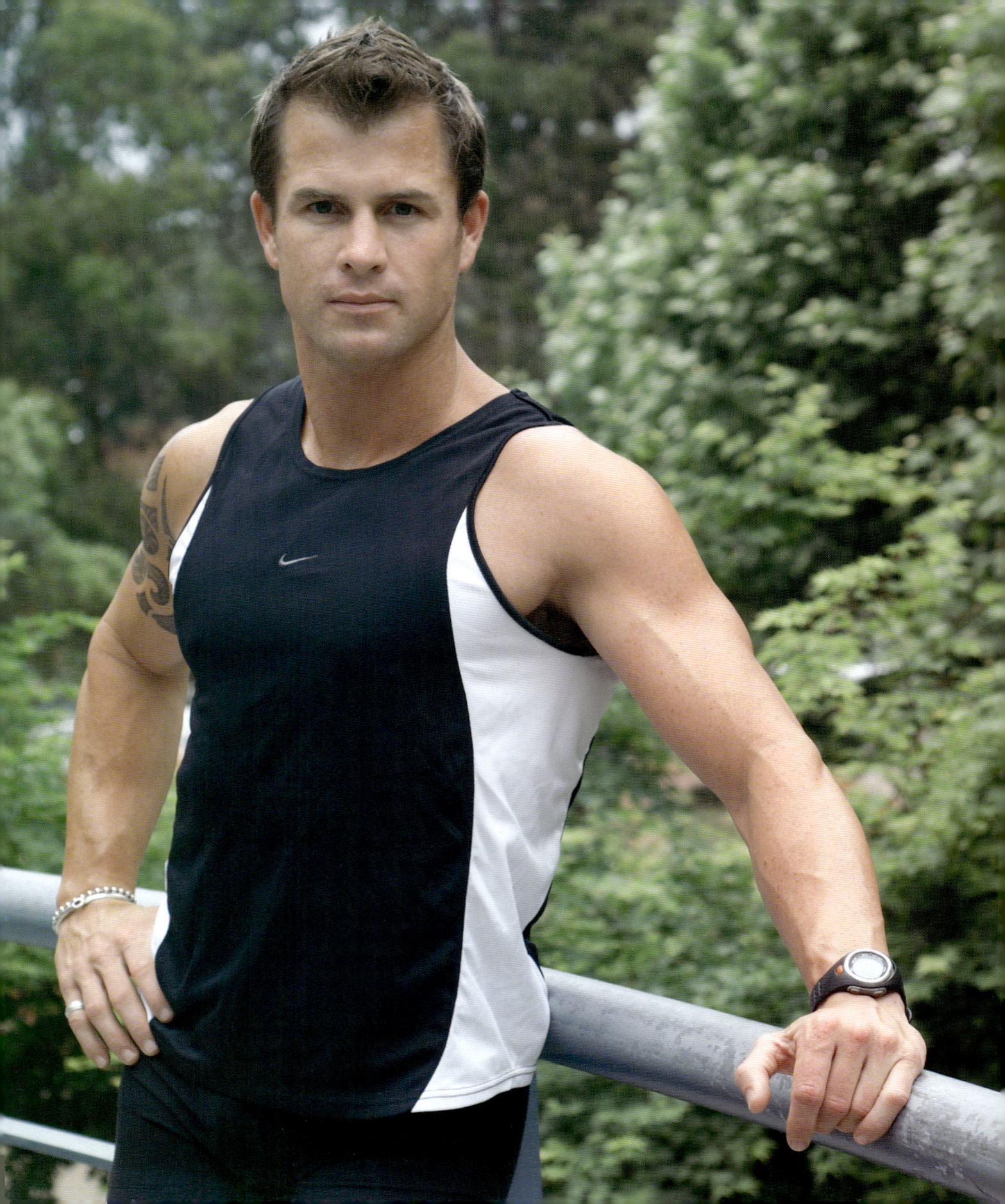

Foreword

The Biggest Loser. What does it mean to you? Well, for a start I can tell you what it means to me.

As a personal trainer, all day, every day, my job is to help people – people who have lost self-esteem, who have lost self-belief but who are ready and willing to commit to transforming their lives. With determination and a positive attitude, they change their lives forever. Their joy gives me the biggest buzz and seeing people develop mentally and physically keeps me motivated and passionate. This is why I love being a personal trainer – seeing people conquer challenges, stay the course and triumph over hardship and adversity.

Maybe that's what you liked about *The Biggest Loser*. All over the world, the show has had an incredibly positive impact on people who thought they could never ever lose weight or change their lives. *The Biggest Loser* shows that anyone, regardless of shape or level of fitness, can completely transform themselves, their bodies and their lives. All you need is self-belief, motivation and support, and that's where this book will help you.

In a straightforward, easy-to-understand way, it explains the training, nutrition and psychology that will help you to lose weight. And you will lose weight – it works! No question. But you have to put your mind to it, set your goals and never compromise or kid yourself because, yes, it's going to get tough. Just remember to focus on the end result and imagine how good you're going to feel putting on clothes you never thought you could fit into, or proudly showing off your six-pack, or going for a run, or knowing that your kids are not embarrassed about you, or being able to go to the beach and look and feel fantastic.

You *are* worth taking your health and fitness seriously: it will save your life. It's that serious. Type 2 diabetes is increasing at an enormous rate and heart disease kills tens of thousands of Australians each year. If you're fit and healthy, the chance of one of these diseases killing you will be dramatically reduced. You won't get a second chance, so your long-term health is vitally important. And, of course, looking good and feeling great come a close second!

Take what you learn from this book and have the courage and determination to apply it to your own life. On the show and as a personal trainer, I want people to understand the value of self-belief and discipline – these are the values of true champions – and that losing weight is about eating less, moving more and being disciplined and committed. There is no easy way.

It's so awesome to see the change in the people I work with. They change their lifestyle, lose weight and then wake up daily with incredible energy and a new found zest for life – it's priceless. These people suddenly have real purpose and direction every day. There shouldn't be a person on earth who wouldn't want to feel that way. Do you want to feel that good? Take responsibility for your life, stand up and know that you can handle all the challenges life throws at you. *You* are in charge of your transformation. Just cut the excuses, believe in yourself and DO IT! You owe it to yourself.

You can do this – I believe in you.

Shannan Ponton

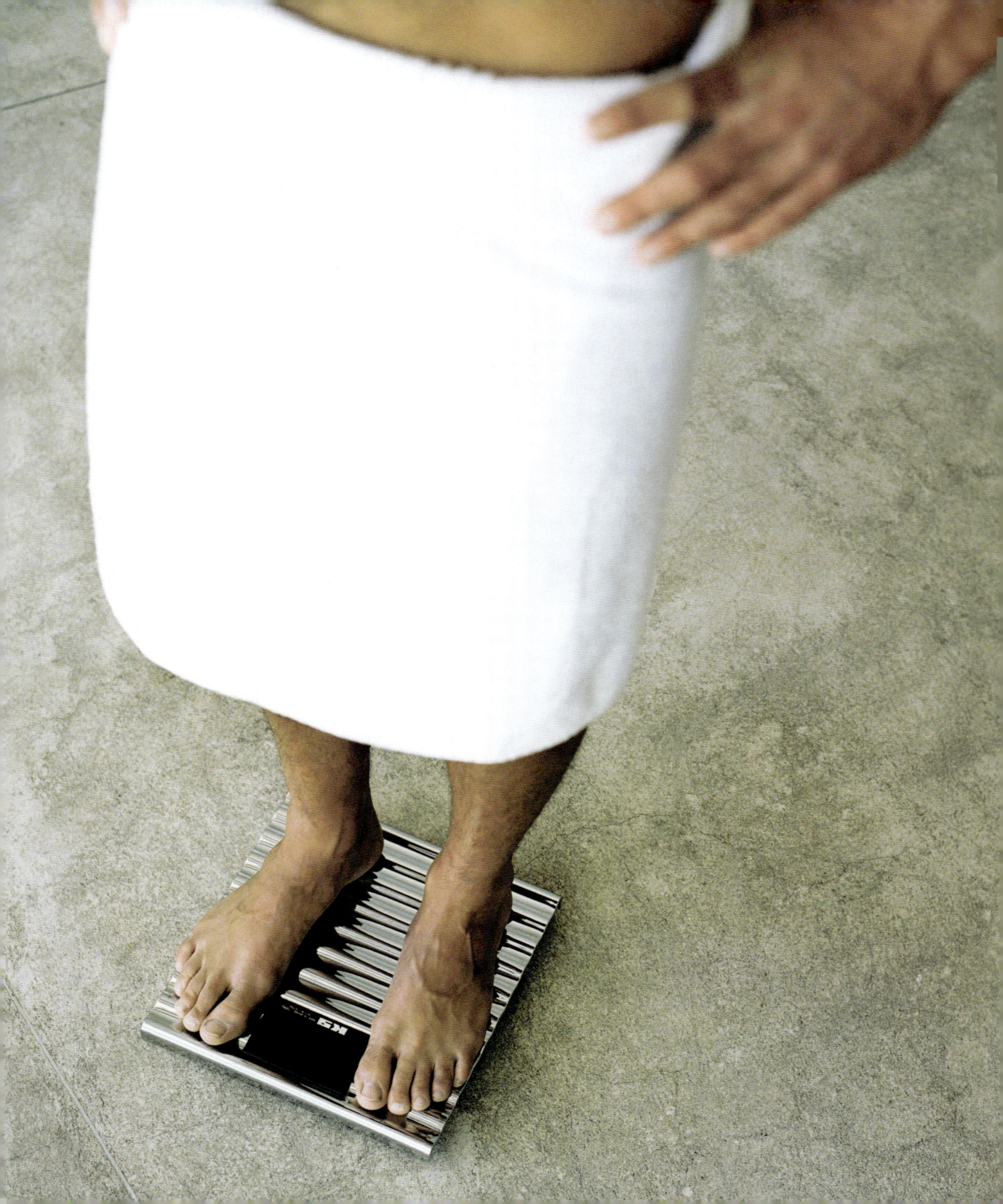

Ready?

Set

Go!

Why are you reading this book?

You've probably picked up this book because you've had enough. Had enough of being overweight and unfit. Had enough of feeling uncomfortable or embarrassed about your weight. Of not fitting into the clothes you would like to wear. Of not feeling attractive. Of struggling out of bed each morning and not having the energy to keep up with your kids. Of feeling like you are missing out on the life you are supposed to live. Sick of dodging cameras and avoiding mirrors. Sick of sitting back and not joining in activities because your weight is a handicap. Sick of not being treated right because of your weight. Or maybe your health is not what it could be and your doctor has told you that your life depends on you losing weight.

That brings you to right now.

You've seen the show and been inspired. You've watched overweight and obese Australians take up the Biggest Loser challenge, commit unreservedly to undertake a major lifestyle change, shed the kilos and get healthy.

Whatever your reason, you've made the right choice. *The Biggest Loser: change your life* offers you all the tools and motivation you will need on your journey to feeling and looking great, improving both your health and your fitness.

So, have you *really* had enough? Are you *really* ready for change – change that takes effort, commitment and hard work, change that will reward you and improve your life more than you have ever dreamed possible?

> 'Dare to dream and you can achieve anything, but you have to want to achieve your goals for yourself – you can't get healthy to please others. YOU are the most important person in this journey.'
>
> **Jo Cowling, Series One**

There are many reasons to lose weight and all are valid. If your main goal is to lose weight for *you*, for your health and wellbeing, to look great and to improve your life, then you will succeed. You need to wholeheartedly want to make a change, because only when *you* are ready can you make the change successfully. Your friends, family and doctor may have talked to you about your weight and your health but until you want to change, you won't be ready and committed.

Ask yourself if you're really ready to lose weight. Have you given it the time and thought the decision deserves? Are you prepared to dedicate the time and energy to make the necessary changes?

Perhaps you've been on diets before and maybe you've lost weight, but not for long. *The Biggest Loser: change your life* is not a fad diet. There is no secret, no magic pill. The Biggest Loser values are based on wellness, physical and mental fitness, health and happiness. The focus is on helping to empower you and motivate yourself to achieve all that you want to achieve – whether that be long-term weight-loss, physical fitness, increased confidence, looking great, feeling happy, or all of the above. You will achieve this through good nutrition and healthy eating, plenty of safe but challenging physical activity, and a positive attitude and never-give-up approach.

This is a long-term change in lifestyle habits, not a diet. You will learn about healthy eating habits and why it's important to get active. It's straightforward, but it won't be easy (but when has anything that's worth something actually been easy?). Good things take hard work, just as learning any new skill takes time and practice. We will show you how to apply the knowledge to your own life. Motivation will be the key to your success.

What will you need and what can you expect?

- commitment
- hard work
- fun
- discipline
- determination
- satisfaction
- reward for your effort
- and the knowledge that your life will never be the same again.

> YOU MAY NOT JUST CHANGE YOUR LIFE; YOU COULD SAVE YOUR LIFE.

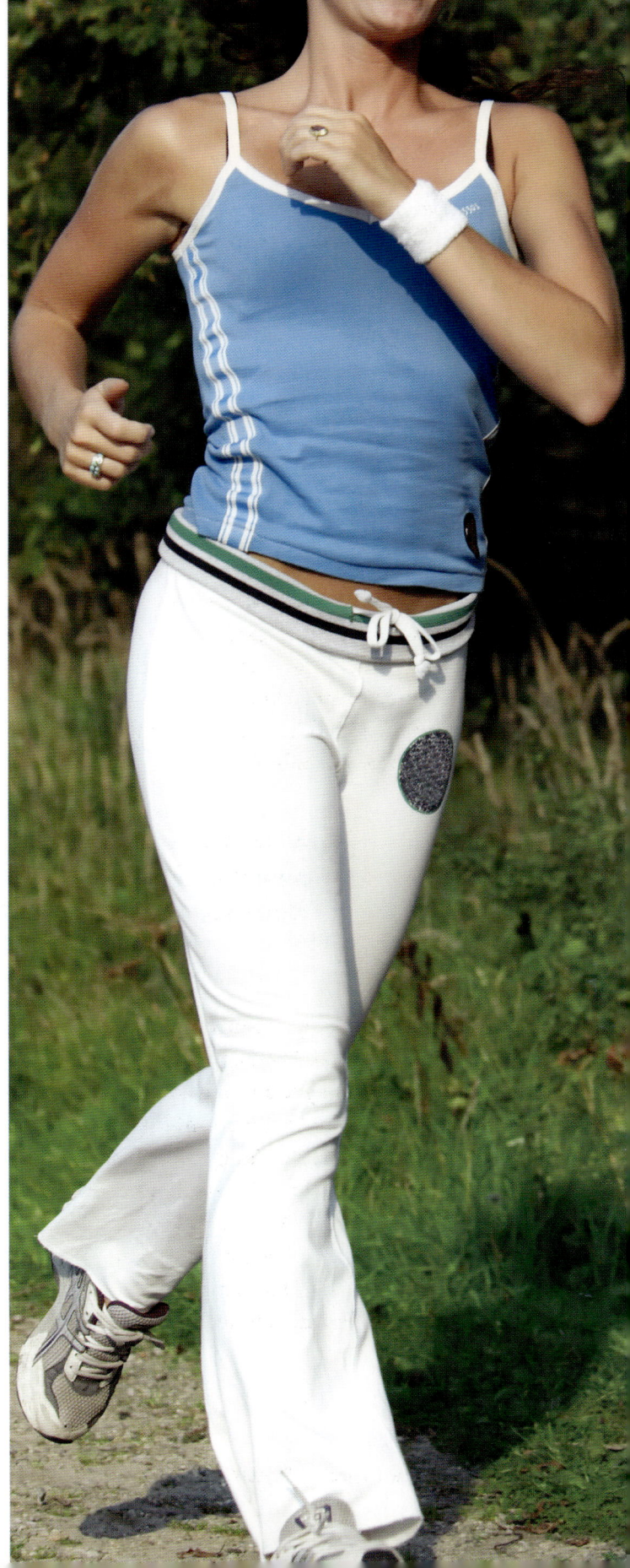

Why lose weight?

You might want to lose weight to look and feel good. Losing weight will significantly improve your health and wellbeing, so it's also about becoming healthy. Be realistic – we're not all meant to be supermodels or body builders, so aim for a goal weight you can live with, for good. Very few of the contestants achieve their goal weights by the end of the show, but they feel so fantastic and have improved their outlook and health with what they have achieved that the original goal becomes irrelevant. If you lose just 5–10 per cent of your weight and keep it off for a year, you will have significantly improved your health and lowered your risk of obesity-related diseases, and you'll look and feel better. So, yes, you may ultimately want to get down to a size 10 or have the buff football-player body you had 10 years ago, but success comes in small steps. Begin with a realistic short-term goal. Achieve that and then review things from there.

YOUR PHYSICAL WELLBEING

Your body is an amazing machine but it needs your help and your respect. If you are overweight or obese, you have an increased risk of heart disease, heart failure, stroke, osteoarthritis, Type 2 diabetes, polycystic ovarian syndrome, fertility problems, sleep apnoea, gallstones, stress incontinence, some cancers (such as colon and breast cancer), pregnancy complications and high blood pressure. Being overweight or obese is also associated with overall poor health, a reduced quality of life and a shorter life-expectancy.

Losing weight has many health benefits. If you achieve a weight that is healthy for you, you will:
- reduce your risk of heart disease, Type 2 diabetes and a range of chronic diseases
- achieve a healthy blood pressure
- lower your LDL cholesterol levels
- stabilise your blood glucose and insulin levels
- have fewer medical expenses and require fewer (if any) medications
- be around to see your kids grow up … and your grandkids.

Type 2 diabetes

Type 2 diabetes is a disease where your body doesn't use insulin properly or becomes insulin-resistant (see page 54) to learn about how insulin works). Over time, Type 2 diabetes can lead to kidney disease, blindness, stroke, heart disease and circulatory problems (potentially leading to gangrene and amputation).

'Before going on The Biggest Loser, I was a Type 2 diabetic. Since losing my weight, I no longer have Type 2 diabetes and am off my medication! My doctor cried when he told me the news.' **Artie Rocke, Series One**

YOUR MENTAL WELLBEING

Another possible effect of being overweight or obese is an increase in psychological problems and negative social experiences (such as discrimination). If you lose weight, you will:
- improve your self-esteem and confidence
- reduce the likelihood of depression
- feel more energetic
- radiate vitality
- look and feel fabulous!

You will also inspire your family and friends to improve their own health.

Ask yourself if your weight stops you from doing things that you really want to do in life. This is about your wellbeing – of body, mind and soul. Everyone deserves a strong sense of wellbeing – and you are worth the effort it takes to achieve this. Change your lifestyle and take responsibility for controlling your life. Be committed to good health and give it everything you've got – this is your life.

AFFIRM YOUR COMMITMENT

Some people find that affirmations keep them motivated and inspired. You've seen the motivational t-shirts worn by the contestants, featuring their very own inspirational mottos. If this works for you, consider some of the following (you can repeat these to yourself each morning, use them during your workouts when the going gets tough and you need inspiration, or make a sign and place it on the fridge, in the pantry or on the bathroom mirror).
- I love and respect myself and my body
- I am in control of my life
- I am strong
- I am committed to my good health
- I am looking and feeling better every day
- I am changing my life
- I can do this
- I am worth this!

Or you may find it useful to stick a copy of your long-term goal or a 'before' photo on the fridge to inspire you every day.

Are you overweight?

Most estimates state that over 7 million Australian adults and one quarter to a third of Australian children are overweight or obese. Australians are some of the fattest people in the world, after the United States. If you're overweight or obese, you are not alone. Our lifestyles of convenience food, energy-saving devices and sit-down leisure options generally result in diets of high-fat, processed foods and an activity level that is sedentary at best. As our resources and leisure options increase, our quality of life is actually diminishing because of poor health. Now is the time to change before you become another health statistic.

Understanding what your healthy weight range is will help you work out how much weight you need to lose. You probably know if you need to lose weight; however, research has shown that men are more likely to think they are not overweight when they actually are, leading to a lack of knowledge about their potential weight-related health problems.

There are a few ways to check whether you are in the healthy weight range or not and also to measure the distribution of your body fat – if you store most of your fat around your abdomen, you are at increased risk of disease compared with people who store it more evenly around the body. Abdominal fat is more 'mobile' than other fat and is therefore more likely to travel and be laid down in your arteries. Use the methods below to work out if you are overweight and whether you are at risk of obesity-associated diseases.

> RESEARCH DEFINES SUCCESSFUL WEIGHT-LOSS AS LOSING JUST 5 TO 10 PER CENT OF YOUR WEIGHT AND KEEPING IT OFF LONG-TERM, UP TO 2 YEARS. THIS SIGNIFICANTLY IMPROVES YOUR OVERALL HEALTH.

WAIST CIRCUMFERENCE

The size of your waist indicates your level of abdominal fat – the classic 'beer gut', 'pot belly' or 'apple shape' – which dramatically increases the risks to your health caused by being overweight or obese. Measure your waist at the narrowest point between your ribs and your pelvis when viewed from the front (and when you are relaxed, not holding your stomach in). You have an increased risk of serious health problems if your waist measurement is, for men, above 94 centimetres, and for women, above 80 centimetres. The health risks substantially increase with waist circumferences above 102 centimetres for men and above 88 centimetres for women.

'I was happy in my own skin and if that meant being overweight, so be it. But then my doctor told me that if I didn't lose weight I would become diabetic. When I realised that I was slowly killing my body, I had to act.'

Jo Cowling, Series One

WAIST-TO-HIP RATIO

The waist-to-hip ratio is a good measure of whether your weight is increasing your risk of obesity-related diseases. Determine your waist-to-hip ratio by dividing your waist circumference by your hip measurement. Measure your waist at the narrowest point. Measure your hips at the maximum point (the widest part of your backside). Divide your waist measurement by your hip measurement. For example, if you have a 90-centimetre waist and a hip measurement of 102 centimetres, your waist-to-hip ratio will be:

$$90 \div 102 = 0.88$$

Waist-to-hip ratios of 0.8 or greater for women and 0.9 or greater for men are associated with increased health risks, including heart disease and diabetes.

BODY MASS INDEX

The Body Mass Index (BMI) is currently the most common way to work out if you're a healthy weight or not. However, it doesn't consider the distribution of fat around your body; it's not suitable for children or teenagers; and there are some variations based on ethnicity.

Your BMI is the ratio of your weight in kilograms to the square of your height in metres (kg/m^2). A BMI greater than 25 is considered overweight (although the result can be skewed if you are very muscular) and a BMI of over 30 is considered obese. Morbid obesity is defined as a BMI over 40. The higher your BMI, the greater are the health risks resulting from your weight (see the table below).

To work out your BMI, divide your weight in kilograms by your height in metres squared. So, a person who is 1.82 metres tall and weighs 90 kilograms has a BMI of 27.2:

$$90 \div (1.82 \times 1.82) = 90 \div 3.31 = 27.2$$

YOUR BMI

BMI	HEALTH	RISK OF OBESITY-RELATED DISEASE
Less than 18.5	Underweight	Low
18.5–24	Healthy weight	Average
25–29	Overweight	Increased
30–39	Obese	Moderate to severe
40 and over	Morbidly obese	Very severe

Why are you overweight?

There are many reasons why you may be overweight. You may eat healthily but have your portion size wrong, you may never have had the chance to learn about healthy eating, you may be overeating as a result of trauma in your life, you may eat well but lead an inactive life, or the extra weight may have just crept on slowly while you were busy doing other things.

For many people, being overweight is driven by more than lack of exercise or eating too much. Overeating and inactivity can stem from not feeling good about yourself or your life, depression, stress, loneliness, relationship issues and other problems.

EMOTIONAL HUNGER

We eat for many reasons and often not just because we're hungry for food. Emotional eating is when you eat (usually a large amount) in response to feeling an emotion rather than actual hunger – eating for comfort. Emotions that trigger overeating vary for every individual, but common ones include:

- boredom
- anxiety
- stress
- depression
- loneliness
- alienation
- avoidance.

> 'I had to confront my own personal demons before I could lose weight. Finding the thing that makes you overeat, choose unhealthy food and not exercise can be difficult but, if you're like me, you have to deal with the WHY first.'
> **Shane Giles, Series One**

Emotional triggers don't always have to be negative, either. You may overeat to celebrate something, to reward yourself for an achievement (even if that achievement is just getting through another day), as a comfort or simply because you're feeling good.

If you are an emotional eater, it is important not to get annoyed at yourself. Emotions are a common trigger for eating. Think about it: ever since you were born food would have been associated with nurturing, love and warmth. You were most likely rewarded and comforted with food during your childhood and food was used to celebrate happy times, and perhaps even to comfort in sad times. However, if emotional eating contributes to your weight gain and has become your main tool for dealing with your emotions, then it's destructive and time to develop a range of non-food responses to the stresses in your life.

Take the time to work out why you feel like eating when you do. Identify your emotional triggers. When you find yourself reaching for food, ask yourself three questions:

1. Am I actually hungry right now?
2. What am I feeling?
3. Why am I feeling that way?

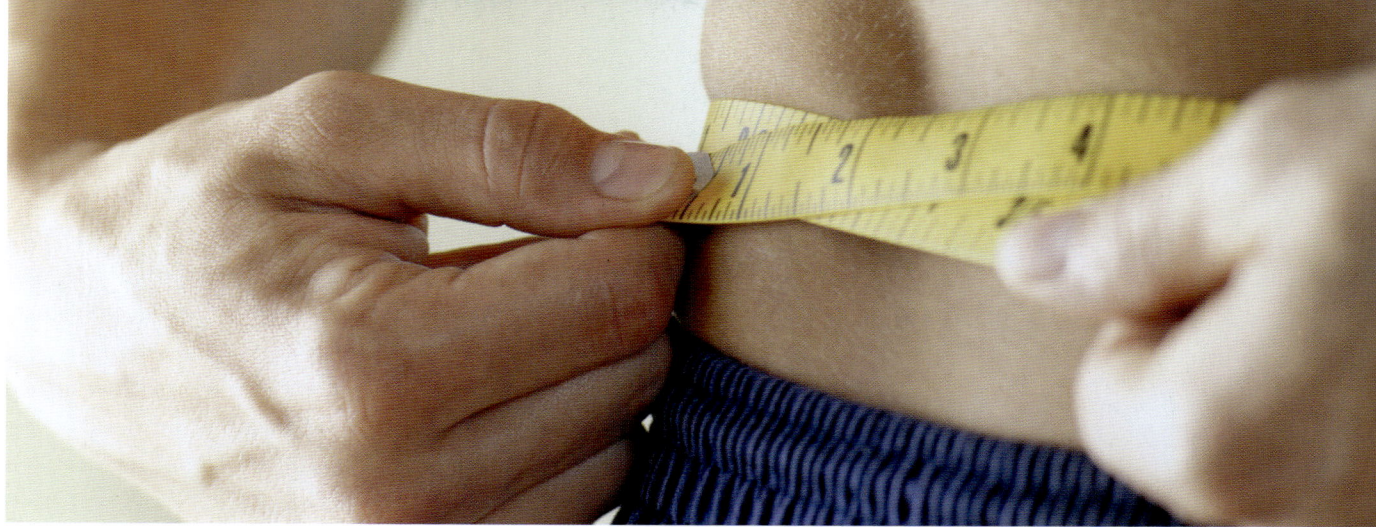

If you're not hungry, don't eat. Grab your food diary (see page 38) or personal journal and write down your feelings, even if it's as simple as 'I'm feeling angry because …' or 'I'm feeling guilty because …'. Emotional eating can be a way of using food to stifle and cover emotions – instead of feeling or acknowledging an emotion, you eat. If this is the case, your weight could be a manifestation of unresolved issues. What's really bothering you?

Keeping note of your eating habits in your food diary will help you become more aware of what your triggers are. Once you know what these are, learn to avoid or change the circumstances that get you emotional eating. You will also learn to recognise when you are truly hungry.

A key factor in long-term weight-loss maintenance for emotional eaters is learning new strategies to cope with your emotions and stress levels. You need to replace your emotional eating habit with a new habit; if you try to stop emotional eating but install no new strategy, you'll return to emotional eating. Consider other things that make you feel comforted. These will keep your mind off food.

Try these suggestions. Go for a walk, call a friend, brush your teeth, chew gum, have a shower, exercise, write – anything that will get your mind off your desire for food. The more you are aware of why you emotionally eat, the more long-term changes you can make.

If stress is your trigger, make changes to reduce your stress levels, whether it be delegating tasks at work or home; taking a regular yoga class; buying a relaxation CD to use at home, in the car or at work; learning to say 'no'; or taking a short walk to think about the things that really make you feel better in the long-term. If, after a stressful day at work, you can't resist stopping off at the takeaway or bakery you always drive past, then plan ahead and take another route home or go for a walk instead.

MEDICATIONS THAT INCREASE WEIGHT

A side-effect of some medications is that they cause you to put on weight, or make it very difficult for you to lose weight. You may not be aware of this and not understand why you're not losing weight when you're doing everything right. Don't give up. Carefully read the information that comes with your medication; if gaining weight is a side-effect, speak with your doctor about available alternatives.

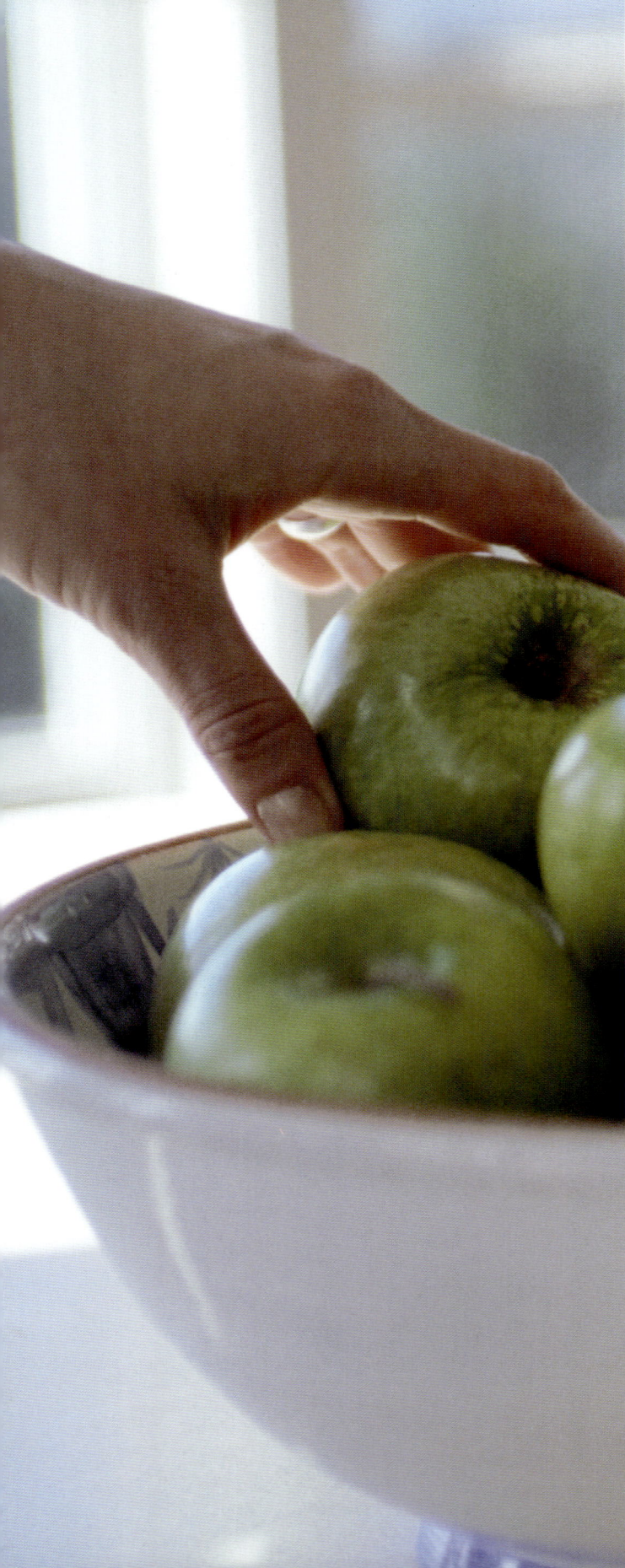

If you overeat because you're bored and there's nothing better to do, *find* something better to do – think about what interests you, what your passions are, what your hobbies are, and do something about them. Join a club, learn a new skill, enrol in a course, become a volunteer. Keep a list of jobs that need doing around your house and, when you're bored, get stuck into one job from that list. If you have absolutely nothing that needs doing, think about someone who might – a family member, an elderly neighbour, a friend, a community organisation. Loneliness can play a part in emotional eating. As cities get bigger, we can become more isolated – other people will be feeling lonely too. When you find yourself reaching for food because you're lonely, choose to do something about it. Organise to see friends, join a sporting team or volunteer for a non-profit organisation. Join a slimming club. Getting out into the community will also help you feel more connected.

'Losing weight feels amazing. I don't know which is greater – the physical joy or the joy of knowing that I beat a demon that has controlled me since childhood. Either way, life is amazing now.'

Adro Sarnelli, Series One Winner

If you overeat when you've achieved something positive, choose another way to reward yourself. Get your hair cut, buy a book or CD or a new piece of equipment that makes it easier to be active or easier to cook healthily. Make your rewards life-affirming, not destructive. (See page 20 for more on rewarding yourself.)

Another strategy if you know you are a regular emotional eater is to include a specific kilojoule allowance for this in your eating plan – for example, 500 to 1000 kilojoules for a treat (but bear in mind that it takes between 30 and 60 minutes of brisk walking to burn off 1000 kilojoules). Include a column in your food diary to write down how you feel when you eat, and also include a space to make notes about how you could respond to this situation differently next time (for example, 'Next time I have a fight with my partner, I will go for a walk, not head to the fridge').

Recognise that medicating yourself with food only works in the short-term and leaves you feeling worse. Believe that you are worth looking after – you deserve to live a healthy life, enjoy a true sense of wellbeing and become healthy at a weight that is right for you. If you have issues that you want to deal with, take a positive step and see a counsellor or psychologist who specialises in weight management.

Sometimes there's comfort in being overweight. Ask yourself what you might get out of being overweight. It can be about safety or it can be a form of protection, or even a form of freedom or rebellion. Is it saving you from having to engage in life, in relationships, taking risks that could mean you fail at achieving things you dream about? Is it an easy excuse so you don't have to be the person you want to be deep down? If being overweight is an excuse for you not to live life to the full, explore your reasons and work out if you're ready to risk changing that.

IS YOUR LIFE CONTROLLED BY FOOD?

Food addiction is like any other addiction – food dominates your thoughts, and your energy is devoted to obtaining it or trying to stop yourself consuming it. You obsess about food and thinking about food controls your life. You look forward to the chance to binge-eat in secrecy, yet hate yourself while you're doing it.

It's not just psychological – certain foods create chemical responses in your brain that can be addictive, so it's possible to be emotionally and physically addicted to food. If you think this is you, you can get help. There are support groups and health professionals who can offer you assistance and support. You are *not* a hopeless case.

Think about how much energy and time you devote to food; imagine what you could achieve if you were able to focus that energy on living your life to the full instead.

How do you lose weight?

Do you want the honest answer? With commitment, hard work and a positive attitude, an attitude that means you forgive yourself when you experience setbacks and get right back up to continue on your journey.

On a physical level, there are two ways of losing weight: eat less or exercise more, or both. To lose weight, you must create an energy deficit – that is, you need to consume less food (energy) than you actually use. You need to eat fewer kilojoules or calories than your body needs to get through the day; this way, your body will use its energy stores to make up the energy deficit.

Understanding this is the basis of successful weight-loss, but clearly there's more to it than that, otherwise few people would be overweight. Your mind is the key – you have to really want to lose weight and you have to deal with all the blocks your mind puts in the way. Successful weight-loss is all about attitude. What gets you up in the morning early so you can go for a walk? A positive can-do attitude and being organised by having clothes and joggers by your bed. What helps you forgive yourself when you eat too much? A positive attitude and an ability to recognise that one setback does not mean you have blown everything.

Part Two of this book explains the Biggest Loser healthy eating and exercise plans in detail. Before you get to that point, it's good to understand how important your frame of mind and attitude will be in your weight-loss. Here, you'll also learn how to create new habits and set goals. This prepares you for the next stage.

To succeed in your weight-loss, you will need to:
- accept yourself and where you are right now
- understand what triggers you to overeat
- break bad habits and learn new ones
- develop a strategy for bouncing back from setbacks
- change your attitude to yourself and learn positive self-talk
- recognise that an all-or-nothing attitude does not help your weight-loss
- be responsible for, and accountable to, yourself
- change your lifestyle.

CHANGE YOUR BEHAVIOUR

Eating a nutritionally balanced diet and exercising are the keys to long-term weight-loss. This isn't a new idea, yet it remains challenging for many people. Why? Because we make poor choices that over time become bad habits, which we then find hard to change. While your current habits and lifestyle have brought you to this point, it has happened over a long period of time. To lose weight, you need to recognise that it will take time to unlearn those habits and develop new responses, so that eventually you will have a new set of habits that support your new healthy lifestyle. Imagine if you decided you wanted to race the 400 metres at the Olympics, but you'd only just started training. You would make it

FAD DIETS

Fad diets negatively affect your health *and* your self-esteem. Most fad diets are nutritionally inadequate and impossible (not to mention unsafe) to continue long-term. Remember, you don't want to diet short-term; you want to eat as healthy as you can long-term.

A fad diet is anything that:
- promises fast, dramatic weight-loss
- promises weight-loss without exercising
- uses the words 'quick' and 'easy'
- needs a hard sell and marketing gimmicks to get your attention
- you have to pay a lot of money for
- promotes an unbalanced diet with unusual food combinations
- emphasises one particular food type only.

Fad diets work in the short-term, because most drastically reduce your daily kilojoule intake (regardless of what food you're eating). You also lose weight because you focus on what you eat and dedicate energy to planning your meals. But many of these diets are far from nutritionally balanced and are not conducive to a long-term healthy eating lifestyle. As soon as you go off the diet, you put the weight back on (and sometimes more), and end up feeling like a failure because of it. Go through this a few times and you'll believe that you're hopeless and can never ever lose the weight. This is not true!

In the diet world, consumers are always drawn to the newest product promising weight-loss — there's usually at least one or two new fad diets each year (which wouldn't be necessary if they actually worked, would it?). But, remember, the best way to lose weight and keep it off is through sensible, healthy balanced eating and exercising. There's no secret or magic pill. You will achieve your goals through hard work and commitment.

'Eating well, hard work and a "Yes I can!" attitude is the only way to tackle weight-loss.'
David Hilyander, Series One

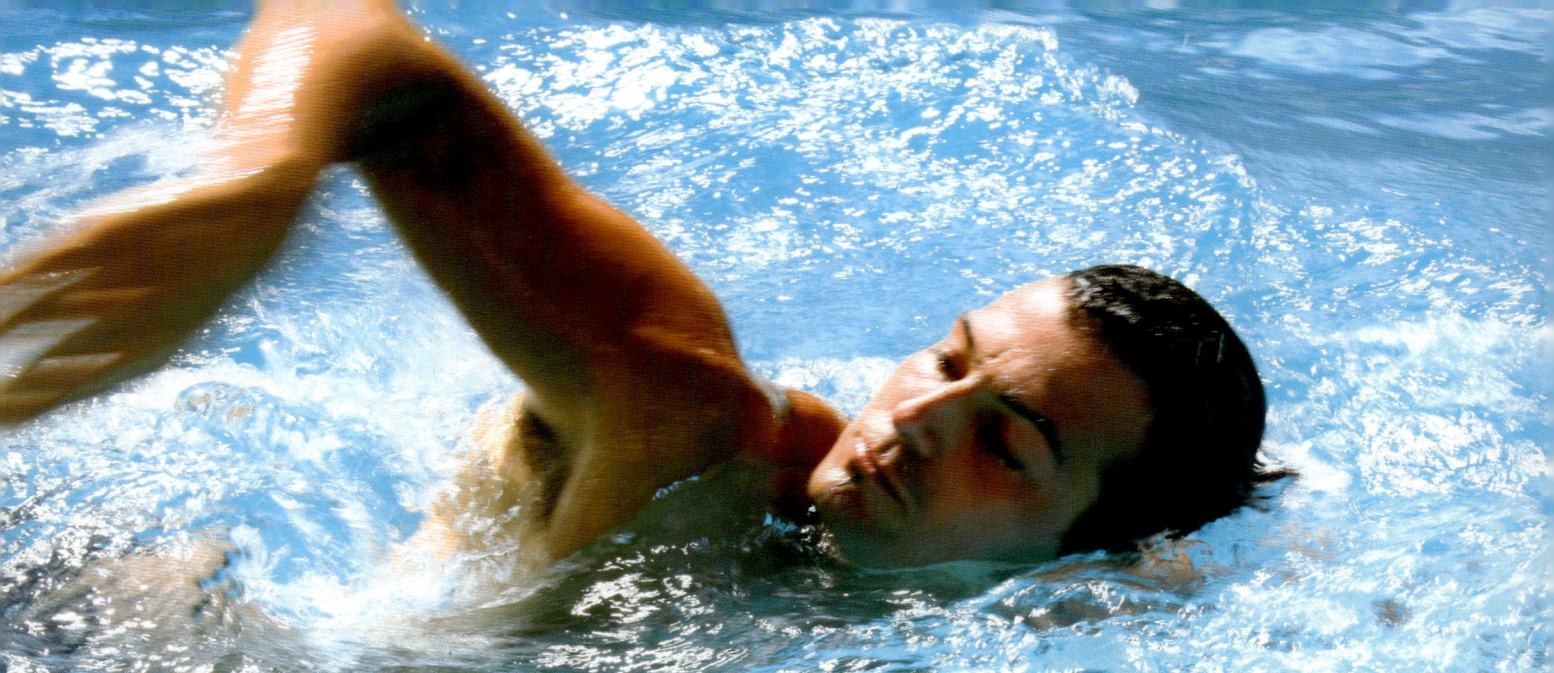

a long-term goal and understand that it would take time, commitment and perseverance. You wouldn't expect to achieve it in a month, nor would you give up when you lost your first race or had your first injury. It is the same with changing your behaviour to lose weight.

Change is always challenging, and successful change takes time. It also depends on what stage of acceptance for taking action you're at. You might be ready to change, you may still be working out whether change is worth it or you may be preparing to change. Perhaps someone has bought you this book, but you do not think you need to change at all. Sometimes it's hard to accept that we have a health problem. We ignore it, procrastinate about it or simply deny its existence. Take the time to work out if you are ready. If you are, then it's time to plan, prepare and then act, recognising that the journey takes time.

> 'I went through most of my life thinking I was just "a little bit" overweight. But one day I walked past the bathroom mirror and saw my reflection – for some reason it was strikingly different to what I usually saw. For the first time in my life, I actually saw my real size, the size people around me had being seeing for years. I was shattered. It was then and there that I realised I had not been living in reality and I had to change what I saw forever.'
> **Cat White, Series One**

The steps to eating and exercising success (on pages 37 and 72) will help you create healthy new habits. Setting goals (on page 18) will show you how to go about it. First, though, are some guidelines for modifying your behaviour.

Change one habit at a time

A total overhaul is likely to be too much too soon. You don't have to change everything at once. Do it step by step – commit to one new habit first and wait until it feels like second nature before committing to the next habit. Commit to being active for 30 minutes five days a week, or to reducing your fat intake by cutting out the hot chips at lunch, or to cutting down your alcohol intake to twice a week, or to getting up 20 minutes early so you can prepare a healthy lunch to take to work. By choosing to focus on one new habit at a time, you make the goal achievable, you'll become more confident as you achieve it and you'll be ready for the next step.

Start small

A dramatic change won't last. You already know this. Small changes make a difference – even just reducing your portion sizes and switching to water or diet drinks only will lower your fat and kilojoule intake. Making a small change in your lifestyle is manageable and will inspire confidence in yourself to make more.

Make one change that will have the most effect

If you're starting by making one change, choose to change the one habit that will make the most difference to your health. If you want to reduce the amount of sugar you eat, don't cut out the cake you have once a week, cut out the can of soft drink you have every day with lunch.

Be patient

You didn't gain weight in a week, so you can't expect to lose it in a week. Don't be in a hurry and don't give up when you fall back into an old habit – remember, you're still learning. Here's a simple analogy. When you were little, you couldn't tie your shoelaces. Your parents did it for you. After a while, they took the time to show you how to tie them, then they helped you to tie them. Sometimes you'd forget so they'd show you again. Then you became so used to tying them that you didn't need help anymore. Now, of course, it's second nature. The same thing applied with learning to drive a car. Did you give up after your first lesson when you stalled in the middle of an intersection? No. So don't give up while you're learning new healthy patterns of behaviour. It takes time and perseverance, and it's completely normal not to get it right straight away.

Be consistent

Modifying behaviour successfully is all about consistency. You need to replace bad habits with good habits, created through repetition. Commit to creating your good habits daily. The more consistent you are, the faster you'll reach your goal. The less consistent, the longer it will take.

Be aware

Often eating is done without thinking – it's mindless. Start to become aware of what and when you eat. Practise eating with mindfulness – that is, pay attention to what and how much you are eating, and what you're doing at the same time. This gives you a chance to learn what triggers your overeating. Do you always reach for food after you've spoken to your mother? Do you always eat when you're watching TV? You need to start by breaking the habit. Speak to your mother when there's no food around; make a rule that you don't eat in front of the TV (or turn it off and only eat while sitting at a table).

MANAGE YOUR ENVIRONMENT

It's difficult to change your behaviour if nothing else changes. Making your home health-friendly will help you create and stick with your new habits. Very few people have a willpower of steel, so avoid having to use yours in the first place – get rid of all the junk food in your house. Restock the fridge, freezer and pantry with healthy food. Change your routine so you eat only at the table.

As well as your home environment, manage other eating occasions. Eating healthily doesn't mean you can never eat out or get takeaway. This is a lifestyle, not a diet of deprivation. The secret is planning ahead – what's the healthiest takeaway you can get? Can you have a healthy snack before you go out to dinner? Any support you can give yourself in learning new behaviours will help make them your habits.

CHANGE YOUR THINKING

Good food and exercise are just as vital for our mental wellbeing as our physical wellbeing – our state of mind drives our choices and influences our decisions. Generally, the healthier you are, the more positive your mental outlook will be and the less likely you'll be to engage in unhealthy habits.

Positive thinking seems a simple-enough concept and yet we often only use it in relation to others and rarely when thinking about ourselves. Throughout our lives we build up our own belief systems according to how we see ourselves, how we interact with the world and how we think the world interacts with us. When everything is going well, it's easy to be positive but when things go pear-shaped we can often descend into a spiral of self-doubt, fear, plummeting self-esteem and uncertainty. Our confidence takes a knock and, once this happens a few times, it can quickly become a negative habit.

Negative thoughts are a self-fulfilling prophecy. Pay attention to your attitude to yourself and to your life. Listen to what you're thinking and what you're telling yourself. How do you talk to yourself? How much negative self-talk is happening in your head? Your internal dialogue significantly affects how you feel, what you believe, and how you behave. Be aware of your negative self-talk and stop it as soon as you hear yourself. It can take time to create new positive thinking patterns and it's easy to slip back into old negative self-talk; when you find yourself being negative, laugh at the thoughts, tell yourself they're not true and replace them with the positive alternative. There is absolutely no reason why negative self-talk should be considered more realistic than positive self-talk. Listen for comments like 'I'm not good enough', 'I'm a failure', 'As if I could ever lose weight – I may as well just give up'. Try to switch them to positive self-talk: 'I am good enough', 'I am learning more about how to get healthy and it may take time to find the things that work for me', 'I am starting to take care of my health' and so on. Avoid using 'should' statements, over-generalising and all-or-nothing thinking.

Choose a positive attitude and start believing in yourself now, as hard as it may feel; don't wait to lose 2, 10 or 30 kilos before feeling good about yourself. This sets you up to fail and perpetuates the negative cycle. Be proud that you are actively changing your life rather than just wishing for change. Remember what you like about yourself and what you are good at. Change your self-talk – start talking to yourself as you would a close friend. Be caring, sensitive, understanding and friendly. You achieve *nothing* by putting yourself down. You are your first and most important supporter, and the positive support you give yourself is essential in helping you to lose weight.

> 'Learn to love and accept yourself for who you are. Only then will you succeed at anything you want to do. When the time is right for you, it will be like a light bulb going on. Don't be afraid to ask for help and don't surround yourself with negative people.'
>
> **Jo Cowling, Series One**

Also listen to how you talk about yourself to others – this can help you realise if you have low self-esteem, lack self-confidence and have a negative self-image. If you're always putting yourself down or being self-deprecating, try to work out why you're doing it. Put-downs do not help you and will sabotage your weight-loss goals. You need to like yourself now, before you start losing weight. You need to believe that you are worth the effort.

Don't underestimate the power of positive thought – your mind is a powerful tool for creating positive change in your life.

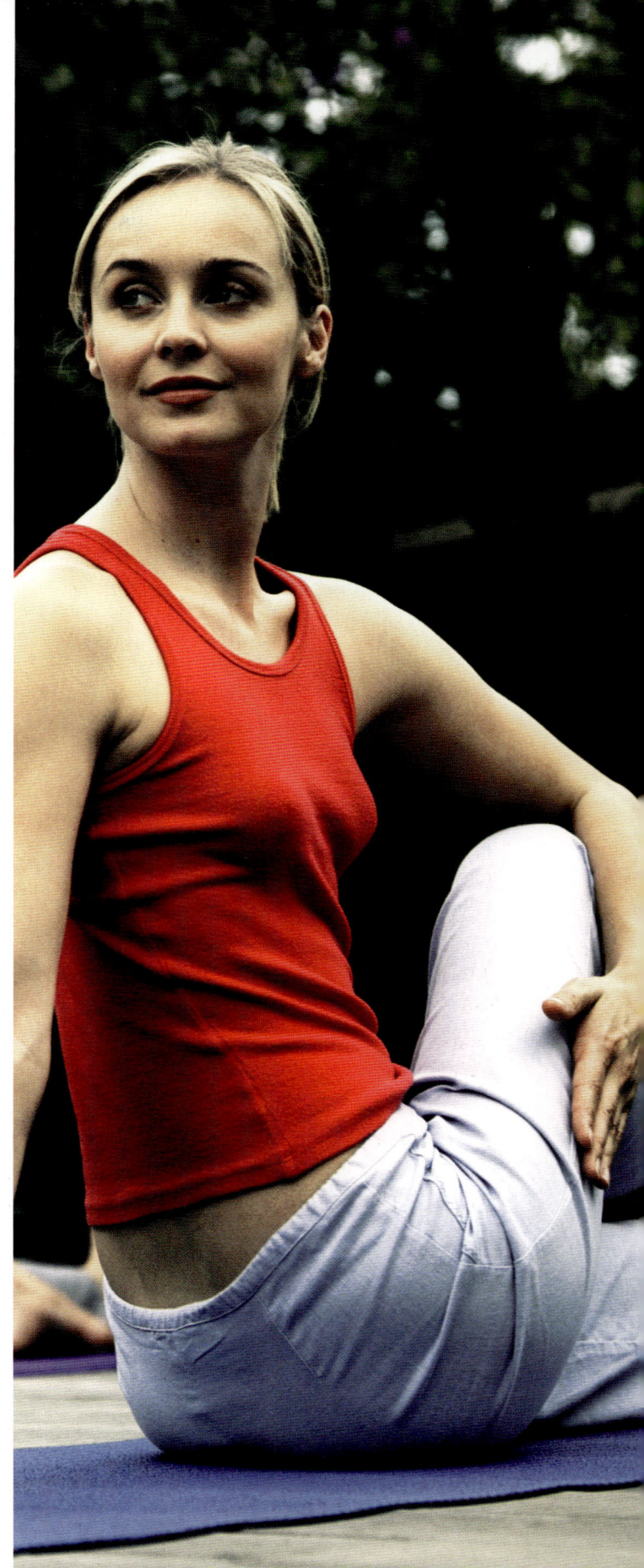

Setting lifestyle and health goals

You achieve success by focusing on and dedicating yourself to a goal. A goal gives you something to work towards. It helps you create a plan, a road map, to achieving what you want. So, where do you want to go? There's no point setting out on a journey if you have no idea where you want to end up. Think about what you want in your life, what you want to change and what you want to be like, physically and mentally. Then follow the steps below and start achieving your goals.

DECIDE ON YOUR LONG-TERM GOAL

Really take some time to work out what you want your long-term goal to be – is it to lose a certain amount of weight; to lower your blood pressure to a certain point; to improve your overall wellbeing; to be able to run 10 kilometres; or to fit back into your wedding dress?

Once you have decided on your long-term goal, visualise it. What will it look like? What will it feel like? What will your life be like? The more feelings you can put into your goal, the more you will be committed to it and the more powerful it will be. The intensity of feeling will strengthen your commitment to the goal and make it more tangible. Your goal must be meaningful to you – how much do you really want to achieve this?

> **MAKE YOUR GOALS SMART**
>
> Specific
> Measurable
> Achievable
> Realistic
> Time-based

MAKE IT ACHIEVABLE AND REALISTIC

To effectively set a goal, it's important to be realistic in terms of what you want to achieve. You need to work with your body type and shape – don't subscribe to the unrealistic ideal body images often portrayed in the media. If you are 180 centimetres tall and currently weigh 120 kilos, it's unrealistic to set a goal weight of 55 kilos, whether it's in one year or five. Instead, pick a healthy weight for your height, a weight you feel you could live with, and then set in place the steps to achieve this goal. To simply improve your health, your goal weight needs to be 5 to 10 per cent from your starting weight, or 6–12 kilograms if you weigh 120 kilograms now.

If you choose an unrealistic goal, you will have trouble committing to it and will most likely give up. If your goal is to improve your health by eating better but you know you can't live without chocolate, cut down to one small snack-size chocolate bar a day rather than a family block. If your goal includes giving up chocolate forever, you're unlikely to stick with it. Even with the best intentions, if you choose an unrealistic goal, deep down you won't really believe you can achieve it. This underlying doubt will undermine your efforts and you'll end up feeling like you can never succeed.

You must believe that you can achieve your goal.

MAKE IT SPECIFIC

Really work out the specific details of your goal. Think about *what* you want, *how* you're going to make it happen and *when* you are going to reach it. What will you need to achieve it – support, time, gym membership? It's not enough to say 'exercise more' or 'eat well'. Say, 'To reach my end goal of losing 10 kilos over six months, I will walk four times a week for 30 minutes and only have one takeaway dinner a week'.

MAKE IT MEASURABLE AND TIMED

If your goal is 'I want to get fit', then it will be very hard to measure. What defines 'fit' to you? If it's being able to walk for an hour or lift a 20-kilogram weight or run 10 kilometres, then make this your goal. You want a goal where you can see and measure the results – how else will you know what you're achieving? Include a timeframe. When do you want to achieve your goal by? What will your milestone dates be along the way?

BREAK YOUR LONG-TERM GOAL INTO MINI-GOALS

Setting short- and medium-term goals not only helps divide the main goal into bite-sized steps, but it also makes you more accountable for your actions and, most importantly, gives you a sense of success and achievement as you reach each goal. Without such steps, plans remain just that – plans that will never be fulfilled because there is no structure to make them happen. Give each step a suitable timeframe so that you can both achieve and measure your success. If your long-term goal is to lose 20 kilos but your mini-goals are to lose 1 kilo every two weeks, then every two weeks you'll know whether you're on track. Achieving your mini-goals will develop your strength of mind, boost your confidence and keep you motivated. They also give you a chance to reward yourself along the way.

You can even use small goals each day – apply them to your exercise workouts so that you are focused on achieving specific outcomes rather than just mindlessly exercising.

> 'Remember to look at your weight-loss in small numbers. I had to lose 70 kilograms and I thought, there is no way I can do this. But then I set my weight-loss goals in 10-kilogram brackets. Once I lost the first 10 kilos, it was goal achieved and onto the next 10 kilos! Take on a "can do attitude", because you CAN do it, you really can – I did!'
>
> **Artie Rocke, Series One**

ADD A REWARD

Remember to acknowledge your achievements on your way to your long-term goal; reward yourself for each mini-goal you reach, be it losing 3 kilos, running for 10 minutes without stopping or not drinking alcohol for a week. Choose life-affirming rewards. Now is the time to stop rewarding yourself with food and alcohol. Reward yourself with something meaningful to you, whether it's a CD, a trip to the movies (no choc-top included), time with a friend, a long, hot bath or just some quiet time to yourself away from the family.

Rewards keep you motivated. Decide ahead of time what your rewards will be for your mini-goals and your long-term goal. Planning your rewards ahead of time will give you something to look forward to, keep you focused and help you create a new habit of not using food as a reward.

FIND THE SOLUTION, NOT THE PROBLEM

You may not be ready to try to discover why you are overweight. That's okay – you don't need to. Take a solution-focused approach to your weight-loss and you'll find yourself achieving your goals. By using a solution-focused approach, you look at what you want to achieve rather than exploring why you might be where you are now – that is, what is the solution to your problem, not why you have the problem in the first place. Consider it a future-focused technique – everything that has happened has been and gone, and now is your time to make a change.

Ask yourself, what do you want in your future? What does it look like? Once you have that end goal in mind, work out what you need to do to get there. Break it down into 10 small manageable steps. Simply achieving one step will increase your confidence and break negative thought patterns and habits. If you achieved the first step when you believed that you couldn't, then what else might you be able to achieve?

Find the solution. One of your steps might be that, if you eat a fried takeaway lunch each day because you always walk past a takeaway shop, you choose to walk back to work a different way. If you know you always give in at the supermarket and stock up on ice-cream and chocolate because you're feeling hungry and craving it, try shopping first thing in the morning after a good breakfast and then decide to avoid that aisle altogether. The last thing you'll feel like is chocolate and ice-cream (or at least you'll have a better chance of resisting the impulse-buy urge).

WRITE YOUR GOALS DOWN

You have to 'own' your goals. If you really want to stay motivated, ensure you are losing weight for yourself and no one else, and that your goals are on your timeframe and no one else's. Write down all the reasons why you want to lose weight. Think about what you want and how to make that happen, not so much why you are where you are in the first place. What would it be like if your problem was solved? What will you notice, what will be different, how will you feel? Move towards your ideal future.

You may want to keep your goals to yourself or you may want to share them. Telling your friends, family and colleagues can be a positive step – not only for their support but also, by verbalising your intent, you are reinforcing your decision to make positive change and are more likely to stick to your plans.

Regularly reread your goals to see your progress. Remember that goals are flexible and you can adapt them at any stage to reflect changes in your life or in your priorities.

Read the example over the page to see how you could structure your goals.

'You don't have to be locked in a house with a bunch of strangers to accomplish your weight-loss goals. If you just decide to take each moment as it comes and do your best in that moment, then your goals will become reality sooner than you think.'
Kristie Dignam, Series One

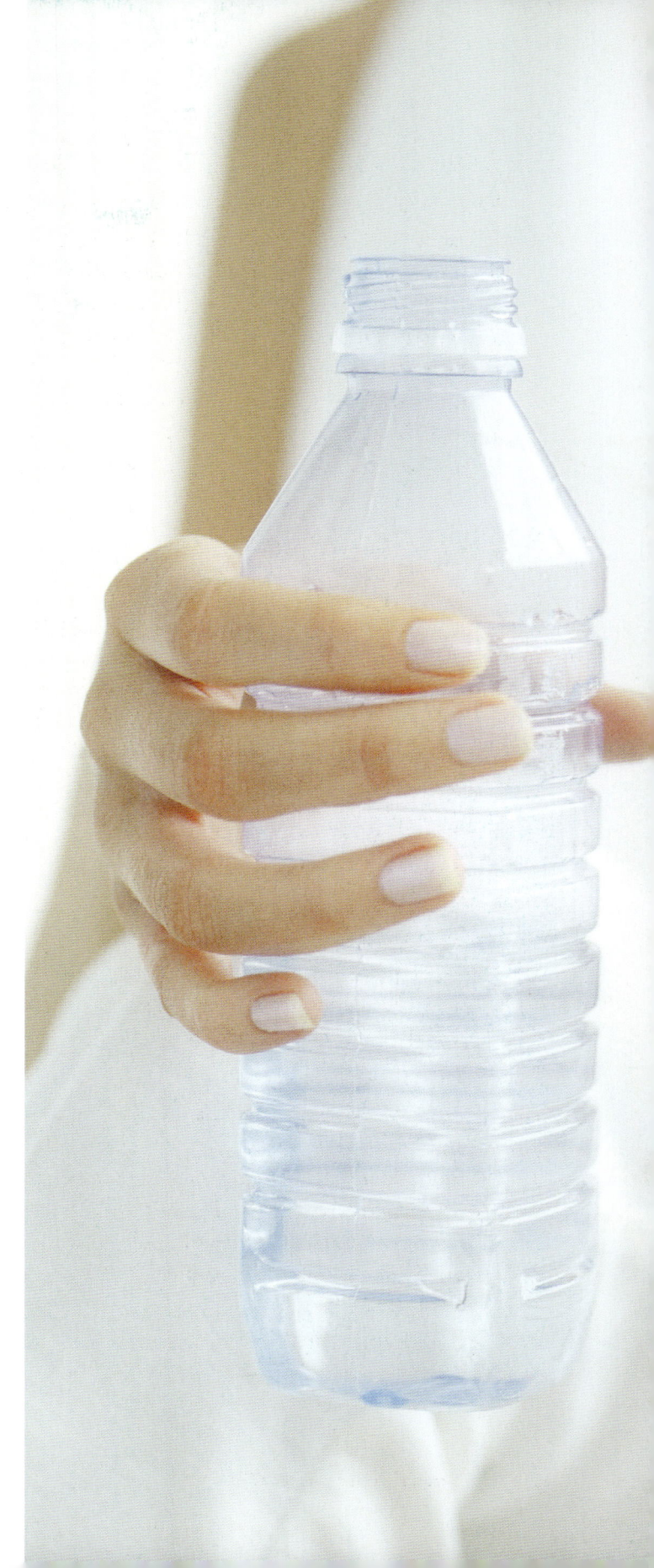

Setting goals

Andy is 42 years old and works as an IT consultant. He is 180 centimetres tall, weighs 100 kilograms and doesn't exercise. He doesn't smoke and relaxes at home with a couple of beers each evening. He never eats breakfast, regularly eats out with clients at lunchtime (often including a glass of wine), and eats home-cooked meals with his family in the evening. He feels lethargic, struggles to keep up with his young children and would like to get fitter and lose 15 kilos. His goal is to weigh 85 kilograms, which is what he weighed when he was 32 years old and swam regularly.

When he decided to lose weight and get fit, Andy worked out his long-term, medium-term and short-term goals. He made them specific, measurable and attainable. He wrote them down, because this would keep him motivated as well as making his ultimate goal more real.

Long-term goals
- Achieve goal weight of 85 kilos
- Be able to have more energy for family life
- Be able to swim freestyle for 1 kilometre without stopping
- Keep up with kids.

Medium-term goals
- Increase my exercise to five sessions each week by introducing resistance training
- Have two alcohol-free days per week
- Eat five to six smaller meals a day
- Improve swimming technique
- Get up early for a swim before work three times a week.

Short-term goals
- Take swimming lessons to improve freestyle stroke
- Swim once a week before work for the first three weeks
- Keep a training diary
- Take lunch to work three days a week
- Eat less food more often
- Stop drinking any alcohol at lunchtime and replace with water
- Eat breakfast at least four out of five workdays.

Next he worked out how and by what date he wanted to achieve his goals. For his short-term goals, he wrote:

- On Monday, investigate local swimming lessons and get the swimming timetable to find out about pool opening hours.
- Go through wardrobe to find swimmers and goggles. Pick a bag to use as a swimming gear bag and add soap, shampoo, towel and other items needed for a swim session.
- Buy an exercise book for my training diary. Write up the columns needed.
- Write a shopping list of the healthy food items we need to buy, based on our new meal plan. Find out if we can get fresh fruit and vegetables home-delivered each week.
- Take healthy snacks such as fresh fruit, low-fat yoghurt and nuts to work to sustain energy levels throughout the day.
- Buy a 2-litre water jug and glass for desk at work. Drink one full jug each day.
- Set aside time to sit down and eat breakfast each morning, either at home or work.

Dealing with bad days

If you have a bad day, the first step is to give up the guilt. Do not beat yourself up about it – you're human after all. There will always be temptations and obstacles in your way, so turn them into positives. Learn from any lapse you may have had. How did it make you feel? What behaviour will you choose in the future to avoid the same thing happening again? Work out how to deal with your triggers, whatever they may be. Start dealing with things directly and find coping strategies that are right for you.

Take it day by day. If you have a bad day (or week, or month) and end up eating too much, or bingeing, or not exercising, *do not* give up. One day does not mean there's no point for the rest of your life. It's so easy to give up but you get nothing and will never, ever be the person you want to be. It's easy to fall back into old bad habits, especially when food provides comfort, but these habits are self-destructive. You can't build a new habit – or change your life – in a day. It takes time, patience and commitment to learn new skills.

> *'My whole attitude to setbacks has changed. I used to turn to food to cope, but now I see a "setback" as an opportunity to learn something about myself or teach myself something new.'*
> **Shane Giles, Series One**

If it works for you, follow the 80/20 rule: if you stay on the path to your goal 80 per cent of the time, giving yourself 20 per cent as room to move, you'll stay committed and still achieve your goal. It may take a little longer but it keeps you on track and it's realistic.

Stop thinking 'all or nothing' or 'good and bad'. Make a resolve *right now* that you will not give up on your new healthy lifestyle, even if you have a lapse for a moment, day or week. Choose not to be discouraged or feel guilty about this; no one is perfect and sometimes you have to miss a workout or you do indulge. Just be confident in yourself that you will resume your healthy eating and exercise plans. And do something as soon as possible that gets you back on track, such as going for a walk or making your next meal extra healthy.

Take this confidence with you on your journey to health and weight-loss. Take small steps and don't rush. Most importantly, stop thinking you can't. It gets you nowhere – except where you are right now. The only failure is giving up on your goal.

Are you ready? You can do this, so believe in yourself.

> *'One of my favourite sayings is "If I could let you taste success, even just for a second, I guarantee you won't give up until you have it". And it's true. If you could feel for yourself what I feel now after losing the weight, you would stop at nothing to make it happen. Anyone can do it, you just need to believe in yourself.'*
> **Adro Sarnelli, Series One Winner**

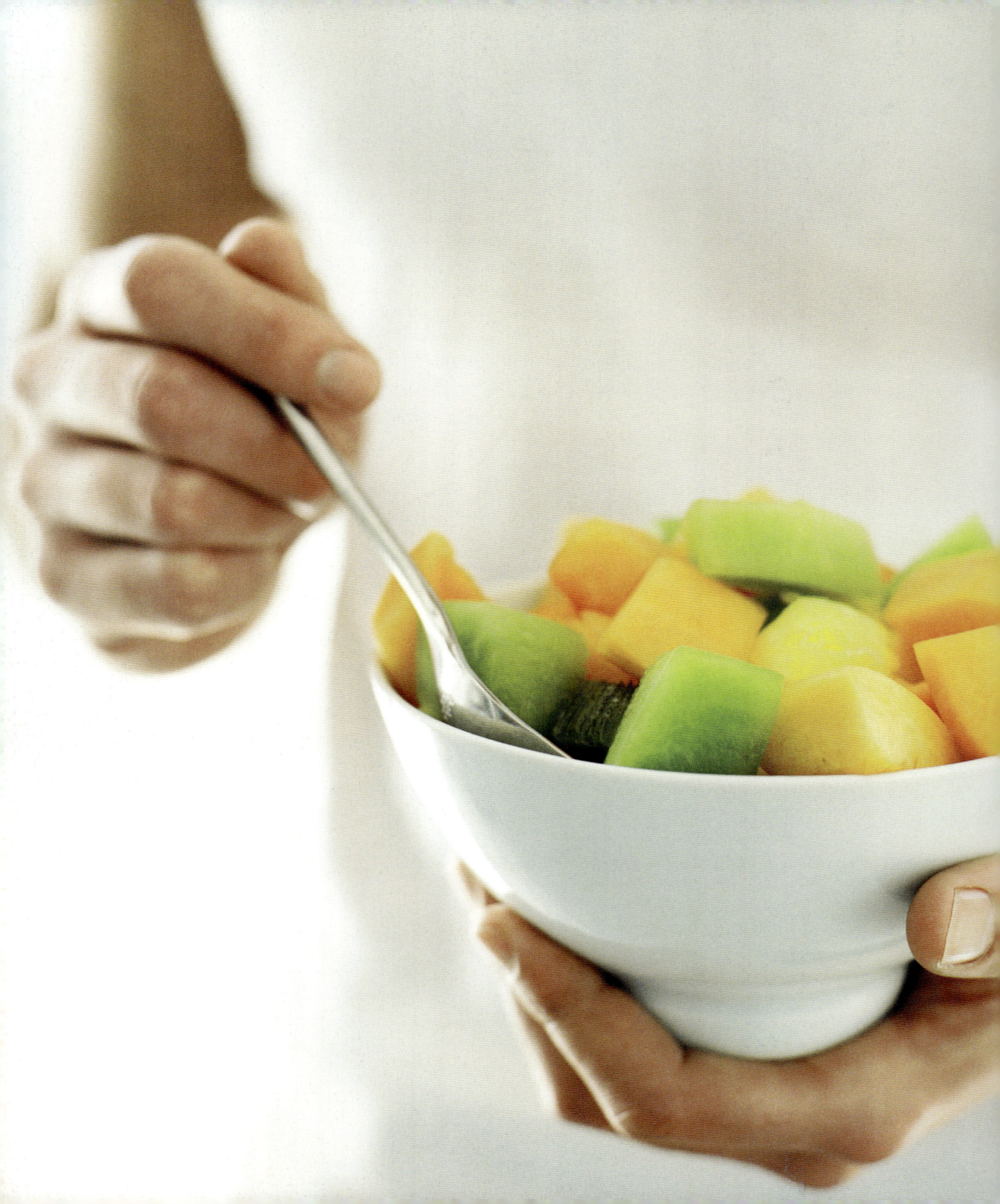

Ready?

Set

Go!

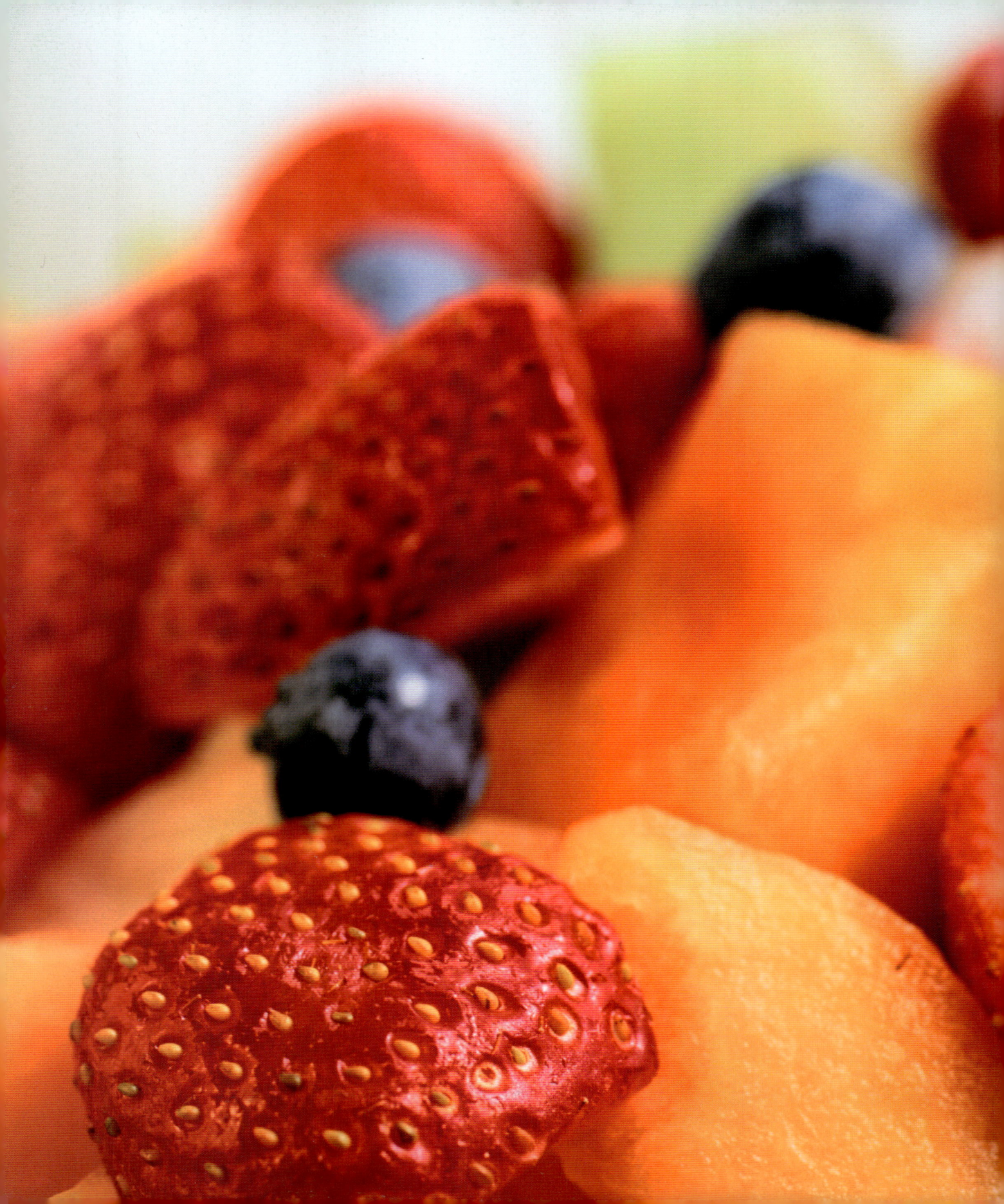

The Biggest Loser Eating Plan

Long-term healthy eating is at the heart of the Biggest Loser philosophy. The Biggest Loser Eating Plan is not a starvation diet. It is a way of eating that you need to be able to integrate into your life. You will be eating healthy foods and moving more. Not only does exercise burn up more energy but it will ensure that the weight you lose will be mostly fat.

How much food do you need?

Our bodies require energy to live, even if we choose to sit on the couch all day. Food provides this energy, which is measured in kilojoules (or calories in the imperial system – 1 calorie equals 4.2 kilojoules). Different types of food provide us with different amounts of energy. For example:
- carbohydrates give you 16 kilojoules per gram
- protein 17 kilojoules per gram
- alcohol 29 kilojoules per gram
- fat 37 kilojoules per gram.

If you are overweight, chances are you're consuming more energy than you're using. If your body gets more energy than it needs, the energy will be stored primarily as fat. To lose weight you need to create an energy deficit – that is, you need to burn up more kilojoules than you eat. If you eat more kilojoules than you use, you'll put on weight. Over time, consuming more energy than you expend (even in small amounts) leads to obesity.

To get healthy and lose weight, the first step is to ensure the kilojoules you consume come from healthy foods – whole, unprocessed, low-fat foods – instead of high-kilojoule, processed foods. The second is to reduce your kilojoule intake and increase your activity level.

> **MAKE THIS YOUR MANTRA:**
> **EAT LESS, MOVE MORE.**

HOW MUCH ENERGY DO YOU BURN?

We all have different physical and metabolic needs and it's good to understand what your body's needs are. Spend the time to work out how much energy you need each day; this way you won't intake too many kilojoules or too few (which can send your body into starvation mode, where your metabolism slows and you stockpile fat).

Your total energy expenditure (TEE) is the amount of energy your body needs to get through the day – it includes the number of kilojoules your body requires simply to support your existence (your resting metabolic rate), plus the energy used to digest and metabolise your food (the thermic effect of food), plus the kilojoules you use up in any activities (your daily activity level).

Working out your TEE using the formula on the next page will be an estimate only. However, it will provide you with an approximate guide of how many kilojoules you use each day, which you can then use to work out how many kilojoules you need to consume to lose weight.

Your resting metabolic rate

Your resting metabolic rate (RMR) is the rate at which you expend energy, even when you sleep. It's the number of kilojoules your body needs to supply energy to all your vital systems so you continue to breathe, your blood circulates, your muscles move, hormones are produced, your body temperature remains stable and all your internal organs continue to function. Your RMR is worth knowing about because it accounts for around 60–70 per cent of your total energy expenditure.

On top of your RMR is the amount of energy you use to process food: eating it, digesting it, absorbing and using nutrients and storing energy. This is known as the thermic effect of food and represents about 10 per cent of your TEE.

Use the following Mifflin calculation to work out your own RMR (using your weight in kilograms and height in centimetres). Or use an RMR calculator available on the internet for an approximation.

Men: (10 x weight) + (6.25 x height) – (5 x age) + 5 = your RMR in calories.
Multiply it by 4.2 to work out your RMR in kilojoules.

Women: (10 x weight) + (6.25 x height) – (5 x age) – 161 = your RMR in calories.
Multiply it by 4.2 to work out your RMR in kilojoules.

So, if you are a woman aged 35, who weighs 80 kg and is 168 cm tall, your RMR would be:
(10 x 80) + (6.25 x 168) – (5 x 35) – 161 = 1514 calories x 4.2 = 6359 kilojoules

Your daily activity level

The activities we do each day affect the amount of energy we burn. Think about what activities you do in an average day and choose a daily physical activity level from the list below.

1.200 = sedentary (little no exercise)
1.375 = light exerciser (light exercise at low intensity a couple of times a week)
1.550 = moderate exerciser (moderate exercise a few times a week)
1.725 = active exerciser (hard exercise at high intensity most days each week)
1.900 = very active exerciser (daily strenuous exercise and physical job)

Now, to work out your TEE, multiply your RMR with the activity level that best represents your current lifestyle (even though this formula doesn't include the thermic effect of food, it is still a good estimate of the amount of energy you use in a day).

So if the 35-year-old woman above is a light exerciser, her TEE would be:
6359 x 1.375 = 8744 kilojoules.

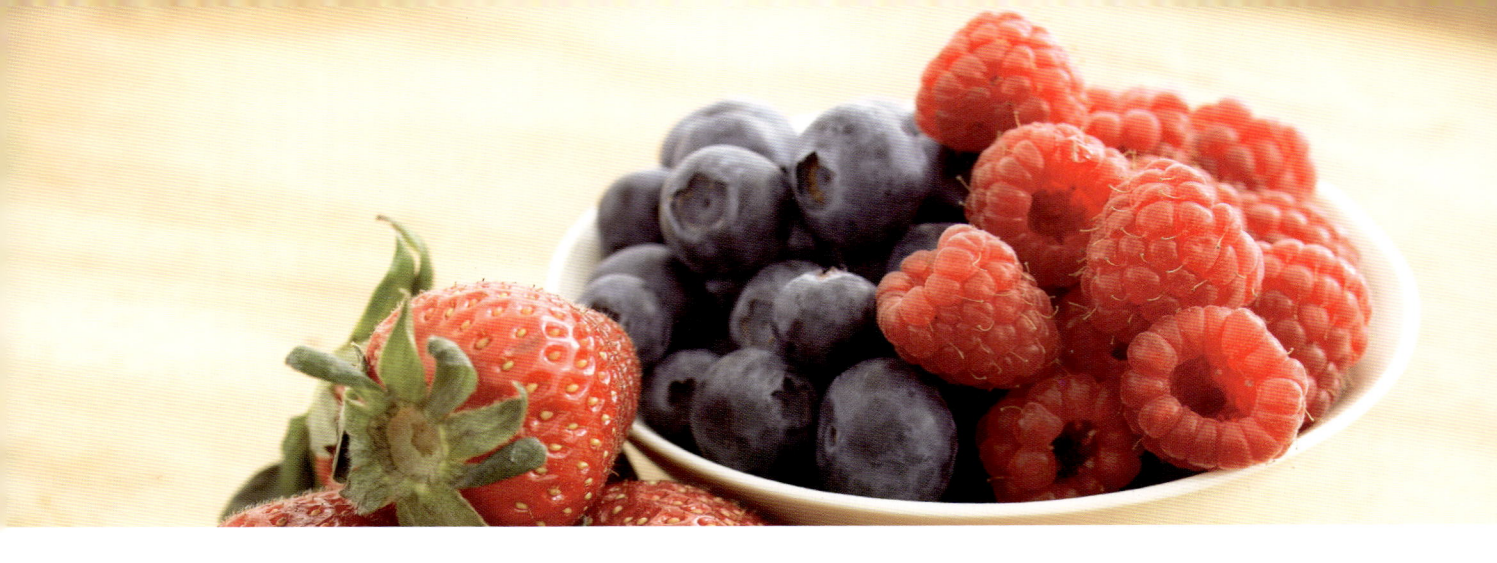

EATING TO LOSE

Now that you have an estimate of how many kilojoules you use each day, you can work out what you want your new intake to be. It takes an energy deficit of approximately 32,300 kilojoules to burn up 1 kilogram of fat so, to lose approximately 0.5 kg each week, you need to reduce your daily intake by 2000 kilojoules or more. If you add exercise into the equation, you'll lose more.

Take your daily total energy expenditure and reduce it by 2000 kilojoules: this is what you need to eat to lose weight. The Biggest Loser Eating Plan offers three daily intake levels, along with the 14-day KickStart Plan. Pick the daily intake level below that is closest to your new daily kilojoule intake.

- 5000 kilojoules (the 14-day KickStart Plan)
- 6000 kilojoules
- 8000 kilojoules
- 10,000 kilojoules.

In Part Three, you'll find sample weekly menu plans for each of the Biggest Loser levels (see pages 102–107). These will help you prepare for your new eating habits. You will also need a few other tools.

Measuring cups and spoons will be useful in your new eating plan. A food scale is optional but it is a good way to keep track of exactly how much you're actually eating. You will also need a weight scale, to weigh yourself, and a measuring tape.

Will you need a kilojoule counter book? No, not necessarily, but using a kilojoule counter book is a great way to learn more about the energy different foods provide. Even if you begin by counting your kilojoules, you'll soon know instinctively what your portion sizes should be and which foods are high or low in kilojoules. The more you learn about what you are eating and the energy you expend, the more flexible you can be with your eating and the more likely you are to keep the weight off long-term. Learning about your body is worth your time and effort – your health depends on it.

If you really can't stand counting kilojoules, that doesn't mean you won't be able to lose weight. Don't give up – it's not all or nothing. Read about the serving sizes below and how to use your household measures (cups and spoons) and your hand to measure them, so you get an idea of what is an appropriate amount of food.

What to eat

The Biggest Loser Eating Plan is based on three well-balanced main meals a day with two to three snacks, supplying you with all your essential daily nutrition requirements. Your recommended daily intake (depending on your kilojoule target) will be:

- 6–10 serves of vegetables and fruit (eat more vegetables than fruit, so 4 of vegetables and 2 of fruit)
- 3–6 serves of protein (lean animal, vegetarian or low-fat dairy protein)
- 3–7 serves of wholegrains
- up to 800 kilojoules per day of 'extras' (oils, fats, nuts, sweets, sauces).

FRUITS AND VEGETABLES

One serve equals 1 cup of raw vegetables or salad, ½ cup of cooked vegetables, ½ cup of cooked dried beans, peas or lentils, one medium piece of fruit (such as an apple or pear) or two small pieces of fruit (such as apricots).

You need to eat a minimum of **six to 10 serves** of vegetables and fruit each day. Eat at least four serves of vegetables and two serves of fruit. Vegetables and fruit supply the most nutrients and are a great source of fibre. Make vegetables the foundation of your eating lifestyle and you will lose weight while considerably improving your health.

In the initial stages of your weight-loss, avoid dried fruit and fruit juice. Dried fruit is high in kilojoules and fruit sugar and is often dried with sulphur. A glass of juice does not equal a serve of fruit or vegetables and will not help you to eat healthily. Juice contains no fibre (so you won't feel full or get the benefit of eating a piece of fruit) and is high in kilojoules.

PROTEIN FOODS

Eat **three to six serves** of protein each day. Choose from animal protein, low-fat dairy protein or vegetarian protein. It is important to ensure that at least two of your serves come from low-fat dairy protein. If you prefer, you can split the protein serves over the day and have protein at each meal.

Animal protein

One serve of animal protein is approximately 65–100 g of meat (a piece roughly the size of your palm) – 2 small chops, 2 slices roast meat, ½ cup of lean mince, 2 eggs or an 80–120 g cooked fish fillet. Animal protein includes meat, poultry, fish and eggs. Choose the leanest meat and trim any visible fat – animal protein can contain considerable amounts of saturated fat. Avoid processed meat such as salami – an easy way to do this is to not buy your meat at the deli. Fish is a great animal protein choice, packed full of healthy omega-3 fatty acids and generally low-kilojoule.

Vegetarian protein

One serve of vegetarian protein is about ½ cup (dried) lentils, beans, chickpeas or canned beans, a piece of tofu the size of your palm, ⅓ cup nuts or ½ cup seeds. Beans and legumes make up the bulk of vegetarian protein and include chickpeas, lentils, black beans, broad beans, kidney beans, lima beans, navy beans, split peas, cannellini beans, borlotti beans and soy beans. Soy beans are made into many other vegetarian protein products such as tofu, tempeh, soy burgers, soy hot dogs or miso, so there is a wide range of vegetarian protein sources available.

Low-fat dairy protein

One serve of dairy protein equals one cup (250 ml) of low-fat or skim milk, 200 g of low-fat yoghurt or two slices of reduced fat cheese. Choose low-fat yoghurt (avoid any flavoured yoghurt that is high in sugar by buying the diet versions), low-fat milk and low-fat cheese. Dairy is a good source of calcium – if you drink soy milk, choose one that is low-fat and fortified with calcium.

WHOLEGRAINS

Eat a minimum of **three to seven serves** each day. One serve equals 1 cup cooked rice, noodles or pasta, 2 slices of wholegrain bread, 1 medium wholegrain bread roll, 1 cup porridge, 1⅓ cups breakfast cereal flakes or ½ cup of muesli. Wholegrains are grains that haven't been refined. This means that they are closer to their original state and retain all their nutrients, vitamins, fibre and goodness. Choose brown or wild rice (not white), barley, couscous, rolled oats, bulgur, polenta, oat bran, wholemeal cereals, wholegrain bread or wholemeal pasta. Avoid eating breakfast cereals that are highly refined; these cereals are usually loaded with sugar.

YOUR EXTRAS

The Biggest Loser Eating Plan allows for up to 800 kilojoules of extra foods each day. This is your chance to select treats or additions to your daily intake. Aim to use 400 kilojoules on a healthy extra and use the other 400 kilojoules for a treat. Choose from good fats such as reduced-fat nut butter, avocado, olives and olive oil, nuts and seeds. Your extras can also include reduced-fat sauces and spreads such as salad dressings, tomato sauce, barbecue sauce and soy sauce, and condiments such as mustard or tomato paste. It is important to avoid denying yourself everything you enjoy because you'll just want to rebel against the restriction. However, if you know that once the packet of chips is open you'll eat them all (100 grams of plain potato chips equals 2265 kilojoules!) or that when you have ice-cream in the fridge you'll eat the whole container, avoid buying these things in the initial stages of your new healthy eating plan. Don't make things difficult for yourself.

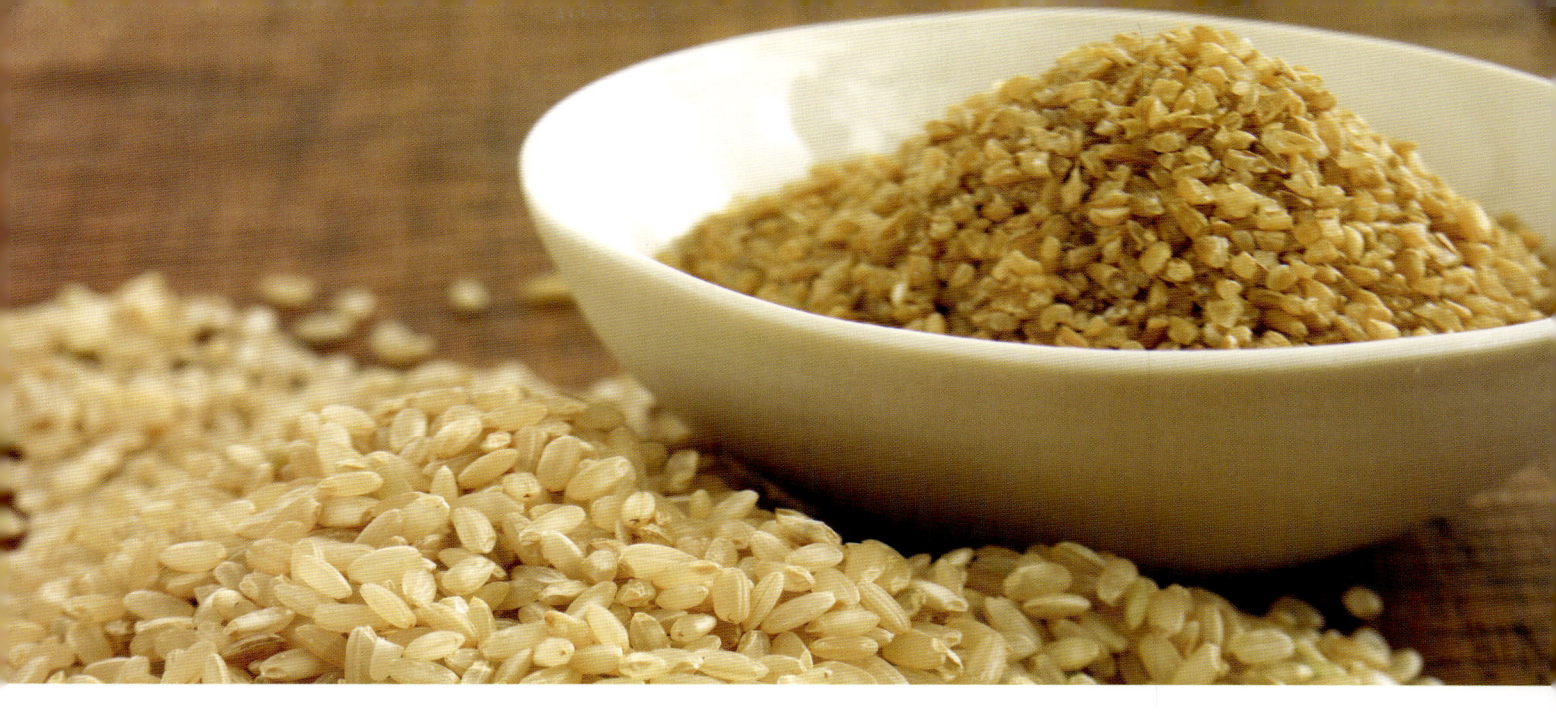

If you are including alcohol in your extras allowance, try to avoid mixers. Instead of mixing with lemonade (375 ml = 657 kJ), choose soda water (0 kJ) with a serve of diet lime cordial (14.5 kJ).

Healthy extras

- 1 (125 g) apple = 270 kJ
- 100 g apricots = 190 kJ
  (whereas 25 g dried apricots equals 176 kJ!)
- 50 g (around ¼) avocado = 445 kJ
- 1 (100 g) banana = 350 kJ
- 100 g grapes = 280 kJ
- 1 kiwi fruit = 205 kJ
- 1 orange = 160 kJ

Treats

- 150 ml red or white wine = 424 kJ
- 1 x 375 ml can/stubby lager = 580 kJ
- 1 x 375 ml can/stubby light beer = 160 kJ
- ½ cup low-fat ice-cream = 340 kJ
- 1 fun-size Snickers Bar = 462 kJ
- 1 fun-size Mars Bar = 401 kJ
- 1 choc-chip biscuit = 243 kJ
- 1 Iced Vovo = 225 kJ
- 1 fun-pack Maltesers = 389 kJ
- 1 fruit Weis Bar = 158 kJ
- 1 English fruit muffin = 574 kJ
- 10 Pringles potato chips = 430 kJ
- 30 ml spirits = 257 kJ

'Remember to stay positive. Setbacks are a normal part of life, but get over it and move on. Don't think that, just because you started the day with an egg and sausage muffin, you may as well finish it off with an entire chocolate cake! Don't deprive yourself of food you enjoy, but eat it in small portions and just as a treat once in a while.'

Harry Kantzidis, Series One

What to drink

It's possible to consume a considerable number of kilojoules from drinks. What you choose to drink can also affect your health, so make wise decisions based on the information below.

WATER

Water is essential for your health – approximately 60 per cent of your body is water. Water forms the base of all bodily fluids, such as blood, urine, sweat, tears and digestive juices, and is involved in almost all bodily functions ranging from circulation to digestion. Water helps your body detoxify, via the kidneys and liver, flushing out toxins and chemicals.

Drinking more water will improve your skin, your muscle tone, your brain function, your bowel function and your overall health. It will help with weight-loss too. Drinking water before you eat will help to regulate your appetite as sometimes thirst is mistaken for hunger. If you don't drink enough water, your body tries to store and retain whatever water it has, setting you up for problems with fluid retention.

The amount that's right for you to drink each day depends on your body, your activity levels, your sodium intake and your state of health, but a safe guide is to aim for **1.5 to 3 litres per day**.

Fruits and vegetables have a high water content, whereas a diet high in meat, fat and dairy provides less water. Most drinks contain water, but it's best to drink some of your daily needs as plain water because some liquids (coffee, tea, cola, cocoa and alcohol) have a diuretic effect and increase fluid loss.

You lose water through the lungs (breath contains water vapour), skin (sweat), urine and faeces (dehydration can cause constipation). Not drinking enough water can have serious effects on your health. If you're dehydrated, you'll probably suffer from:

- thirst
- headaches
- tiredness
- a dry mouth
- light-headedness and dizziness
- muscle weakness.

ALCOHOL

Alcohol is the most commonly used drug in Australia. It can be a pleasurable and relaxing part of life but moderation is the key. If over-used, it significantly contributes to weight gain. Alcohol offers 'empty' kilojoules – energy that doesn't make you feel full and that has little or no nutrient value. Alcohol can reduce the level of nutrients within the body and, due to the high sugar content, can be a contributing factor to obesity. It also:

- slows your fat metabolism (hence the 'beer gut')
- weakens your resolve (so you're more likely to over-eat and choose unhealthy foods)
- increases your kilojoule intake, especially when mixed with soft drinks or juices.

Because of its antioxidant properties, some alcohol (such as red wine) can help to reduce the risk of some types of cardiovascular disease.

In Australia, the recommended guidelines are no more than two standard drinks per day for women and four for men, and at least two alcohol-free days each week. To lose weight it's best to reduce your alcohol intake further. A standard drink is any drink with 10 g alcohol – a 30 ml shot of spirits is a standard drink, as is 100 ml wine or 375 ml mid-strength beer (3.5 per cent). Check the label if you're unsure; the label will always state the number of standard drinks in that one bottle or can.

If you're going to indulge every now and then, drink alcohol with food (it helps to reduce the alcohol absorption). Make your first drink non-alcoholic and kilojoule-free (such as water) and drink a water between every alcoholic drink. Finish each drink before refilling so you can keep track of how much you're drinking. Try not to overload your liver: drink in moderation and aim to have at least two alcohol-free days each week to reduce your chance of alcohol-related damage or dependency. Count any alcohol as part of your extras allowance as a way of reducing your total daily kilojoules.

COFFEE AND CAFFEINATED DRINKS

Any coffee-lover knows that to go without feels like a terrible sacrifice, so don't give up coffee if you don't want to, but drink it in moderation. Coffee contains the drug caffeine, which over-stimulates the brain and central nervous system. Your adrenal glands are stimulated so your body produces more adrenalin, turning on the 'fight or flight' response in your nervous system.

In small doses it can make you feel refreshed, increase your heart-rate, improve concentration and create a feeling of alertness with a burst of energy. In larger doses, however, it can lead to insomnia, shaking hands, anxiety, headaches, dehydration and, once the caffeine buzz has died down, even lower energy slumps and fatigue, which could have you craving high-sugar snacks. It can also reduce the body's absorption of vitamins and minerals. Caffeine takes between 4 and 7 hours to be cleared from your body, so avoid it in the afternoon if you want to sleep well that night.

Ideally, you should consume no more than approximately 300 ml of caffeine each day. One cup of instant coffee contains between approximately 60 and 100 ml caffeine; a cup of freshly brewed or espresso coffee between 80 and 300 ml; a cup of black tea between 10 and 90 ml; a 375 ml can of cola approximately 40 ml; and energy drinks from about 40 ml and upwards.

If you're going to include coffee in your lifestyle, aim to limit yourself to one or two cups each day. Choose good-quality coffee and really savour the flavour. If you're buying a coffee, walk to a café that's at least 5 minutes away.

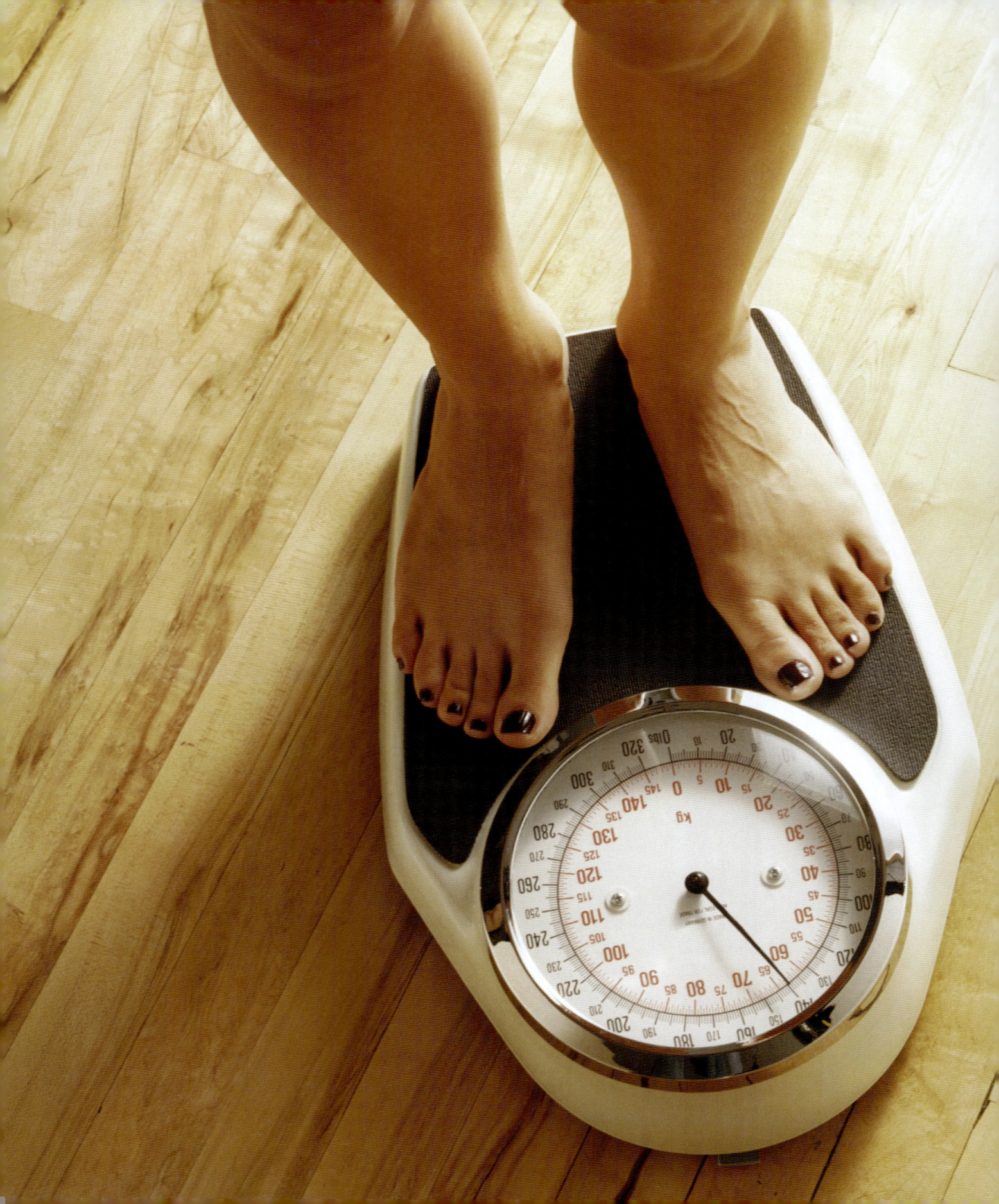

10 Biggest Loser steps to weight-loss success

Everyone is different but there are a number of steps that you can take that will help and support you in your weight-loss journey. If you're feeling overwhelmed, choose one or two steps to begin with, then slowly incorporate them all into your life.

1. Be accountable
2. Change to healthy food
3. Get organised
4. Eat breakfast
5. Eat three to six meals each day
6. Reduce your portion sizes
7. Manage where and how you eat
8. Get moving
9. Ask for support
10. Change your attitude and be committed

THE BIG WEIGH-IN

When and how often should you weigh yourself? On *The Biggest Loser*, weigh-ins are weekly and a real goal to work towards. Weigh yourself on the same day each week at the same time – the best time is first thing in the morning before you eat or drink anything. Write your weight in your food diary.

Some people find that weighing themselves every day works better – it keeps them accountable. Bear in mind, though, that your weight will fluctuate daily (often due to water retention) and you need to ensure that if it's not the reading you want, you don't get disillusioned and head straight to the fridge. If your mood is driven by what you weigh each morning, choose to weigh yourself weekly instead. Remember that this is a long-term lifestyle change; it's not going to happen overnight.

If you don't have scales or prefer not to weigh yourself, that's fine too. A tape measure will give you a good indication of your body's change in your fat stores. Measure your waist (at the narrowest point for women and the belly-button level for men), hips, thigh and upper arm when you first begin your new eating plan; note the measurements in your food diary. Each week, measure the same areas and continue to record it in your food diary. Think of your weight-loss in centimetres – you lost how many centimetres this week?!

1 BE ACCOUNTABLE

Self-monitoring is one of the key factors in long-term weight-loss. Self-monitoring keeps you honest. If you want to be successful in your weight-loss, you must be accountable to yourself for your actions. If you are not honest with yourself, you won't be successful. Self-monitoring also makes you conscious of your behaviour.

To be accountable, write a list of your health and fitness goals (see page 18); keep a food diary; keep an exercise/training diary; write in a personal journal; and commit to creating at least one good habit that supports your good health. You can do all of these or start with just one or two.

Don't underestimate the power of support systems such as your family and friends or a weight-loss group to keep you accountable. If you have to weigh yourself weekly at a weight-loss group, or if you have a friend waiting for you at the corner every morning at 6 a.m. to go for a walk, you will be more accountable. There are also many online weight-loss groups to help you.

Food diary

It may seem a time-consuming task, but keeping a food diary is an important tool in your weight-loss journey. It will keep you accountable and aware. It's about assessing where you are right now, without beating yourself up about it. It makes your eating habits concrete and tangible, and helps you think about what you're eating and why.

Initially a food diary (which can be as simple as an exercise book) is a good way to see what and how much you actually eat. You may think that you eat relatively healthily but, when you write down everything you eat in a day, you could be surprised! Be honest – if you cheat, you are only fooling yourself. The diary is a way to stay true to your goals, and also see where and when you might struggle. It also helps you become more aware of what may trigger overeating or unintentional eating.

It is important to include absolutely *everything* that you consume – food and drinks. If you're unsure what to include or want some easy ready-made diary printouts, there are many available for free on the internet.

Keep a diary for three to five days before you start the Biggest Loser Eating Plan. This will help you work out your problem areas, such as what you eat most and when. Then, once you start the plan, you can maintain the diary to see how well you stick to it, when you might have problems, and how your eating patterns change.

If you like things simple, all you need are four columns in your diary: *the date*, *the time you eat*, *exactly what you eat and drink*, and *how it was prepared* (don't just say 'bread', say 'three slices of white bread, toasted, with about a teaspoon of salt-reduced margarine'). If you like counting kilojoules, include a *kilojoules* column. You can also include how much you weigh each week.

If you know you are an emotional eater, then you will benefit from a more extensive food diary. Include a column 'How do I feel and why?'. You could also include columns such as 'Activity' and 'Ate alone/with others', so you can note whether you ate in front of TV, or while working, or at the table with friends or family. You will become more aware of your patterns, habits and triggers. If you are really keen, start a personal journal – this will help you uncover any underlying problems or unresolved issues that are leading to your overeating. (See pages 8–9 for more information on emotional eating.)

Your food diary will keep you focused on your goals and help you to become conscious of what you are putting into your body. You can't fool yourself when it's in black and white on the page before you. Your food diary will be the road map to your weight-loss – you can refer back to it to see how much you have achieved.

2 CHANGE TO HEALTHY FOOD

Now you understand that you lose weight by consuming less energy than you use. But not only do you want to lose weight, you want to feel *healthy* and improve your overall wellbeing! To do this, ensure the kilojoules you consume come from healthy foods – whole, unprocessed, low-fat foods – instead of high-kilojoule, processed foods. Wholefoods are those that are close to their original natural state – think of them as more *alive*. They provide your body with a higher ratio of nutrients to kilojoule intake. Wholefoods don't include added sugar or fat, or food additives. Wholefoods make you feel full and improve your digestive health. Processed foods are often energy-dense, which means that you get a lot of kilojoules for not much substance – you will have eaten more kilojoules before you feel full and you won't get many nutrients.

Use your food diary, shopping lists and shopping receipts to examine the types of food you are currently buying. How many items are processed and refined? How many come pre-packaged rather than fresh? How many bottles of soft drink are you buying each week?

Look in your pantry, fridge and freezer: clean out all the junk food. Be ruthless! If it's not there, you won't be tempted. Not everyone has willpower of steel, so be kind to yourself and make things easier by removing the temptation.

Go to a fresh food market if you can. Not only is it usually a more enjoyable experience than pushing your trolley through crowded shopping aisles, but also the produce will be fresher (and most likely cheaper!).

Choosing healthy foods and making that choice a life-long habit will help you remain at a healthy weight for the rest of your life.

> 'I was overweight because of bad management: I badly managed my body, my food, my activity and my lifestyle. In changing that, I learnt to appreciate and control myself, to live life rather than just be alive, and to see my health and body as more important assets than the house.' **Adro Sarnelli, Series One Winner**

READING NUTRITION LABELS

To help you choose healthy food, read nutrition labels. The nutrition information panel on food lists the energy (kilojoules or calories), protein, total fat, saturated fat, total carbohydrate, total sugar and sodium content of the food (see page 53 to find about more about nutrition). You'll see two columns – one is the amount per serve (an amount determined by the manufacturer) and the other is per 100 g (or 100 ml). The panel may also show the amount of iron, calcium, potassium and fibre the food contains.

Reading the nutrition information panel helps you compare products, so you can pick ones lower in fat or sugar. It also helps you work out how much fat or sugar you've eaten during the day.

Also read the list of ingredients. They are listed in order of quantity, so the first ingredient makes up more of the food than the last ingredient. If the first ingredient is sugar, that means the bulk of that food is sugar.

3 GET ORGANISED

It's easy to let things slide when you lead a busy lifestyle, but if you really want to change your life and your health, you need to make that goal a priority. This means setting aside time and energy to do what is required to get – and stay – healthy. If you really want this, you can make it happen.

Learn how to get organised, how to manage your time better and how to say 'no' to things that will not benefit your health goals. Your health is important and you need to support yourself on your weight-loss journey. If you 'never have the time to exercise', see what you can cut out of your day. Can you turn off the TV and go to bed so you can get up earlier in the morning for a walk? Can you reduce your TV watching by 30 minutes a day or get up in every ad break? Can you avoid scheduling any early morning work meetings that interrupt your exercise time? Can you walk the kids to school? If you *really* want this, you can make the time to get organised.

Planning ahead also saves you time, money and stress.

'I don't eat junk food or chips anymore, but of course I still sometimes crave these foods, so my strategy is to be prepared. I always carry a supply of nuts and tuna around so that if I get caught out and about, I have healthy food I can snack on. I also always try to eat every 3 hours so that I don't reach that starving stage where I know I'd reach for the first bad thing I see.'

Cat White, Series One

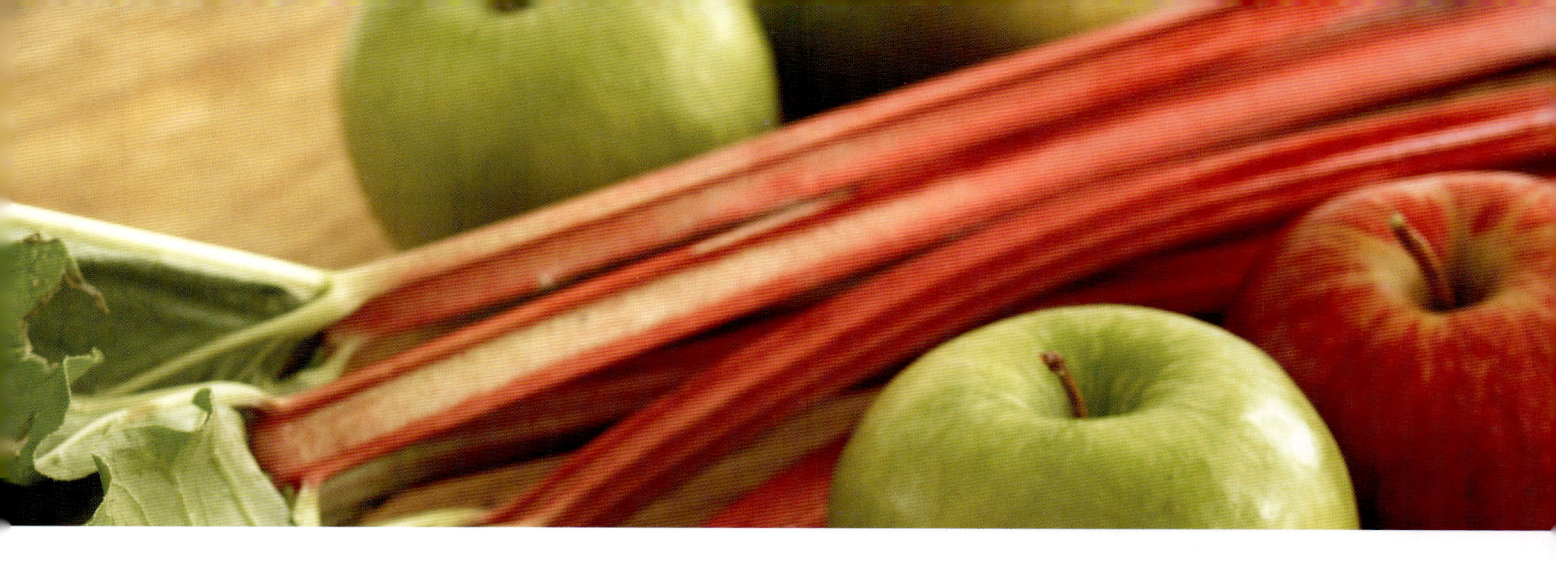

Shopping

We often buy the same food week in, week out and cook the same meals. Worse still, we decide what the weekly meals will be while cruising the supermarket aisles. We can lose interest in what we eat and it can reinforce our bad habits. Look back through your food diary to see any monotonous patterns. In your new healthy eating lifestyle, try to buy one new item each week, something you haven't tried before – it could be new herbs or vegetables, a new low-fat cheese, or a grain you haven't cooked before.

Keep a shopping list – shopping lists will save you time and hassle, and make you less likely to impulse-buy. Make sure it's handy in the kitchen and that there is always a pen next to it. Try to shop in the mornings when you're less likely to crave food and over-shop. Never shop when you are hungry. Avoid the junk food aisles – if you sail straight past them you're avoiding temptation without even trying.

Choose seasonal fruit and vegetables; this will save you money, ensure you get fresh produce and give you variety year-round. Frozen vegetables are also nutritionally good options.

Planning meals

Most people lead busy lives and it's easy to just pop into the supermarket or takeaway on the way home from work and pick up a quick and easy dinner. But consider this: eating is an essential part of your day, every day, and your health relies on it, so don't you think it's worth a little forward thinking?

Planning your meals helps you control your kilojoule intake. It saves you the time and energy of having to decide what you're going to have for dinner while you're on the way home from work. You will have healthy food on hand and be less likely to resort to high-kilojoule takeaways. It will also mean fewer trips to the supermarket during the week so you'll save money too.

By planning ahead, you can keep to your daily kilojoule limit. For example, if you know that you're going out for a special lunch, then plan to have a light meal for dinner. You can also plan to ensure you have healthy food at work for snacks or lunches.

It sounds like a lot of effort, but consider trying a weekly menu plan (use the menu plans in Part Three as inspiration). Get the whole family to contribute their requests for the week then stick it on the fridge. Shop to the menu plan and aim to stick to it.

4 EAT BREAKFAST

You will have heard many dietitians and nutritionists say that breakfast is the most important meal of the day. It is. Your body hasn't had any fuel since the night before; you need to refuel so you have the energy to get through the day. Eating a good breakfast will kickstart your metabolism and give you more brain power. Research has shown that people who eat breakfast are less likely to be obese or suffer from heart disease. Eating breakfast will also improve your performance at work in the morning.

A healthy nutritious breakfast ensures you get a good serve of your required daily fibre and important nutrients like iron and calcium. You are more likely to eat good food than unhealthy food at breakfast time (not many people crave pizza or chocolate first thing in the morning).

If you're running short of time, do not skip breakfast. Missing breakfast will not help you lose weight and, come morning-tea time, your energy will have slumped and you'll be ready to dig into high-sugar, high-fat snacks. Instead, set your alarm for 10 minutes earlier to give you time to make a quick breakfast. Alternatively, keep your breakfast food at work.

If you really don't feel hungry in the mornings, you can slowly train your body to eat breakfast. Begin with a small piece of fruit and then, over time, move to a smoothie, toast, muesli or porridge – your body will thank you for it, especially when you no longer need to reach for the sugar snack mid-morning. Another strategy is to eat your evening meal earlier so that you wake up hungry.

A good breakfast includes wholegrains, protein, including dairy, good fat and fruit or vegetables. Think poached eggs on wholegrain toast with mushrooms, or muesli with yoghurt and fruit and nuts. Try almond or peanut butter on wholegrain toast with a piece of fruit to follow.

5 EAT THREE TO SIX MEALS A DAY

Skipping meals will slow down your metabolism and keep you hungry, making you more likely to choose unhealthy food when you do eat. Some of the contestants on *The Biggest Loser* had been eating one meal a day, yet they were still considerably overweight. It's very difficult to get your necessary daily intake of vitamins and minerals in one meal a day.

Skipping meals lowers your blood sugar, leading to energy slumps, whereas eating regularly helps to keep your energy levels constant by releasing glucose slowly into your bloodstream. You will be less likely to crave unhealthy foods or get so hungry that you'll consume any food in sight. If you eat three to six healthy meals a day, you won't feel deprived and you'll regulate your appetite (and be less likely to impulse-eat).

Because you need to think about your overall wellbeing, not just losing weight, it's really important not to skip meals. Eating regularly will give you more energy, better concentration and fewer cravings. Eating a healthy morning and afternoon snack is an important part of the Biggest Loser plan – aim to eat every 2 to 3 hours.

> ## MEAL REPLACEMENTS
>
> If you decide to use some form of meal-replacement product at some point in your weight-loss journey, it is vitally important that you choose one that is nutritionally complete, meeting all the daily nutritional requirements (some over-the-counter products do not). It is best to visit an accredited practising dietitian for personalised advice. Think of it as an investment – you'll spend money on a service for your car, and you and your health are more important than your car!

6 REDUCE YOUR PORTION SIZES

Remember the energy balance: if you want to lose weight, you need to eat less energy than you use. If you want to maintain weight, you need to consume the same amount of energy as you use. You gain weight when you consistently eat more than your body needs. Often this happens unconsciously through large servings.

If you have worked out your total energy expenditure (using the formula on page 29), you will have an estimate of how many kilojoules you need to eat each day to lose or maintain your weight. If you're not counting kilojoules or weighing food, use your hand:

- one serve of protein would be approximately the size of your palm
- one serve of wholegrains or vegetables would be the size of your fist.

Eat smaller portions of food and you will automatically reduce your kilojoule intake. You need to train yourself to eat less. Some people find it difficult to leave food on the plate. If this is you, buy a new set of smaller plates and bowls. Don't be tempted to go back for seconds; put any leftovers away and enjoy the convenience of having them for lunch the next day. Also reduce the size of any drinks that contain kilojoules.

7 MANAGE WHERE AND HOW YOU EAT

Set the scene when you eat – eat at the table, set it nicely, savour the smells and the way the food looks. Remember that food is good for you – it's not naughty or bad, and you need it – so it's worth taking the time to enjoy your meal. After all, you've just spent time cooking it. Value the food you prepare as it gives you life and energy. Enjoy the preparation and the eating – instead of watching that cooking show on TV, why not spend a little more time in your own kitchen?

EATING OUT

Eating is an essential part of many social activities, and biggest losers don't have to give that up. It's about becoming conscious about your choices. There are many ways to manage eating out.

- If it's up to you, choose a café or restaurant that you know serves healthy wholefoods, not a fast-food takeaway restaurant. If you know you can't resist over-ordering at your favourite restaurant, go somewhere else.
- Try not to arrive at the restaurant absolutely starving. Ensure you've had a light snack beforehand or a bowl of steamed vegetables, salad or vegetable soup – this will help to reduce your appetite and make you less likely to over-order.
- Move some of your social occasions to breakfast or brunch. It's easier to order a healthy meal, such as an omelette, smoked salmon or poached eggs on multigrain toast with mushrooms and tomatoes (avoid the hash browns), and you won't be tempted to eat three courses.
- Take your time to order what you want. Don't rush into an unhealthy choice and don't feel pressured to order three courses just because your companions do.
- It's okay to ask the waiters how dishes are prepared. More and more people are eating healthily and cafés and restaurants cater to this.
- Choose an entrée serving as a main course, or choose two entrées instead of a main and dessert and order a bowl of steamed vegetables or a side salad.
- Choose a dish that has grilled vegetables or some lean protein with complex carbohydrates. The simpler the better.
- Stick with food that has been steamed, grilled or poached and avoid anything fried, battered or covered in a creamy sauce.
- You know what not to order – avoid the fries or potato wedges.
- Remember what it feels like to be over-full, how uncomfortable that can be. When you feel as though you've had enough, stop eating, even if it means leaving something on your plate.
- Share your dessert or opt for a fruit platter.
- Keep an eye on your alcohol intake and remember to ask for water.
- Enjoy the occasion – remember, someone else is doing the cooking and washing up.
- If possible, walk to and from the restaurant!

If you don't feel ready to go out, invite friends over and cook for them. And don't give up on your new healthy eating plan if you have a big night out. One night of unhealthy food or overeating does *not* ruin your plans for the new you. Just start again straight away at the next meal.

Consider how you actually eat. Do you wolf down your food, half-chewed, without savouring the flavour? Fast eaters will overeat before their bodies send the 'I'm full, stop eating' signal (it takes approximately 20 minutes before your brain registers that the stomach is full). Eating slowly and chewing your food thoroughly improves your digestion. Chewing is actually the first stage of your digestive process: enzymes in your saliva combine with the mechanical process of chewing to break food down so that when it reaches your stomach, it can be easily broken down further and released into the small intestine, where it's then even further digested and the nutrients properly absorbed.

By eating slowly and taking the time to chew, you will avoid digestive problems such as bloating, indigestion and constipation. Your health relies on your body absorbing the nutrients in your food. You will also eat less if you eat slowly. This will help you feel comfortable with the reduced portion sizes that you will now be eating. If you struggle with eating slowly, try putting your fork or spoon down while you're chewing. Pick it up only when you've finished that mouthful. Set your oven timer for 20 minutes and try to spread your meal out over this time. By eating slowly and savouring your meal, you will feel as though you have eaten a satisfying amount. Sometimes when a meal is rushed, it's hard to actually remember eating and the brain doesn't register any fullness or satisfaction.

Remember, break out of the all-or-nothing mentality. Aim to spend every meal at the table but, if you're used to eating every meal in front of TV, why not begin with eating two or three meals a week at the table with friends or family, chatting and enjoying the meal. Soon you will want to spend most meals at the table.

8 GET MOVING

This book isn't just about losing weight, it's about getting healthy. And it's very hard to get healthy if you don't move your body. Exercise has many benefits and if you don't include it in your weight-loss plan, you'll find it very difficult to maintain your weight-loss long-term. Not exercising means that you must eat less to maintain your weight-loss, which can be challenging.

If your weight-loss plan focuses solely on limiting your food, you'll get frustrated at the deprivation and may give up. Adding exercise and incidental activity to your lifestyle will allow you to take a more relaxed and realistic approach to food. Exercise also energises you, improves your overall health, creates a positive mood and reduces stress. (See page 66 for some quick tips on how to get moving.)

> 'My life right now is so very different to the "old Artie" – I'd hate to think what he'd be like now. My approach to food has changed, I count kilojoules and I exercise every day. That's my life and I'm so happy for it.'
>
> **Artie Rocke, Series One**

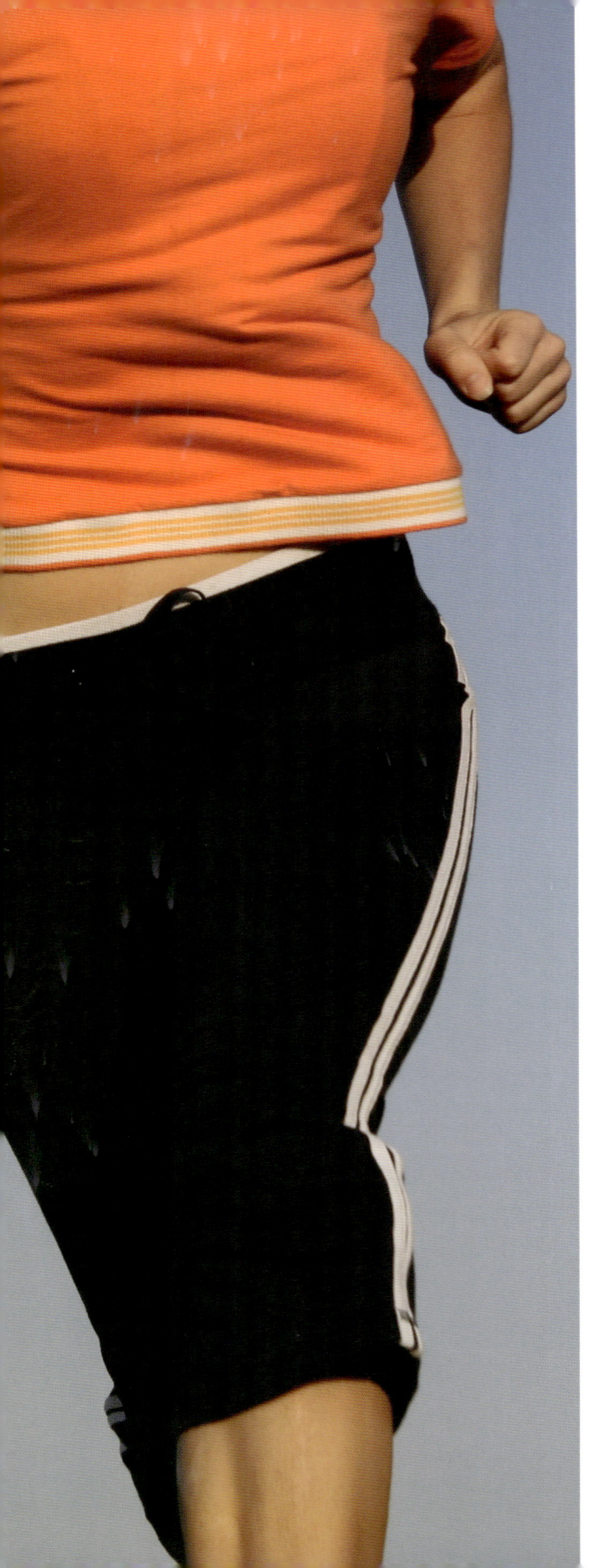

9 ASK FOR SUPPORT

One of the important factors in long-term weight-loss is a strong support system. This can take many forms – you need to find what works for you.

If they are supportive, enlist your entire family and friends to help you lose weight and get fit. Positive encouragement along the way will motivate you. Let the people you care about know what you're doing and what your goals are. You will also inspire them to make changes in their lives.

Pay attention to the people in your life; are there any who might not be able to support you in losing weight and getting healthy? It may be unconscious behaviour, but some people in your life may act as saboteurs, whether it's by tempting you with unhealthy food or complaining when you get up early. If you change your life, their relationship with you – the way they interact with you – may also change in some way and that can be challenging to deal with at first. Be kind but assertive – let them know how you feel, what your goals are and how they can support you in reaching them.

Find a weight-loss buddy; it could be a friend, family member or someone from a weight-loss group. You will be accountable to each other and this will make you more likely to turn up for the gym session or the morning walk. You can swap recipes and craving-busting solutions. Your buddy will also be there for you if things get tough, because they will understand – they are going through the same experience.

Join a community weight-loss group. This can both keep you accountable (especially when you know you'll be weighing in each week) and provide support, friendship and encouragement. Or you can go online and find support there. There are many internet weight-loss support groups, including a Biggest Loser group (visit www.biggestloser.com.au).

Adding a competitive edge can often help in weight-loss, particularly for men, so start your own Biggest Loser weight-loss competition. Do this with friends, work colleagues or family (or even advertise in the local paper). Organise weekly activities to support your daily exercise and organise a weekly weigh-in. Share your short- and long-term goals.

Professional support is always a good option: consider seeing an accredited practising dietitian who can help individualise the Biggest Loser Eating Plan for you; a weight-loss counsellor for assistance with your eating and exercise plan; or a counsellor or psychologist to motivate you and help resolve any underlying issues.

Know that you are not alone. Other people are going through what you're going through and feel like you do, and working together will make achieving your goals more enjoyable.

10 CHANGE YOUR ATTITUDE AND BE COMMITTED

A positive attitude is an essential driver for successful weight-loss. You learnt about positive self-talk and setting goals in Part One. You can choose to have a negative or positive attitude towards losing weight and getting healthy, and that choice will most likely affect your chance of success. If you think of following this plan as self-denial and deprivation, it's unlikely that you'll succeed, but if you think of these new changes as an opportunity to improve your health, empowering yourself, learning new skills, then you will succeed.

Remember these points:
- Change your self-talk – no more putting yourself down, getting angry or frustrated at yourself.
- Accept and forgive the times when you indulge or slack off. Follow the 80/20 rule: if you follow a healthy lifestyle 80 per cent of the time, with 20 per cent room to move, you'll lose weight and stay committed. Let go of the all-or-nothing mentality.
- Develop a positive self-image – you need to like yourself now, not put it off until you lose weight. If you don't like yourself now, will you really care enough to make the changes to improve your health and wellbeing?
- Changing your lifestyle isn't all hard work and deprivation; you'll have fun, probably meet new people and feel great about yourself – remember that if it gets tough!
- Stop the self-criticism; start praising yourself.
- Make your good health non-negotiable. This is *your* life.

'What does it feel like to have lost weight? Incredible! It's amazing how you can change you life with a little discipline and determination.'
'Big Wal' Milberg, Series One

The KickStart Plan

This 14-day plan has been devised to help kickstart your weight-loss – not only will it improve the health of your body and digestive system, it will strengthen your motivation to continue your lifestyle change. The KickStart Plan will help you to lose weight and give you more energy to get out and exercise.

The KickStart Plan provides both a menu plan and an exercise program for two weeks (see page 92 to find out more about the exercise program). It's a relatively low-energy diet (but not a very low-energy diet) that achieves safe weight-loss at a mildly fast rate for the first two weeks. It's nutritionally balanced and tasty, with a daily kilojoule intake of approximately 5000 kilojoules. The KickStart Plan is an optional stage – you can just move straight to one of the LifeStyle kilojoule intake limits if you prefer. If you have any medical problems, see your doctor before undertaking it.

It's not a detox plan; however, in the first week of the KickStart Plan (especially if you have previously eaten mostly processed, high-sugar, high-fat food), your body may be detoxing slightly – your liver will be working hard to release all the toxins you have been storing. Ensure you drink plenty of water (at least 2 litres a day). Try not to take on too many activities during the two weeks if you are feeling a little tired. Alternatively, you may feel full of energy for the first time in a long time. Enjoy it – this is the start of the new you! You are improving the state of your physical, mental and emotional health. Any side-effects (such as tiredness, pimples or headaches) won't last long and your renewed health and wellbeing at the end of the two weeks will be worth it.

SAFE RAPID WEIGHT-LOSS

There is growing evidence to support the idea of safe rapid weight-loss; however, this requires close medical supervision. Sometimes it's necessary to lose some weight rapidly, such as before surgery, to achieve improved health or to lose enough weight to allow mobility. The KickStart Plan is not a very low energy diet (these diets, often called VLEDs, usually limit daily intake to around 3500 kilojoules or less), but you may still experience fairly rapid weight-loss, especially if you have a high starting weight or are very active. The key to any safe rapid weight-loss is to ensure your diet is still nutritionally balanced and that you remain in contact with your healthcare professional. You also need to be aware that the rate of your weight-loss will slow down after the initial phase and that, unless you follow up with a healthy long-term weight-loss plan, the initial weight-loss will not be sustained.

PREGNANCY

Don't choose a restrictive weight-loss diet if you are pregnant; it's normal to gain weight during pregnancy. Pregnant women have an increased need for energy (an additional average need of 1800 kilojoules on top of their daily intake) and this is even higher during lactation (an extra 2500 kilojoules a day). Aim to eat well by making better food choices. This will keep you healthy, benefit your baby, and limit your weight gain to what your body needs during your pregnancy.

You will be eating three meals and two snacks a day, but the portion sizes will be reduced so you may feel a little hungry at first. Remember, this is just for two weeks.

For your successful KickStart Plan:

- prepare for the plan by going shopping with the KickStart shopping list (on pages 84–86) the day before you begin
- clear the house of all high-fat, high-sugar food (ignore any complaints from other family members)
- have your food diary ready
- plan ahead – if you are at work all day, take your snacks and lunch with you
- have a quiet two weeks – try to avoid social occasions that involve rich food, cigarette smoke and alcohol. Take this opportunity to do different activities, whether you have picnics in the park or trips to an art gallery or the movies.

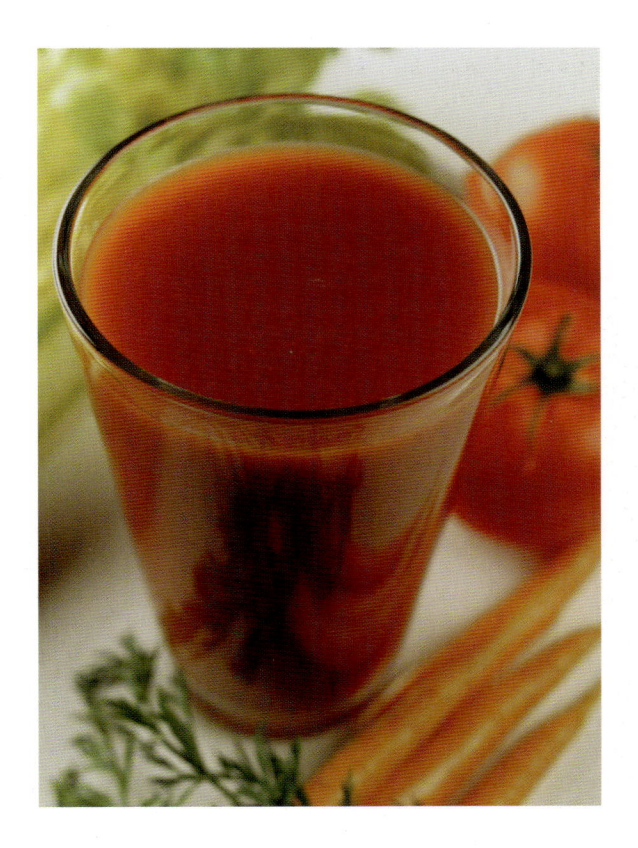

The LifeStyle Plan

Once you have completed the KickStart Plan you're ready to begin your new lifestyle of healthy eating and exercising. Part Three contains sample weekly menu plans for each of the daily kilojoule intake levels (6000, 8000 and 10,000 kilojoules). It also includes 60 delicious, healthy and easy-to-make recipes. Follow your sample weekly menu plan and then mix and match with some of the recipes (their nutrient breakdown, including kilojoules, is always included to help you work out your kilojoule intake). You will also now move on to the first of the two six-week LifeStyle Plan exercise programs (see page 108).

During the next three months, focus on creating new habits and continuing positive self-talk, even if things get difficult. You'll be feeling fitter and healthier than you possibly have in years. Enjoy this and remember to praise yourself for the commitment and focus you have shown.

MAINTAINING YOUR WEIGHT-LOSS

Research shows that people successful at maintaining their weight-loss over years follow a low-kilojoule, low-fat eating program balanced with exercise. That is, they don't fall back into their old behavioural habits and they continue to eat healthy food, consuming less energy than they expend.

You now understand what healthy food is and you have steps to take to support you in long-term weight-loss. If you follow the Biggest Loser Eating Plan, you should lose weight. Many people, especially if they're overweight, eat more than 10,000 kilojoules a day. By simply reducing what you eat currently by between 2000 kilojoules and 4000 kilojoules per day, you'll lose between 0.5 kilograms and 1 kilogram a week. You may lose more than this initially, but this is a typical amount to lose. Half a kilogram is equivalent to a tub of margarine and quickly adds up over the weeks. Don't feel disheartened if you're not losing the big numbers that the Biggest Loser contestants did – not many people can have personal trainers and assistants to make sure every daily task is organised so they only have to focus on losing weight and exercising.

Once you are losing weight your weight-loss may plateau. Once again, don't be disheartened by this – it's very normal. As you lose weight, your body requires fewer kilojoules. In the long term, your RMR reduces as your body weight decreases, so slowly reduce the number of kilojoules you consume to continue to lose weight (move to the daily kilojoule intake level lower than your current one), or increase the amount or intensity of physical activity you do. The good news is that your appetite gradually reduces over time as well. If you have lost about 10 per cent of your starting weight and you take a look in the mirror and decide you look great and feel much better, then this may be the right healthy weight for you and it's time to move into maintenance.

Once you've followed the Biggest Loser eating and exercise plans for three months and continued to eat healthy meals based on the Biggest Loser recipes and menu plans, you'll be feeling and looking great. However, after three months you may be feeling a bit flat about your exercise or want to try

CHILDREN

Children and teenagers require large amounts of energy because they are growing and developing rapidly. Regardless of whether children are overweight or not, their energy should come from healthy wholefoods, because these contain higher levels of the vitamins and minerals required for healthy development. Children should not be on a restrictive diet without supervision from a heath professional; however, the Biggest Loser recipes and guidelines are suitable for children. Persevere in offering your children healthy foods including vegetables, fruit and low-fat dairy for their snacks instead of highly processed bars and junk foods.

something new. Don't revert to your previous lifestyle. Now is the time to see a personal trainer and an accredited practising dietitian to personalise your health and fitness goals for the next 6 to 12 months.

Maintain your weight-loss long-term by:
- eating breakfast
- continuing to self-monitor
- keeping your eating consistent across weekdays and weekends (no huge splurges on the weekends)
- eating low-fat foods and monitoring your fat intake
- avoiding over-the-counter diet products
- planning meals
- remaining physically active
- weighing yourself weekly so you can catch any weight-gains early
- enjoying your life.

The good news is that research into successful long-term 'losers' has shown that maintaining weight-loss becomes easier over time. Your new eating plan becomes habit, and requires less attention, effort and time. It becomes your new lifestyle and along with that comes all the benefits: increased self-confidence, improved physical and mental health, and considerably more energy for life.

Eat well, stay active and enjoy!

'You can change your life by consciously eating well and exercising regularly. I was once 188 kilos and, no doubt, close to a heart attack or stroke. By the end of the show, I was 112 kilos and felt great. Now I have more energy to play with my boys (and my wife!). I am a "Big Loser" and proud of it. Remember, if I can do it, anyone can. Oppa!'

Harry Kantzidis, *Series One*

OTHER WEIGHT-LOSS OPTIONS

People suffering from obesity sometimes require a little extra help. If you find yourself struggling, see a doctor to discuss your options.

PRESCRIPTION DRUGS

Prescription drugs to aid in weight-loss and appetite control are available and may be right for you. See your doctor to find out what would help. These drugs complement a healthy eating and exercise plan; they do not replace it. They should only ever be used under medical supervision and as part of a long-term treatment strategy.

SURGERY

When your health is severely affected by your weight, obesity surgery may be an option to discuss with your doctor. Options generally exist in two categories of surgery. The first category is restrictive procedures (generally called gastric banding), which reduce the amount of food you can comfortably eat. The second category is called malabsorptive procedures; these procedures change the digestive ability of your body, meaning you can't absorb or digest food very well so it passes through your system. Sometimes the two approaches are used together.

Some procedures are performed by key-hole surgery whereas others require open surgery. Obesity surgery is *not* cosmetic surgery; it involves major operations and comes with all the complications and risks of major surgery. There may also be an emotional aspect to your obesity that will not be dealt with by the surgery; this is something you need to consider.

Long-term medical and nutritional supervision is essential to prevent digestive or nutritional complications after surgery.

If you think you may require surgery, see your doctor who will refer you to a qualified bariatric surgeon.

What is healthy eating?

Our bodies get all the nutrients they need from eating a balanced diet consisting of macronutrients (carbohydrates, protein and fat) and micronutrients (vitamins and minerals). You need macronutrients in large amounts and micronutrients in smaller amounts.

CARBOHYDRATES

Carbohydrates (often called 'carbs') are the body's preferred energy source; the body breaks them down into glucose, which fuels our cells to make energy. There are three different types of carbohydrates: sugars, starches and dietary fibre. Dietary fibre is sometimes also considered in a category of its own, separate from the other two types of carbohydrates.

Sugars

Known as *simple carbohydrates*, sugars are easily and quickly absorbed into the bloodstream, causing a rapid rise and fall in blood sugar levels, which can lead to energy slumps. Glucose is also an indicator of blood sugar levels (hyperglycaemia occurs when blood sugar is high, hypoglycaemia occurs when blood sugar is low; high blood sugars are a feature of impaired glucose tolerance and can lead to diabetes). Naturally occurring simple carbohydrates are found in fruit (as fructose), fruit juices and vegetables, and in milk and yoghurt products (as lactose, which is the only sugar of animal origin). Refined simple carbohydrates (added sugars) include white and brown sugar, corn syrup, molasses and honey; they can be found in biscuits, soft drinks, chocolate and nearly all processed food and refined snacks.

Sugar is a source of energy for the body. A little sugar can be useful because it provides a quick 'energy hit' and can add flavour to wholegrain products; however, sugar in its simple form (for example, white and brown sugar) contains no vitamins or minerals and so counts as 'empty' kilojoules. It's easy to get a lot of sugar in your diet: a 375 ml can of soft drink contains about 10 teaspoons of sugar per serve – that's a lot in one go! Consumption of sugary soft drinks has been linked to increasing numbers of overweight and obese children. Sugar is not the only reason for obesity but it does increase the kilojoule content of foods without adding any nutritional and satiety value.

Starches

Known as *complex carbohydrates*, starches have a more complicated molecular structure than sugars, which means the body needs longer to break them down and digest them. This leads to a slower rise in blood sugar levels. Complex carbohydrates can be found in a natural or refined state. Natural complex carbohydrates (the best choice for good health) include wholegrains, wholemeal pastas and breads, root vegetables, bananas, oats, barley, corn, nuts, legumes and brown rice. Refined complex carbohydrates include white bread, white flour, white rice, white pasta, processed cereals, pizzas, biscuits and cakes.

UNDERSTANDING GI AND GL

The concepts of the glycaemic index (GI) and the glycaemic load (GL) have gained considerable attention in the past few years. What do they mean and what effect could they have on your weight-loss? First you need to understand how your body uses glucose.

Your body's cells run on energy created from glucose (blood sugar), which is created when you eat and digest carbohydrates. The rate at which glucose is released into your blood directly affects your energy levels. Insulin, a hormone created by your pancreas, regulates your blood sugar and helps to carry the glucose from your blood into your cells where it is burned up to produce energy. Any glucose not used becomes glycogen, which, once the storage areas in the liver and muscles are full, gets converted to and stored as fat.

If you have too much glucose in your blood (high blood sugar) from eating too many refined carbohydrates, your body has to produce a lot of insulin. The higher your insulin levels, the more your body tries to send the glucose to the cells. Some people become resistant to the effects of insulin over time and their body makes more and more as it tries to bring the blood sugars down. Too much insulin also stimulates the conversion of glycogen from the liver and muscle stores to fat. This situation is known as insulin resistance or impaired glucose tolerance and is the first step to developing Type 2 diabetes.

The glycaemic index measures the rate that carbohydrates are digested by the body, based on carbohydrate samples of 50 grams. High-GI foods are quickly digested and absorbed by the body, creating a rapid rise in your blood sugar levels. Low-GI foods are more slowly digested and enter your system gradually, resulting in a slower rise in your blood sugar levels.

Low-GI foods can also be high in fat, and complex carbohydrates can be high GI, so it's best not to slavishly base your eating around GI. The glycaemic load index is a more appropriate measuring tool because it tests the GI based on portion size rather than the set 50 g. It considers the *amount* of the carbohydrate you're eating as well as its GI (so, even though watermelon has a high GI, you would not normally eat enough of it to get a rapid, large increase in your blood sugar levels). GL better indicates the total effects of food on your blood sugar levels.

Other things that affect blood sugar include:
- fat, which slows the rate of your stomach emptying, leading to a more gradual increase in blood sugar levels
- protein, which also slows the rate of your stomach emptying, so consuming protein with every meal can give you a slower rise in blood sugar and longer lasting energy to get through the day
- fibre, which may slow your rate of digestion and give a slower rise in blood sugar levels
- food particle size, because a smaller grain is more quickly digested, creating a sudden rise in blood sugar, whereas a larger grain takes longer to be absorbed (for example, choose wholegrain bread over white bread for a slower energy release).

Dietary fibre

Fibre is only found in plant foods. Fibre cannot be digested by the body and therefore passes fairly quickly through the digestive tract, collecting toxins and other waste as it goes. Because fibre is bulky and decreases transit time, it helps to keep you regular, decreases blood cholesterol, controls blood sugar levels, improves nutrient absorption and reduces the risk of colon cancer. It's also a key factor in controlling your appetite and, because dietary fibre needs more chewing, it helps you feel more satisfied after eating (so you eat less).

You need about 30 g fibre a day for good digestive health; fibre intake needs to be supplemented with sufficient water to avoid constipation. Low fibre intake over a long period of time can increase your risk of a range of health problems, including constipation, diverticulitis, haemorrhoids, hiatus hernia, varicose veins, obesity, diabetes and colon cancer.

Ideally you should increase your fibre intake through food. It's not difficult to increase fibre intake – switch to a high-fibre breakfast cereal; eat wholemeal bread and brown rice instead of the white varieties; add an extra vegetable to every meal; and eat one or two pieces of fruit every day. Try adding a source of bran, from wheat or oats, to your breakfast cereal. If this isn't possible, fibre supplements are available. If you need a supplement, choose one that is low in or free of sugar. Take it between meals and away from any medications (its binding effect may reduce their efficacy). Increase your water intake and start with a small fibre dose, then gradually increase it. Try natural supplements such as psyllium husks or LSA (a mix of ground linseeds, sunflower seeds and almonds, which is also a good source of protein and essential fatty acids).

There are two types of fibre: soluble and insoluble.

Insoluble fibre doesn't dissolve in water but binds to it and has a bulking effect; this helps the body to efficiently and quickly remove substances such as toxins and bile salts that are needed to make cholesterol from the bowel (reducing your risk of cancer). Even though fibre is indigestible, it is fermented in the gut, producing nutrients for the cells of the intestines. This process improves your intestinal health, reduces the risk of bowel cancer and prevents constipation. Sources of insoluble fibre include wholegrain cereals, wholegrain breads, wholemeal flour, wholemeal pasta, brown rice, legumes and pulses, oats, some fruits (especially those with edible seeds), some vegetables, dried beans, nuts and seeds.

Soluble fibre dissolves or breaks down in water and is also important for good intestinal health (it protects and soothes the intestines and creates the right environment for 'friendly' bacteria). Sources of soluble fibre include fruits (citrus, apples, pears), vegetables, oat bran, oats, barley, flaxseed, psyllium husks, lentils, peas, dried beans and soy products.

The truth about carbs

Carbohydrates are the basic fuel for your body, like petrol for a car. Despite their tarnished name over the past few years, carbohydrates are not 'bad' and will not sabotage your weight-loss if you choose the healthy versions (choose complex, unrefined, low-GL carbohydrates). If you don't eat enough carbohydrates, you may suffer from nausea, constipation, fatigue, irritability, headaches, bad breath and an inability to concentrate.

PROTEIN

Second only to water in the body's cells, protein makes up 20 per cent of your body weight. The average daily general requirement for health is 0.8 g per kg of body weight. Protein builds and repairs your body's tissues such as muscles, skin, blood vessels and hair. It makes enzymes, hormones and disease-fighting antibodies, helps balance fluid in your body and is essential for healthy growth.

Protein is made up of amino acids; these are your body's building blocks. When protein is eaten, it is digested and broken down into the individual amino acids. These amino acids are then reassembled by the body to renew its tissues (from hair, skin, nails and eyes to internal organs, especially the heart).

There are 20 amino acids: your body produces some of these (called non-essential amino acids) and needs to get the remaining ones (called essential amino acids) from food. Because of this, there are two types of protein: complete and incomplete. Complete protein is found in most animal foods (dairy, meat, fish, eggs) and from soy products (such as tofu). Complete proteins can be high in fat, so choose lean meat and low-fat or skim dairy foods. Incomplete protein, which lacks at least one essential amino acid, is found in the vegetarian sources of protein (such as legumes, grains, nuts, seeds and fruit). For vegetarians and vegans, eating a balanced combination of incomplete proteins over each day (such as including both grains and legumes) will help to provide your body with complete proteins.

Protein is an inefficient source of energy for the body; your body converts energy more efficiently from carbohydrates and fats. If you follow a high-protein, low-carbohydrate diet, you put extra stress on your kidneys. If you want to follow a very high protein diet, it is recommended that you have your kidney function checked first. Eating too much protein and too few carbohydrates may also increase your risk of muscle wasting (as your body will burn muscle tissue for energy), digestive disorders and bowel cancer.

FAT

Fat is energy-dense, containing 37 kilojoules per gram (more than twice the kilojoules contained in a gram of protein or carbohydrates). Fat is essential for our body because it transports fat-soluble nutrients such as vitamin A and E; aids our nerve function and the structure of cells; manufactures hormones; protects the internal organs; provides insulation; and creates energy. It also adds flavour and a nice 'mouth feel' to food.

Cholesterol

Cholesterol is part of the cell membrane of every animal cell, so all animal products contain cholesterol regardless of the fat content. There is good cholesterol (high-density lipoprotein, or HDL), which protects against heart disease, and bad cholesterol (low-density lipoprotein, or LDL), which can clog your arteries. High LDL cholesterol levels are implicated in heart disease. Your body needs good cholesterol for tissue repair, hormone production (notably oestrogen and testosterone), vitamin D synthesis, and for the structure of the myelin sheath coating brain cells. The majority of the body's cholesterol is made by the liver; not much cholesterol is absorbed from the diet. A key determinant of how much cholesterol your body makes is the amount of saturated fat you consume.

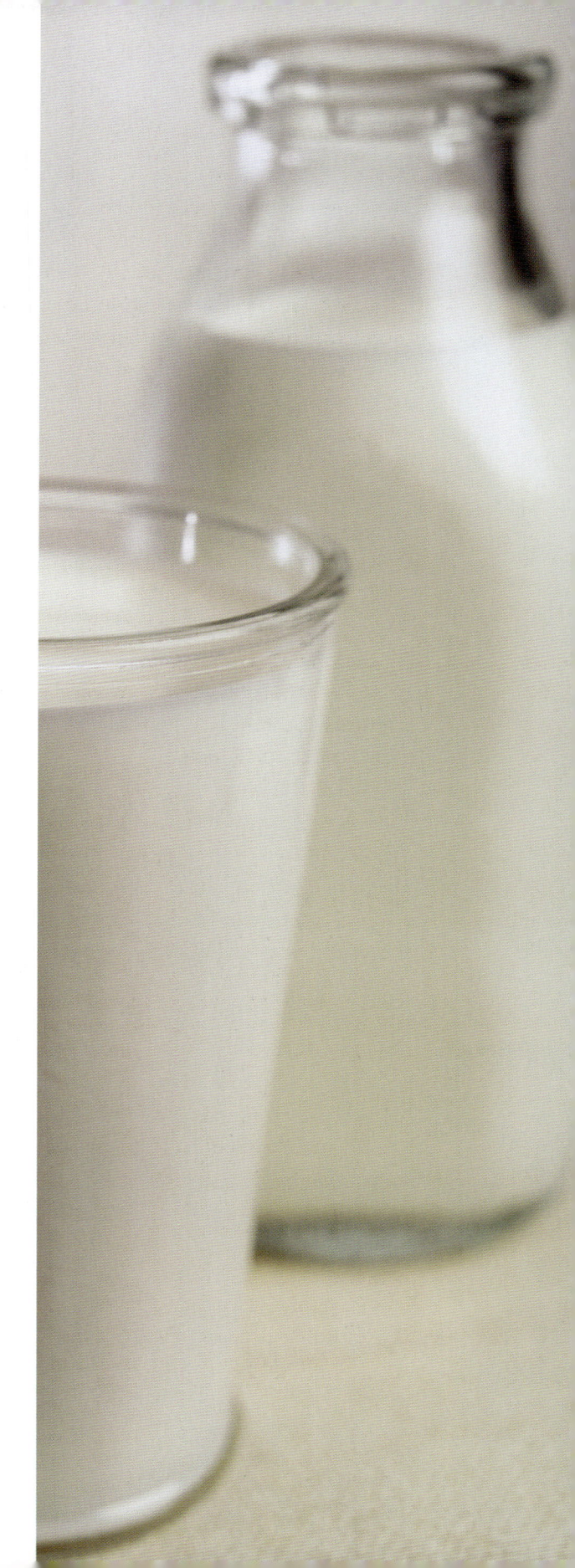

Saturated fats

Saturated fats are considered the bad fats and are usually found in animal and dairy products, and palm and coconut oil. These fats are usually solid at room temperature and are less likely to go rancid than other fats. They are very stable when heated and add the 'crunch' to biscuits and other such products, which is why saturated fats are used in cooking and food processing. Most deep-fried and commercially prepared foods are high in saturated fats. Saturated fats can raise the body's bad cholesterol levels, clog your arteries and increase the risk of heart disease, obesity and diabetes. Limit your intake of saturated fats to lose weight and improve your health.

Unsaturated fats

These good fats are categorised into monounsaturated and polyunsaturated fats, which usually come from plant sources and fish. Sensitive to light and heat and usually liquid at room temperature, unsaturated fats become rancid more easily and are less suitable for frying. They tend to lower the cholesterol levels in the body.

Monounsaturated fats (also called omega 9) are found in olive oil (and olive-oil margarines), canola oil, peanut oil, avocados and nuts such as cashews, almonds and peanuts. These fats reduce the level of bad cholesterol while increasing good cholesterol in the body.

Polyunsaturated fats are found in fish, fish oils, flaxseed oil, legumes, wholegrains, some nuts, and seeds. These fats include the essential fatty acids omega 3 and 6, which can't be created by the body. Essential to the body, these fats must come from what you eat. They help to form cells; transport and metabolise cholesterol; and release chemicals called prostaglandins that have anti-inflammatory, cholesterol-lowering effects, reduce blood pressure and relax your muscles. Omega 6 is found in safflower oil, evening primrose oil, sunflower oil, cottonseed oil, soy oil, sesame oil and nuts and seeds. Omega 3 is found in linseed oil, pumpkin seeds, wheatgerm, walnut oil, dark green leafy vegetables and seafood, especially cold-water fish such as salmon, tuna and sardines.

Trans fatty acids

These unsaturated fats (also known as hydrogenated fats) have undergone processing to make them stable and solid at room temperature and resistant to heat, light and air, mainly to reduce spoilage. This processing means they now affect your body like saturated fats, increasing your risk of heart disease and raising the bad cholesterol, while lowering good cholesterol. They occur naturally in some meat and dairy products, but are also found in some margarines, peanut butter, baked goods, biscuits, cakes, muesli slices and other processed food – basically in almost anything that requires oil to be reheated. However, manufacturers in Australia are limiting the use of trans fatty acids, and consumption in Australia is lower than in the US or UK. When reading ingredients on processed foods, look for vegetable oil, vegetable shortening or hydrogenated oil as this may indicate the presence of trans fatty acids.

VITAMINS

Essential for good health, vitamins don't supply any energy in the form of kilojoules but do aid the body in extracting energy from the macronutrients. They are essential for growth and vitality and play a key role in digestion, elimination and immunity (through their disease-fighting abilities). Your body can't make vitamins so eating a healthy, well-balanced diet is essential. (As some vitamins can be stored in the body, extremely high doses can cause toxicity, so if you take supplements, do so under the supervision of a health professional).

Vitamins come in two main groups: water soluble and fat soluble.

Water-soluble vitamins (such as vitamins B and C) are mostly found in plant/vegetable sources rather than animal sources. They are easily lost in cooking and processing (the fresher your fruit and vegetables, the higher the vitamin content), and, as they are not stored within the body, a constant supply is needed from the diet to maintain optimal health.

Fat-soluble vitamins (such as vitamins A, D, E and K) are found in the fat component of animal and plant foods. Different foods contain different levels of vitamins – for example, nuts, seeds and wholegrains are high in vitamin E, whereas plant foods contain vitamin A in the form of beta-carotene (the orange in carrots and pumpkin). Fat-soluble vitamins can be stored by the body so we don't need as regular a supply as we do water-soluble vitamins.

MINERALS

Minerals play a vital role in creating a healthy body and mind. Minerals provide no kilojoules but help the body create and use energy. The body can't make minerals so it's important to ensure your diet contains sufficient minerals. The amount of minerals in food depends upon the mineral content of the soil it's grown in. If mineral levels in the soil are low, then the amounts in the food will be low.

Minerals create healthy bones and blood, ensure the healthy functioning of muscles and nerves, activate hormonal and enzyme production, and are used in almost every physiological process of your body. They help in weight-loss because they play a key part in metabolic reactions – some minerals help the body use glucose for energy rather than converting it to fat.

A well-balanced diet including lots of leafy green vegetables, wholegrains and lean meat will help you get the necessary levels of minerals.

> YOU NEED AN ENERGY DEFICIT TO LOSE WEIGHT – THAT IS, YOU NEED TO BURN MORE KILOJOULES THAN YOU CONSUME. MAKE THIS THE FOUNDATION OF YOUR WEIGHT-LOSS AND CHOOSE YOUR KILOJOULES FROM HEALTHY FOOD.

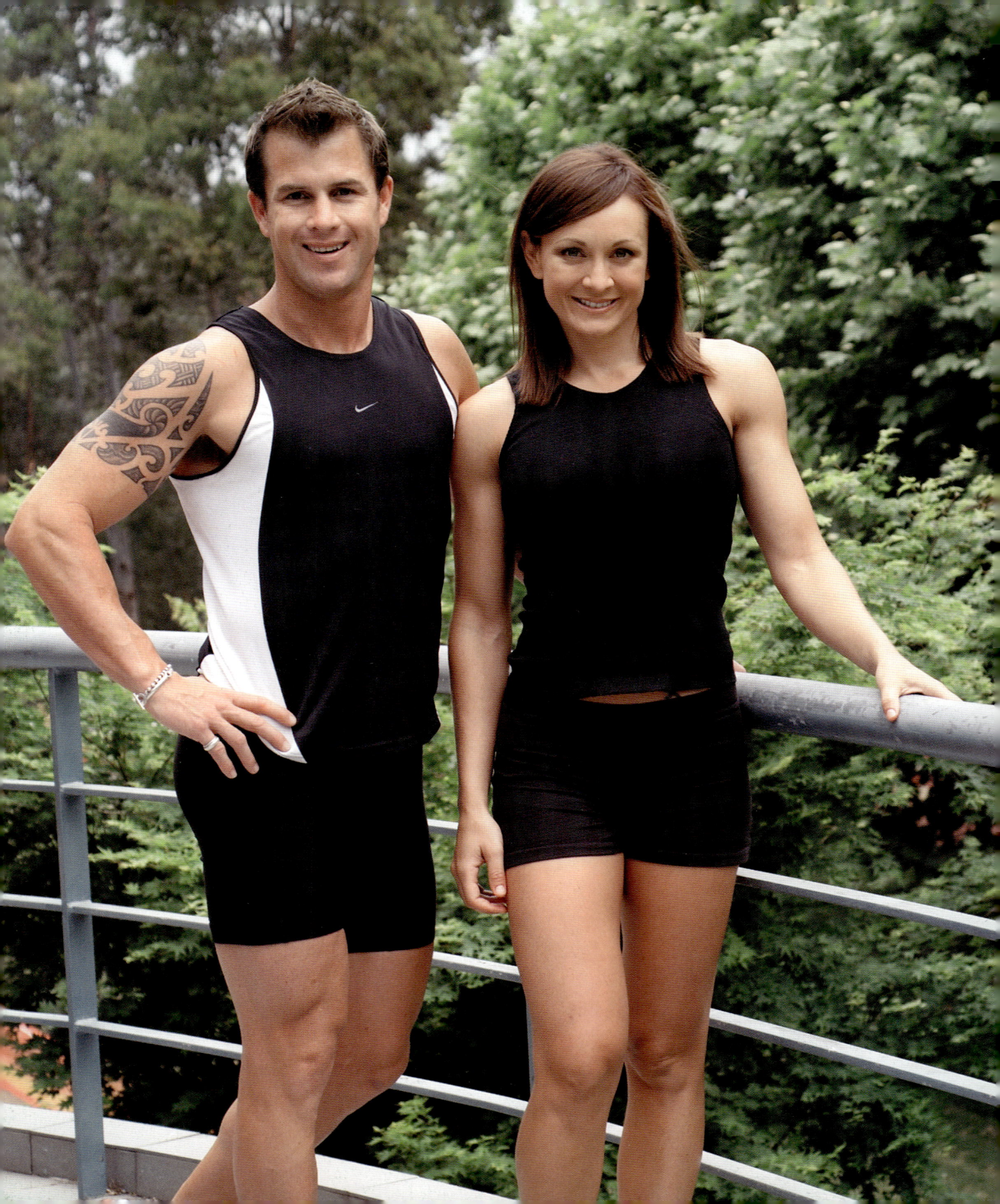

The Biggest Loser Exercise Plan

The number-one thing most people want when beginning an exercise plan is change. Change from feeling tired and unmotivated. The biggest step towards this change is committing to do something about the way you feel, and you did this when you picked up this book. The Biggest Loser Exercise Plan is do-able and sustainable, and will help you achieve long-term weight-loss and good health, with the added bonus of looking great!

Why exercise?

If you've seen the show, you know how hard the contestants work to get fit. Yes, it's hard work but, as the Biggest Losers will confirm, the results are well worth it. Every contestant felt an improved sense of health and wellbeing, and a renewed energy and passion for their lives, and so will you. Of course, you're not expected to work out 5 hours a day like the contestants on *The Biggest Loser* – that was a competition. You have work commitments, family, kids to look after, friends to catch up with and a life to live, so that's just not feasible. You need something that you can maintain – and enjoy – for the rest of your life, and this exercise plan will set you up for that.

By regularly exercising, you're committing to *your* health and wellbeing. We invest time and energy into managing our finances, our families and our property – we also need to make that investment for ourselves. The best way to create more time for your future – that is, a longer life – is to invest in yourself and your health *now*. If this isn't a good enough reason to put down the remote and get moving, what is?

Maybe you didn't like sport at school and haven't played any since – that's okay. Developing a healthy lifestyle doesn't mean you have to suddenly become a keen footballer or runner. First, all you need to do is get moving, then, knowing that exercise will make you look and feel better, why not try it? Experience the adrenalin rush of a decent workout, the buzz afterwards at your sense of achievement and the gradual changes as your fitness levels improve and your weight reduces. This could be yours before you've even had breakfast!

'I always knew it would be great to fit into nice clothes when I had lost weight, but I didn't realise that was just the tip of the iceberg. Now I don't creak when I get out of bed and I never groan when climbing stairs. My moods are constant and my energy levels are just through the roof. I still don't love training but I love the wonderful feeling I get when I have finished a tough session. I can honestly say that I feel younger than I have in years.' **Kristie Dignam, Series One**

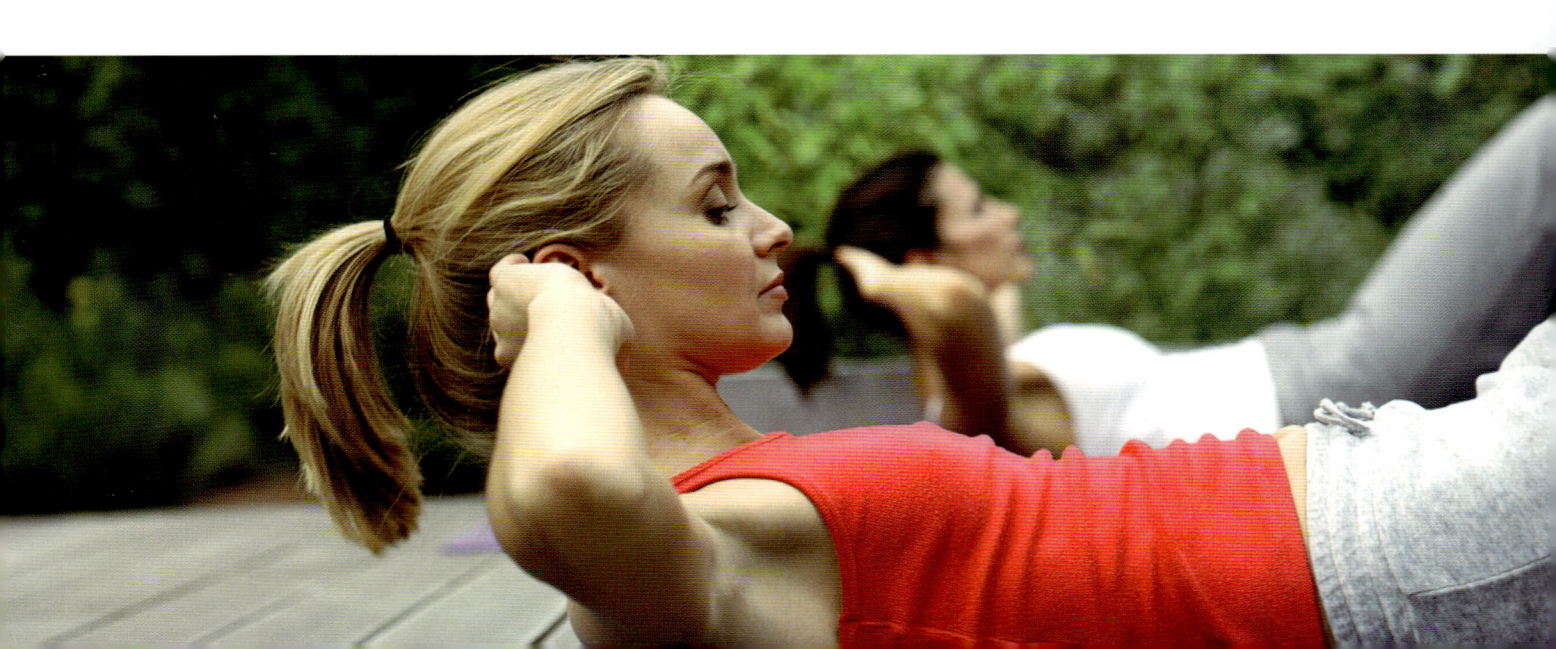

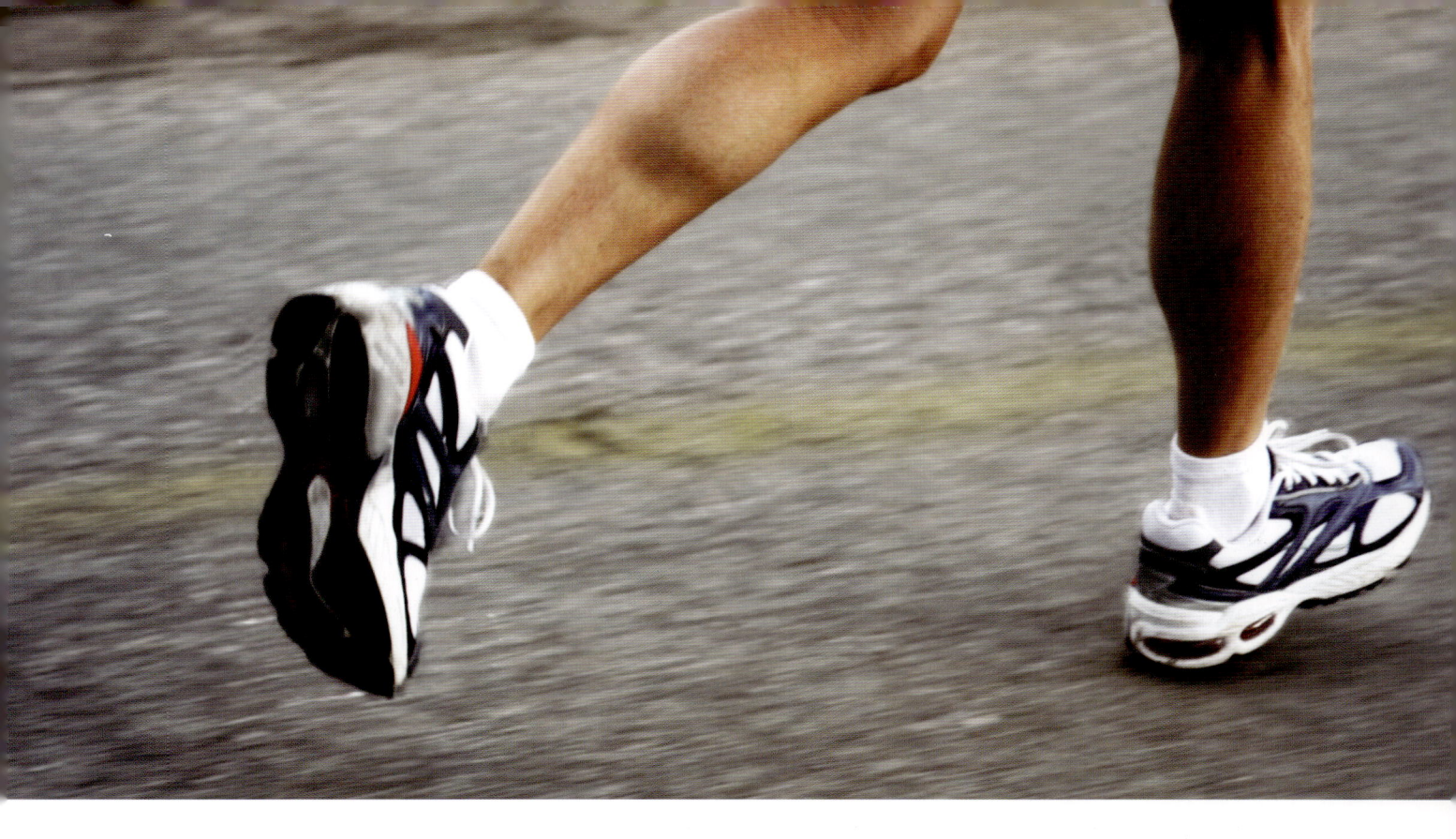

THE BENEFITS

A common mistake people make is to assume that by not seeing instant weight-loss, no progress is being made. Whatever your reasons for exercising there are numerous advantages to getting moving regularly. Weight-loss is one benefit; here are some others:

- improved sleep
- improved libido
- increased metabolism
- higher self-esteem
- reduced risk of cardiovascular disease, stroke, diabetes and osteoporosis
- increased energy
- reduced likelihood of depression and its effects
- improved lung capacity
- healthy blood pressure.

Exercise will have a positive effect on your daily life. The fitter you become, the easier life gets – you'll have more energy for everything from picking up the shopping, dancing the night away or chasing your grandkids. If you exercise regularly, you will:

- feel stronger and be stronger
- be less stressed
- breathe more easily (and be less likely to snore)
- fit into your favourite clothes
- keep up with your kids
- have more 'you' time
- receive compliments about how great you look
- be more flexible and have better balance.

The Biggest Loser programs

The Biggest Loser Exercise Plan aims to help you create good habits and to get you moving and burning fat. To do this, especially if you are new to exercise, you'll need to commit yourself to moving more, trying lots of different activities and persevering if things get tough.

The Biggest Loser Exercise Plan consists of three programs, spanning over three and a half months. It's split into smaller, more manageable programs to help you focus on step-by-step goals. This makes each stage more achievable and less overwhelming, and helps you stay accountable. Where will this plan lead? To a lifetime of enjoyable exercise, good health and overall wellbeing.

All three programs in the plan have been specifically designed to be undertaken anywhere. Other than scouting your local area for a few hills and the odd step or bench, you don't need much more, so give it a go! You don't have to join a gym to get fit and feel great. However, you can do all the programs at a gym if you are currently a member or want to become one, and included is an optional specific gym workout if you want it. Results can be quicker when you work out at a gym, especially if you have a personal trainer to support and guide you. See pages 70–71 for tips on what to look for when joining a gym.

The Biggest Loser Exercise Plan is intensive and some days will be harder than others. This is why you need to listen to your body and learn to understand whether it's your mind that simply can't be bothered getting out of bed, or whether physically you do need to rest. Rest is vital and each week includes a rest day, but allow yourself additional rest time if you really feel you need it.

'When I started this journey, I never thought I would actually learn to like – let alone love – training. Yet now I have set myself so many training goals. I'm hoping to run a mini-marathon and I'm also very interested in body building. Who knows, I could be on the stage competing in no time!' **Cat White, Series One**

WHAT'S YOUR LEVEL?

The Biggest Loser Exercise Plan works at three different levels: beginner, intermediate and advanced. Choose the beginner level if you have exercised regularly for less than three months or not at all. Choose intermediate if you have been exercising for between three months and one year. Choose advanced if you have trained consistently for one year or longer.

Fitness and strength improve over time, even if you don't see any immediate results – muscles take time to adapt and grow and the heart gradually works more efficiently. By taking on these programs, you will increase both your knowledge and fitness – when you feel ready for a new challenge, move up to the next level. Before beginning one of the programs, read through it thoroughly and look at the exercises so you fully understand the program and what's required of you.

THE KICKSTART PLAN

Begin with the 14-day KickStart Plan, designed to get you moving and into the habit of regular exercise, as well as eating healthily. Two weeks isn't long and by the end of it you'll be used to making time for exercise in your daily life. You'll also start noticing differences in your fitness and weight.

This plan prepares your body for the LifeStyle Plan by getting you out walking 20–55 minutes each day (depending on your level), six days a week. No matter what your fitness level, it's important to begin steadily before moving onto either of the follow-up programs. During this KickStart period, you'll discover what time of day works best for you and you'll have explored your local area for varied walking, running and cycle tracks, playgrounds and hills, all of which you'll use in the coming weeks.

Go to page 83 to see the full KickStart Plan.

THE LIFESTYLE PLAN

Once you've completed the KickStart Plan, it's time to get a little more serious and head into the LifeStyle Plan, two six-week programs that will burn fat, build lean muscle, increase your overall fitness, get you looking great, and set you on the path to long-term health and wellbeing.

These two programs ask you to commit to one hour of exercise each day and one rest day per week. The program structure consists of 50 per cent cardio and 50 per cent resistance training. The format is flexible so that you can fit it in a busy life – you can choose to exercise outdoors, at home or in a gym, and add your own preferred alternatives such as yoga or aerobics classes.

Because these programs incorporate resistance training, they run for the optimum time of six weeks each. In the first two weeks you'll master the exercise techniques so that your body becomes used to the movements. The second fortnight works on your coordination and firing the muscles effectively. The final two weeks are when your muscle fibres adapt and your strength builds.

Go to page 97 for the LifeStyle Plan programs.

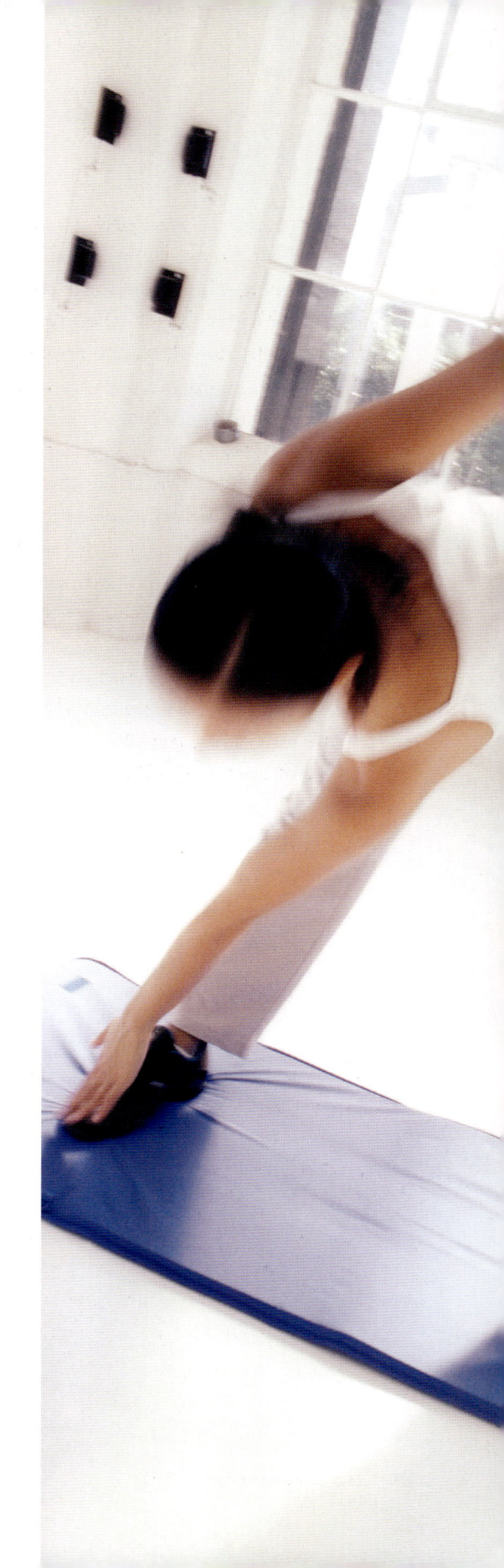

Where do you start?

Change occurs gradually. Creating a mindset for a new, improved you is a huge process – just considering it is a great first step! If it's been years since you've exercised and you're feeling overwhelmed, just remember this: sometimes it's just a matter of getting off the couch. Don't head out the door to try to run 10 kilometres if you haven't exercised for months or years. Begin with small changes in your incidental activity each day. Just making small changes in your daily life can help you burn more energy and improve your health – you'll increase your resting metabolic rate, keep your muscles moving and have more energy. Increase your incidental exercise during the day by trying these tips:

- Take public transport to work – walking to and from the station or bus stop equals extra exercise (and you'll probably save money too).
- Ask a friend to walk with you a couple of times a week. It's a great way to catch up and exercise at the same time. Choose different routes and include hills to maximise the effects and ensure you don't get bored.
- Hide the remote. (Go on, try it!)
- Dust off your bike and go for some early morning rides.
- Take a healthy lunch to work and then go for a walk.
- Arrange to meet a friend for a coffee or juice and pick a café that's 15–20 minutes walk from home – that's 30–40 minutes of exercise without even thinking about it.
- Walk or ride to work – begin with once a week and then try to increase it.
- Take the stairs not the lift or escalator.
- Hang your clothes out on the washing line rather than using the dryer.
- Take your kids to the park and kick around a football, throw a frisbee.
- Walk your dog; walk a friend's dog.
- Buy a pedometer and measure how many steps you take in a day. Set goals to gradually increase this.
- Walk over to a colleague's office rather than emailing or phoning.
- Park in the furthest corner of the car park.

'Trust me, just move your butt! Walk, walk, walk! You are not going to get healthy sitting on your backside, so get off it and start moving. Do it for yourself; no one else will.'

David Hilyander, Series One

Before beginning any exercise program, it's a good idea to visit your doctor. This is especially important if you are particularly overweight or have suffered from injuries in the past. However, don't let the fact that you can't get in to see your doctor for two weeks stop you from getting active. You can start walking now, even if it's just a slow walk around the block each day.

Getting a medical check-up will provide you with key information about your current state of health and give you a benchmark to start from. A standard check-up may consist of a blood pressure reading, weight reading and a blood test to gauge your cholesterol and glucose levels. This baseline check-up will be a great way for you to see how far you will come in three months. This is also the time you can, if you feel comfortable, see a personal trainer or get a personal assessment done at a gym. The trainer will test your general level of fitness and flexibility and take your body measurements. You can also take your own measurements (measure your upper arm, thigh, waist and hips). Get yourself assessed again in three months after following the Biggest Loser exercise and eating plans to see the rewards of your hard work!

HOW FIT ARE YOU?

Gyms and some doctors offer specific fitness testing, but you can also create your own test. Pick a local walk and keep going at a steady, fast pace for exactly 10 minutes. Stop at 10 minutes and gauge how far you have walked by noting a landmark (such as a tree or park bench). Record it and make a note of how hard you are breathing along the way on a scale of 1 to 10, with 1 being your resting rate of breathing and 10 being when you are unable to speak and your breathing is fast and shallow (see the intensity level indicator on page 108). Use this exercise as your starting point to chart your progress. Repeat the walk after you've completed the KickStart Plan and see if, in the 10 minutes, you walk further and breathe more easily. Return to this simple test at any stage along your exercise journey as a measure of how your cardiovascular fitness is improving.

There are two other simple tests you can do that test your upper body and abdominal strength. Count how many push-ups you can do in a minute (it's fine to do them on your knees) and then how many crunches (sit-ups) you can do in a minute. (See pages 134–142 for the correct technique for these exercises before you start.)

WHICH EXERCISE IS BEST?

Basically, no one exercise is better than another. What it comes down to is that *any* exercise is better than none. You need to find something that you enjoy, or at least something that you can stick with. All the types of exercises described over the page can be done as part of or in addition to the Biggest Loser programs.

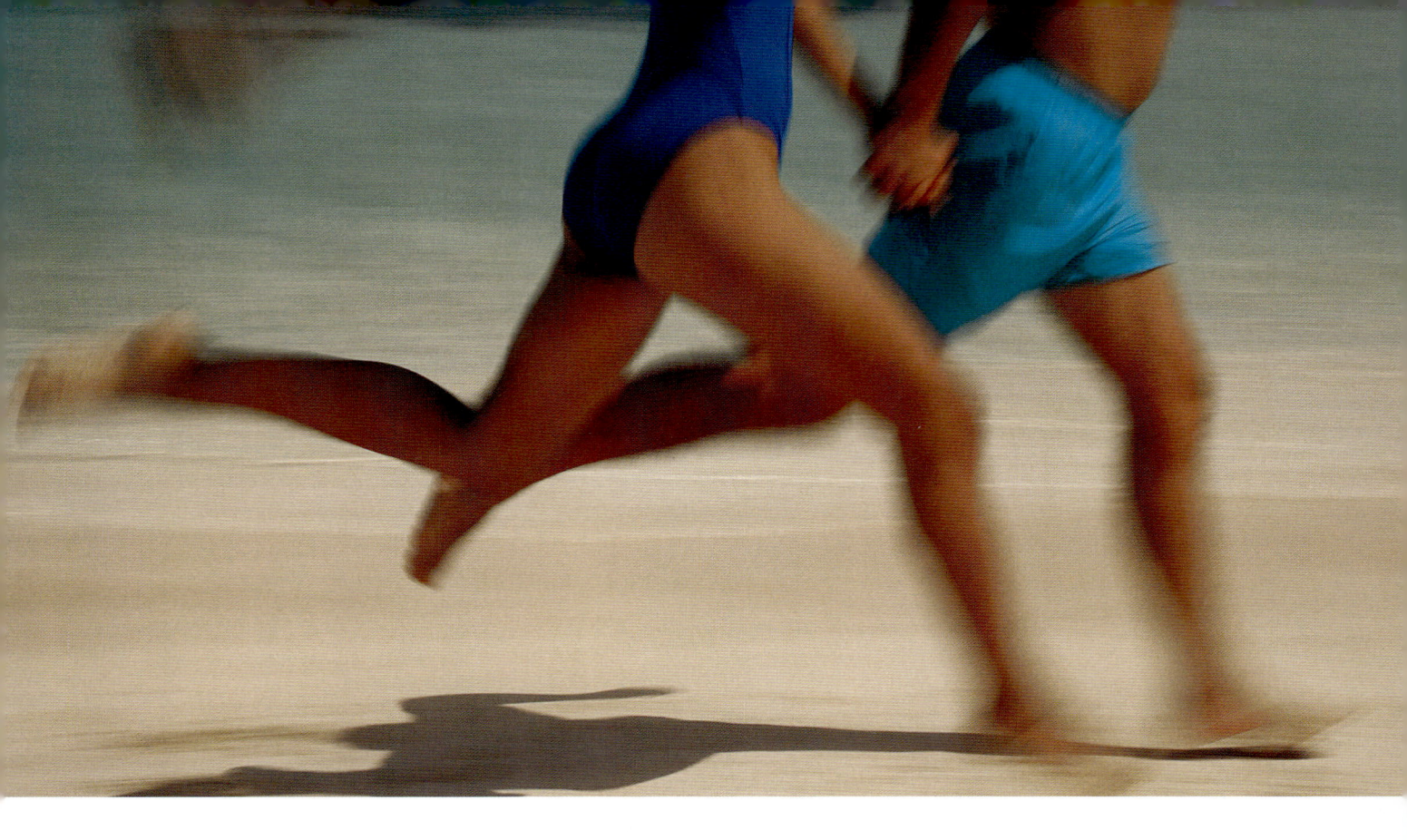

Walking

This is the easiest starting point for any exercise program – it's free, achievable and can be done every day. Vary the pace, change the route (include some hills when you're ready) and choose to walk alone or with your weight-loss buddy.

Swimming

Swimming is good cardiovascular exercise and, because it's non-impact, it's useful if you're overweight as it puts less pressure on your body. However, for this same reason, it's not as good for dramatic weight-loss or substantially improving muscle tone compared with weight-bearing activities. Swimming gradually builds up strength and mobility after injury or illness. You don't have to be limited to swimming laps; visit your local swimming pool to see if they offer lessons to improve your stroke, deep-water running classes (a good fat-burning option) or aqua-aerobics classes. If you don't feel comfortable wearing swimmers, try to bear with it – others will be feeling the same and your health and fitness are more important than what others think (anyway, soon you'll be feeling fabulous in your swimmers!).

Aerobics

A higher intensity workout guaranteed to get your heart-rate up, aerobics is a great way to burn excess energy in a fun environment. Check out your local gym timetable for a variety of classes, which usually run several times each day and last approximately 55 minutes. Some coordination is required but aerobics is generally suitable for any fitness level and can be included in your fitness program.

Cycling

Another exercise great for improving aerobic fitness, cycling is a non-impact form of exercise, making it gentle on the joints. Get your bike out of the garage, get it serviced and start riding to work, or go to spin classes at the local gym. Spinning and cycling are excellent fat burners and a great way to tone your thighs and backside.

Running

Running is a fantastic way to improve your cardiovascular fitness and take your overall fitness to the next level. It's a fast way of burning calories but, because it's also an intense, high-impact workout, you need to introduce it gradually to your weekly routine. If running is new to you, the best way to begin is to do a run-walk, or timed interval training. Don't worry if you think it might look odd – it doesn't, and you're improving your fitness. Start with a brisk walk to get the heart-rate up and then break into a jog for a minute or two. Ease back to a fast-paced walk and then try the jog again. Time each element so that, over a few weeks, you gradually increase the jog and reduce the walk until you can keep jogging consistently. A good starting point is to walk for 1 minute, then run for 1 minute. As your fitness improves, increase the intervals to 1-minute walks and 2-minute runs, then 3-minute runs and so on. From here, work on your speed and make it a jog-run – add some faster runs into the jog to keep challenging the body. Running is also a great stress release and, beware, it can be addictive!

Sport

Visit your local sports facility to see what team sports they offer. You may have always wanted to try volleyball or tennis or indoor cricket; well, now's your chance to give a new sport a go. No experience is necessary, just plenty of enthusiasm. Ask a friend to come with you if you're not sure about going by yourself.

Dance

Dance classes are a fun, social way to get moving and can be a good addition to any exercise program. Most dance classes don't require you to have a partner and are a great way to make friends. Look up local dance schools or CAE courses offering beginner, intermediate or advanced classes in all forms of dance from Latin, funk and jazz through to capoeira, ballet and belly dancing.

Yoga

Yoga complements an exercise program perfectly as it gently improves your strength and flexibility while also calming your mind and body. It won't burn a lot of fat but it will help you get back in touch with your body, which is great – especially if you've been caught in a cycle of body-hatred. Your local gym or yoga centre will run beginner classes where no experience is necessary. Yoga is suitable for any fitness level (all practices can be modified) and can be done every day. It will also help you relax and de-stress, and it balances your bodily systems, which improves your overall health.

> **SHANNAN'S TRAINING TIP**
>
> Be patient and ease into your training, especially if you're a first-time exerciser. There's no point getting so sore that you can't finish the full week's program.

THINKING OF JOINING A GYM?

One common reason people are put off joining a gym is apprehension about what to expect. Do I have to be fit before I can join? Will everyone stare at me? How do I know what to do once I get there? Will it be full of body-builders lifting massive weights who will think I don't belong there? Will I know how to use the machines? You don't have to get fit before you go to a gym – you're going to the gym to get fit. Gyms are designed to help you get awesome results. They are full of great equipment to reshape your body and help you lose weight, and most offer an array of classes to suit any shape, fitness and coordination level. And, of course, there are always fitness professionals to support you and really personalise your workout.

But, for a first-timer, a gym can be a potentially intimidating experience and it's quite normal to be apprehensive or nervous. However, you can overcome this, especially once you know what to look for, what to ask about and how to make the most of the facilities on offer. Here are some useful tips on how to go about joining a gym:

- Check out the gyms in your area. There are probably a few so visit several and get a feel for each one. Explain that you are unfamiliar with the gym and would like a tour. Gyms usually have trainers and consultants who are happy to walk you through the place and explain it all.
- Most gyms offer a complimentary session or trial period where you can try some classes and the equipment. Use this opportunity to test-drive their facilities.
- Spend a little time in a gym and you will soon see that people of all shapes, sizes, ages, economic backgrounds and abilities use them. There is no norm other than wanting to feel good and becoming strong and healthy. They can be social and a great way to meet new people. Remember that you're all there for similar reasons, and you deserve to be there just as much as everyone else.
- Ask a gym staff-member to talk you through the group exercise timetable so that you understand the format, intensity and types of classes they offer. Find out if you can try some out and bring a friend along too. One of the great benefits of participating in a group exercise class is that you are committing yourself to one full hour of exercise. You can completely switch off from your day and allow the instructor to guide you and motivate you through the next hour without having to think at all. Simply focus on the music and the moves – these classes are a fun option.

- Gyms are at their busiest before and after work (6am–8am and 6pm–8pm). Visit before or after these peak times for a quieter (and possibly less intimidating) experience.
- Book in for a fitness assessment. This service is part of your membership and is a one-on-one session with a gym instructor in a private room, usually taking about an hour. This will help you work out what your fitness, strength and flexibility levels are. You can also be weighed and measured and have your percentage of body fat taken, but feel free to decline if you feel uncomfortable with any of these options. An assessment often includes some or all of the following:
    - blood pressure reading
    - aerobic fitness evaluation where you may spend 10 minutes on a stationary bike
    - body-fat reading
    - measurements of your waist and hips
    - flexibility test, also called the 'sit and reach' test, where you sit on the ground with your legs straight out in front and reach forward along a marked line
    - upper body strength test, where you perform as many push-ups as you can in 1 minute (it doesn't matter if you just do one)
    - abdominal strength test, where you perform as many crunches as you can in 1 minute.

  There is no pass or fail with these evaluations. They are never compared with anyone else's and are strictly confidential. You can ask to refer back to them at any time. They just help to show the areas you need to work on and also highlight where your strengths lie.
- Book in with a personal trainer – not only will they be able to devise a program especially for you, but also they will help you navigate the equipment and weights that can appear initially very overwhelming. This service can be beneficial at any stage of your training, whether you are brand new to exercise or have been training by yourself for years and need some more information to take things to the next level.
- Finally, remember that moving out of your comfort zone will always be a bit challenging. Once you get through those first few initial visits you'll know your way around and feel right at home. Your health is worth putting up with the unknown!

7 Biggest Loser steps to fitness success

You've worked out your starting level for the Biggest Loser Exercise Plan and know more about the programs that you'll be following. You've learnt about positive thinking, goal-setting, eating well and now exercising. The seven steps below will help you set up your exercise routine and reach your exercise goals. Integrating these steps will help you to create new healthy habits. During the three and half months while you're on the Biggest Loser Exercise Plan, there may be times when you falter or lose motivation; return to these steps and remember how far you have come.

1 Be accountable
2 Ask for support
3 Create good habits
4 Set achievable goals
5 Inspire others
6 Mix it up
7 Choose a positive attitude

1 BE ACCOUNTABLE

In Part One you wrote down your health and fitness goals. You are accountable to these goals and, if you struggle with motivation, remind yourself of what they are. Keep them in a visible place and remember why you want this so much!

Training diary

Make yourself responsible for the steps involved in getting fitter by keeping a training diary. Just like your food diary, it will be a key support for you – not only will your training diary show your achievements in black and white, it allows you to incorporate setbacks and schedule modifications when you need to.

First of all, use your training diary as just that, a diary. Put in all your scheduled workouts at the start of the week and plan your other commitments around them. Second, after each workout write the details down in your training diary: each cardio session, the intensity you worked at, the time it took and how you felt; every resistance session, including any weights you used and the number of repetitions; and your general energy level and experience of the day's exercise. This will help you work out how and when you should increase your intensity and weights.

Your training diary will help you understand your exercise strengths and weaknesses, allowing you to adapt your training plan and respond to any problems quickly and effectively. Are you better at training in the mornings or evenings? Are you skipping sessions or cutting them short as the week goes on? By charting your progress, you'll be able to see how much you have improved, and there's nothing more motivating than that! Remember it's all about consistency and, above all, be honest with yourself.

2 ASK FOR SUPPORT

Tell people about your plans. Share your hopes and your goals, and ask for the support of your friends, family and colleagues in achieving these. Also, by saying it out loud, you are taking responsibility for actually doing it – your friends will call you on it if you don't. Seek professional support too if you think it will help you reach your goals.

> ### FINDING THE RIGHT PERSONAL TRAINER
>
> Consider whether you would prefer training with a male or a female. Ask around for personal recommendations and find out why a particular personal trainer (PT) is considered good. Most PTs specialise and have particular areas of expertise, from rehabilitation, post-pregnancy, weight-loss, building muscles, to sport-specific skills. In hiring a PT you're not looking for a friend – you're looking for someone who will motivate you, challenge you and guide you towards your goals. Watch them train others and see if they have a good rapport with their clients. As in most things you generally get what you pay for, so make sure your PT is qualified, insured and has a suitable level of experience for you.

3 CREATE GOOD HABITS

Get into an exercise routine so you know what you are doing for the week ahead – commit to the schedule so you don't waste energy thinking about if and when you should exercise. Organise yourself so you plan your life around the goal of good health. Find the time of day that suits you best and stick to it, whether it's cold, raining or hot. If you have to cut a session short one day, make it up over the week. The discipline of keeping your training habit will increase your self-esteem and help you to realise that you are capable of a lot more than you originally believed.

Try getting into the habit of exercising in the morning if you can. You won't have to deal with missing an evening exercise session because you've been held up at work or for another commitment. So get up a bit earlier and fit it in first thing so you can revel in the sense of achievement before you've even sat down to breakfast!

> ## SHANNAN'S TRAINING TIP
>
> Training is a metaphor for life. The harder you train and the more disciplined you are, the more capable you become at dealing with life's challenges. You strengthen your character and your resolve as you strengthen your body. People will respect you more – *you* will respect you more.

4 SET ACHIEVABLE GOALS

You read about setting goals earlier in the book. Set small achievable goals and challenges for yourself. Breaking your ultimate goal into smaller goals will keep you from feeling overwhelmed. Your exercise mini-goals might be something like if last week in your cardio walk-run workout, you ran for 3 minutes then walked for 1 minute, this week try running for 5 minutes with a 1-minute walk. If you ran on the treadmill for 12 minutes at level 8, get onto it and try 12 minutes at level 8.5. If you did three-quarters of an aerobics class last week, this week the whole thing is yours. If you did three sets of 10 on the bench press at 20 kilograms, this week aim for three sets of 12.

5 INSPIRE OTHERS

Encourage a friend or relative to exercise too. Not only will this make the whole program more fun, but also it's the perfect way to encourage each other. Make it into a friendly competition: if one of you doesn't make it out of bed for an early morning training session, that person buys lunch! In this small way you are now changing your world. People will be attracted to your new positive and ambitious energy and will look to you for inspiration. Stay committed and watch your influence spread.

6 MIX IT UP

Variety is essential so try many different exercises. Keep your workouts varied and interesting by introducing new ones when you feel yourself getting bored. If you try something for the first time and don't think you like it, have another couple of tries – once you've mastered the basics, it may become much more fun. As you get healthier, try activities and sports that you once dreamed about trying but didn't have the confidence for. Every time you try something new, you expand your comfort zone and increase your confidence.

7 CHOOSE A POSITIVE ATTITUDE

Failure is a mindset. Don't let knock-backs or disappointments stop you in your tracks and send you to the fridge. One small hiccup doesn't mean you should give up forever – remember to let go of that negative self-talk (see page 16 for more about positive thinking). Instead, learn from setbacks and move forwards. If you sustain an injury, modify your program to allow that body part to rest while you still keep moving. If you are tired and can't be bothered, focus on the bigger picture and remind yourself of your goals – there is a good reason you're doing this. The more effort you can put in early on, the quicker you'll see great results; this will motivate you to continue. If a busy time at work upsets your schedule, modify and re-plan your day so that you can still have that time out to exercise. Prioritise and re-prioritise each time you are faced with a setback to ensure you keep going. Remember, your health is non-negotiable.

Most important of all – commit to being honest with yourself.

> ### SHANNAN'S TRAINING TIP
>
> If there's one thing I've learnt, it's that training is *all* about consistency. If you miss a workout, don't forget about it! No excuses! Re-plan your week so that you can make it up. Consistency is everything and you must be disciplined and committed to succeed. 'Systems don't fail people, people fail systems' – you don't have to be one of them!

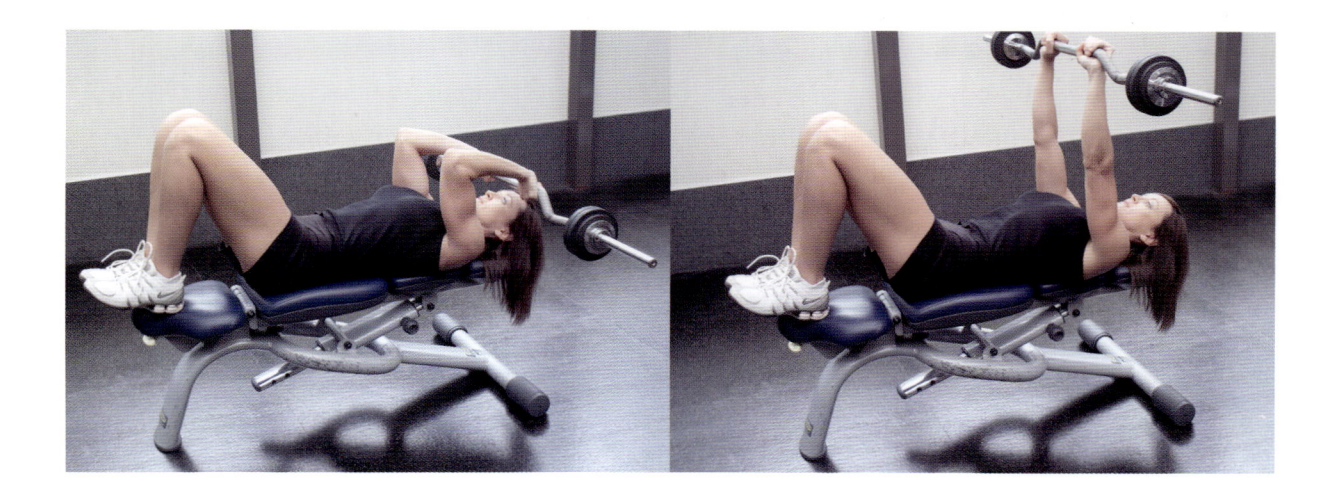

What else do you need to know?

Before you move on to the exercise programs in Part Three, there are a few other things you need to know to help you get the best out of your training.

SAFE EXERCISE

It's important you know how to push yourself but also when to stop. Begin with a visit to your doctor before starting an exercise program. Once you've started the program, make sure you listen to your body. If you feel faint or dizzy at any time during exercise, or your breathing becomes uncomfortable, slow down immediately, stop and sit down with a glass of water.

It's normal for muscles to be tired after exercise. Often a good stretch and some movement such as a walk will help ease any tightness. If there's an imbalance in the muscle soreness (that is, only one side of your body is sore) or you experience any joint discomfort, monitor it (note it in your training diary). If it persists, contact your health professional.

FOOD AND EXERCISE

Some planning needs to go into the timing of your meals when incorporating an exercise program into your day. Just as you don't want to be working out with a full stomach, nor do you want your energy levels to flag halfway through a power walk. As a general rule, it is ideal to eat smaller meals more often to sustain your energy levels, and on the Biggest Loser Eating Plan you should not go longer than 3 hours without eating. This will assist your workouts and keep your energy levels stable. Before an afternoon training session, it's a good idea to eat a high-energy snack (such as a banana) at least an hour before you begin.

Exercising first thing in the morning is great for a number of reasons: first, you achieve your exercise goal for the day before it's really even started. Second, because you won't have eaten since the night before, your body will use stored energy (your fat deposits) instead of the energy provided by a recent meal. This works well for low-intensity exercise (at between 50 and 60 per cent heart-rate) but for high-intensity workouts, have a piece of fruit or a smoothie up to an hour beforehand to avoid possible dizziness or limited training improvement (without this sustenance, your body may not be able to keep up with the energy demands).

After exercising try to eat a well-balanced meal, rich in nutrients, protein and carbohydrates, within 2 hours. Eating during this timeframe maximises the protein uptake into the tired muscles, giving them the best chance to develop and grow. Also at this time the body is three times more likely to store carbohydrates in your muscles as protein, rather than converting them to fat and storing them in your fat tissue. This will increase your recovery rate and allow you to train harder next time.

ESSENTIAL WATER

We are all aware that we need to drink water regularly as part of a healthy lifestyle, but how much is enough? We lose around 2.5 litres of water a day. In order to balance this loss we need to consume around 8–10 glasses of water and eat plenty of foods with a high water content such as fresh fruit and vegetables. Thirst is an indicator that the body is *already* dehydrated and in need of water. The most effective method of maintaining fluid levels is to sip water regularly throughout the day. Always having a water bottle to hand is a simple way of making this happen. Exercising increases our expenditure of water through sweat and therefore it is important to drink a glass of water prior to working out, sip small amounts regularly during exercise (around 150–250 ml of water every 15 to 20 minutes) and follow up with several glasses afterwards.

WARM-UPS AND COOL-DOWNS

Warming up and cooling down are essential before and after each exercise session; stretches are included in the Biggest Loser Exercise Plan (see pages 130–133). A warm-up prepares the body and mind for the workout ahead, gradually increasing the blood flow to the working muscles and lifting your heart-rate. It should consist of 5–10 minutes of gentle movement with a gradual increase in intensity followed by a brief stretch of the major body parts (the quadriceps, hamstrings, calves, back and chest).

Warming up before exercise:
- raises your heart-rate so your body is prepared for physical exertion
- speeds up nerve impulses so that your reflexes are enhanced
- reduces muscle tension
- sends oxygenated blood to the muscle groups
- reduces your risk of injury, particularly to connective tissue such as tendons
- increases your flexibility and joint mobility.

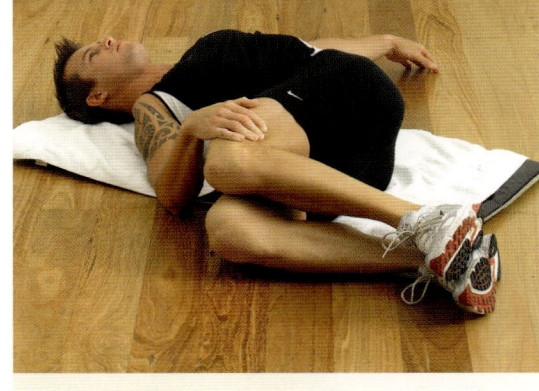

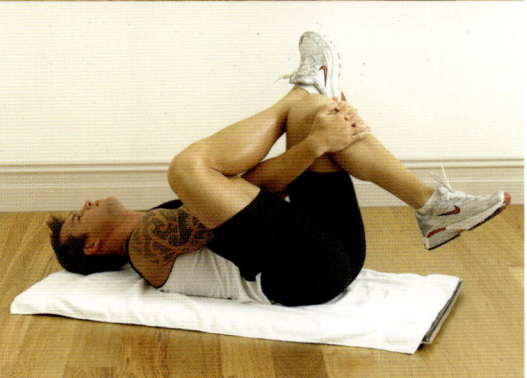

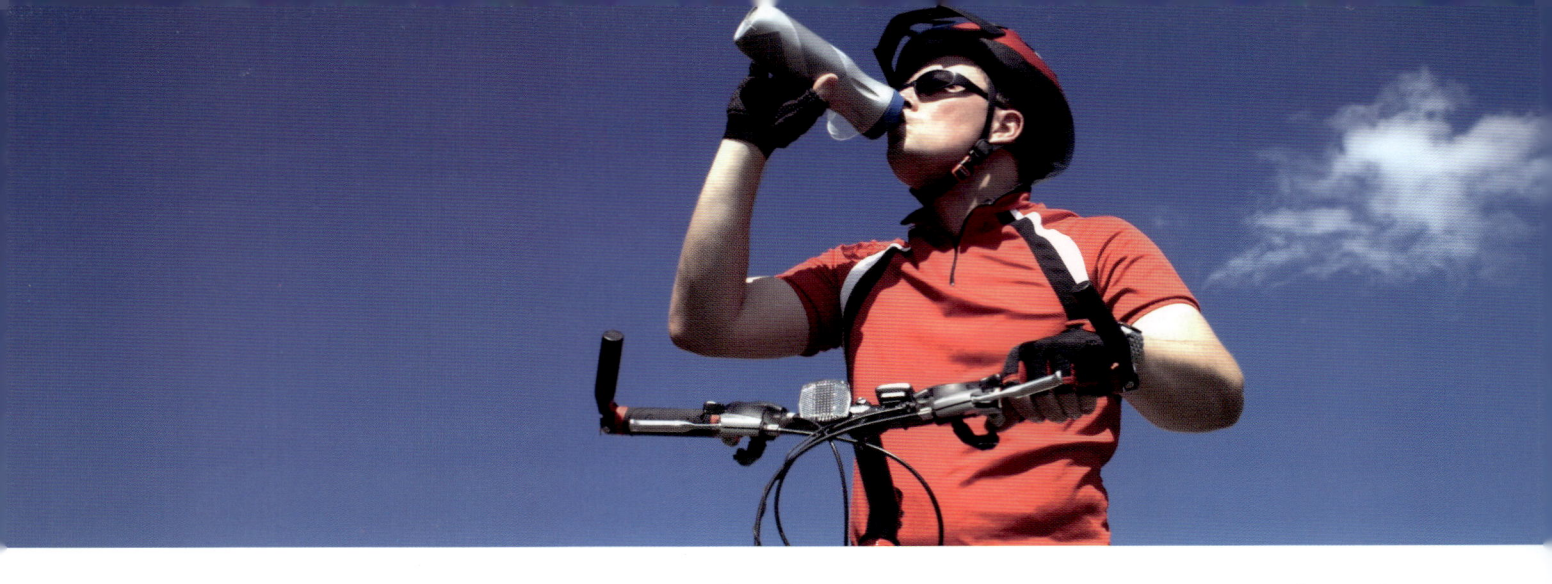

At the end of an exercise session, you need to allow the heart-rate time to return to normal. Avoid stopping suddenly because it can cause dizziness. Simply reduce the intensity at which you are exercising bit by bit, allowing your body to slow down gently. It's vital to stretch well at the end of the session. Your muscles have been working hard and need gentle stretches to lengthen again and help prevent injury. Hold each stretch for 15–30 seconds and perform them while you're still warm for maximum benefit. Continue to stretch through the day to release tension and improve your flexibility.

Cooling down after exercise:

- helps the heart-rate, breathing and blood pressure gently return to normal
- improves flexibility
- reduces your risk of injury
- removes waste products from muscle tissue (such as lactic acid) and helps to reduce any soreness.

TOOLS OF THE TRADE: HEART-RATE MONITORS

If you are new to exercise, it can be daunting to work out what level you should be training at, or to walk into a gym and try to figure out what to do. Each piece of cardio equipment is asking you for what level, speed and incline you wish to work at and yet, how do you know what's right for you? A heart-rate monitor is an inexpensive tool that can help gauge the intensity at which you need to train for your age and fitness level. It consists of two transmitters: one is a narrow strap worn around the torso underneath your top, close to your heart, and the other is a wrist-watch. The first transmitter measures the rate at which the heart is beating (your heart-rate) and sends a signal to the wrist transmitter. By keeping an eye on the wrist-watch as you exercise, it's easy to increase or reduce your intensity.

If 1 is your resting heart-rate and 10 is what we call your maximum heart-rate – that is, the highest number of beats your heart can sustain per minute – a beginner should aim to work between 6 and 7 during their first few months of cardio exercise. So, once you've worked out your 60–70 per cent target heart-rate, simply program the number into your heart-rate monitor, start the equipment and go. You can then elevate the speed of your training as you go to ensure your heart-rate remains in its target zone. A heart-rate monitor takes the guesswork out of exercise and gives you the confidence to know what you are doing.

To work out your target heart-rate, you need to find out your maximum heart-rate. Use this formula to do so:

$$220 - \text{your age in years} = \text{maximum heart-rate.}$$

To then work out your target heart-rate, you simply need to work out 60–70 per cent of your maximum heart-rate.

For example, imagine you are 45 and have just begun a new exercise program. You want to lose weight and improve your cardiovascular fitness but aren't sure how hard to push yourself when you exercise. This is what you do:

$$220 - 45 = 175$$
$$(60 \div 100) \times 175 = 105$$
$$(70 \div 100) \times 175 = 122.5$$

Therefore, your target heart-rate zone is between 105 and 122.5 and to achieve your weight-loss and fitness goals you will need to maintain your heart-rate within the given range for around 20–40 minutes.

If you are an intermediate exerciser, try to work at 70–80 per cent of your maximum heart-rate. Advanced exercisers can aim for 70–90 per cent. Basically the fitter you become, the harder you can push your cardiovascular system. Remember, the harder you work the more fat you burn!

Work out your maximum and target heart-rates and note them in your training diary. Keep a record to see how long you sustain your target heart-rate each time you go for a walk or run. Some days you'll have more energy and you may feel you can keep going or take the level a little higher, others will be tough and it will be hard to get through. It doesn't matter. Write it all down so that you can re-cap at the end of each week and clearly see how you went.

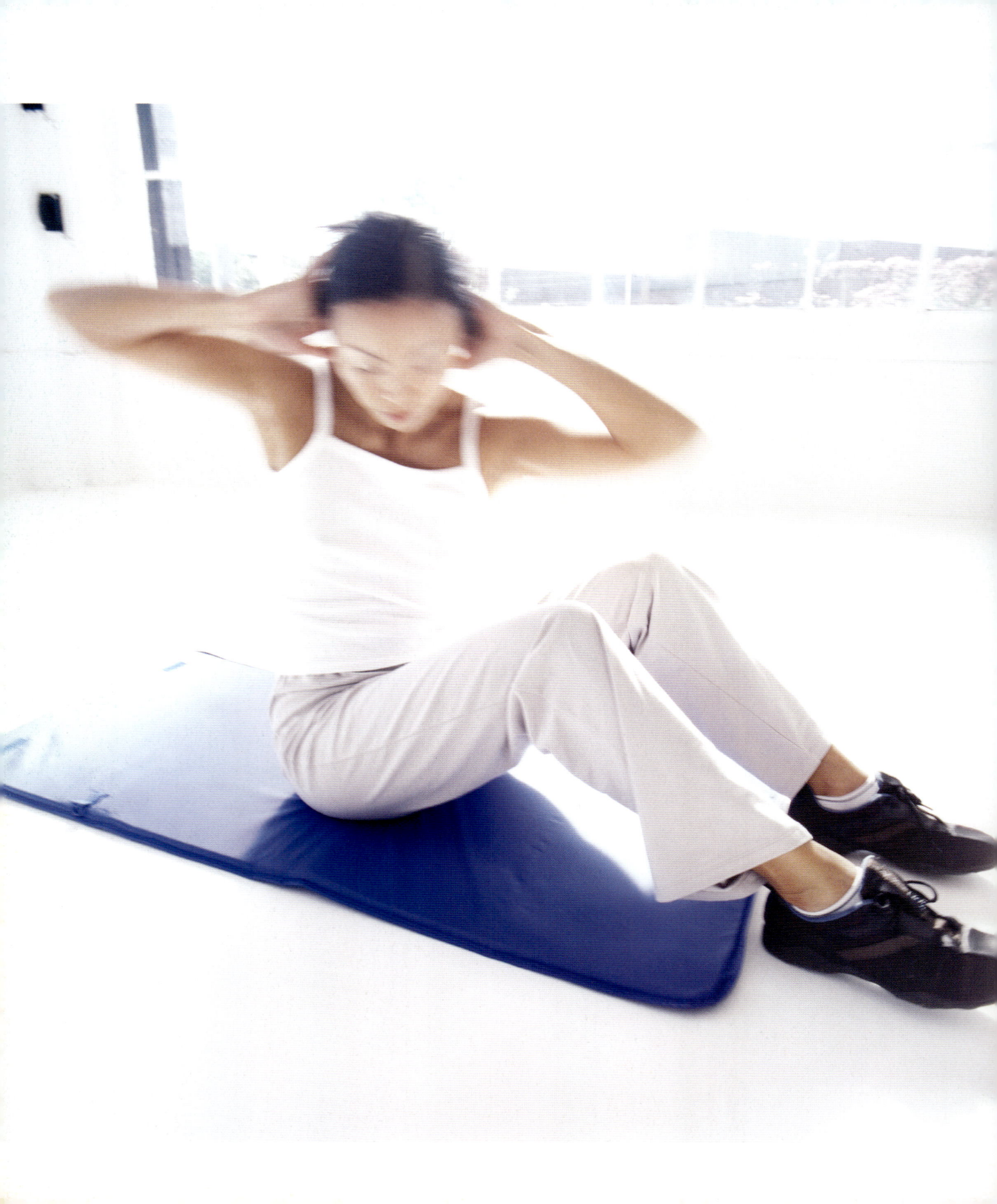

Ready?

Set

Go!

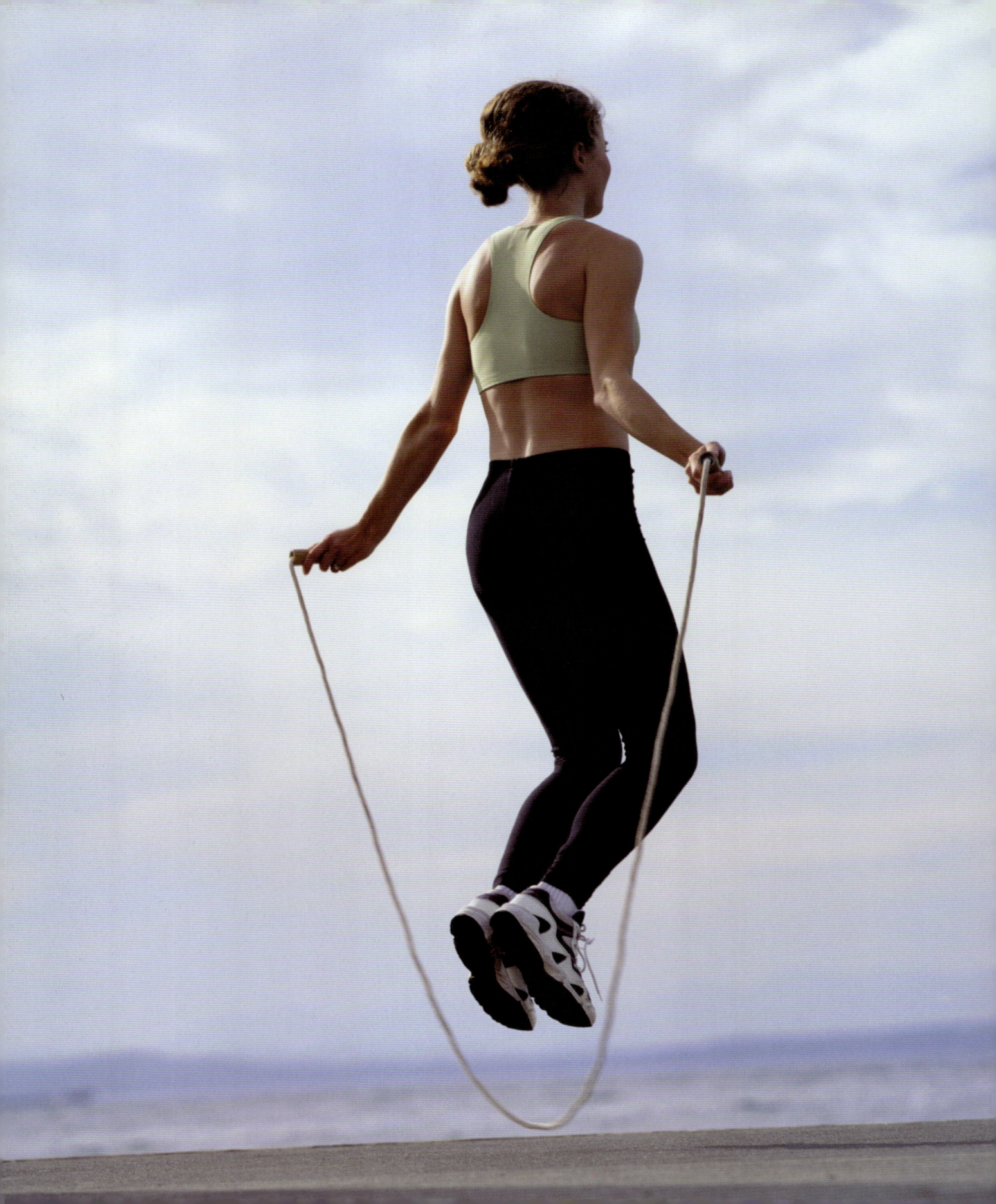

The KickStart Plan

You now have the knowledge and inspiration to change your life – it's time to put it into action! You'll begin with the KickStart Plan, creating new eating and exercise habits, and within two weeks you'll be feeling better than you've felt in a while. The differences you'll notice in these two weeks will motivate you to continue. Take what you've discovered about yourself – your goals, your dreams and your positive attitude – and go!

Eating

As outlined in Part Two, the KickStart Plan includes a relatively low-energy diet that will help you safely begin to lose weight in the first two weeks. It's nutritionally balanced and tasty, with a daily kilojoule intake of approximately 5000 kilojoules.

If you find that you're getting too hungry on this plan, don't give up. Just move to one of the LifeStyle menu plans at a higher daily kilojoule limit. That way you'll still be eating healthy, nutritious food and probably still will be consuming fewer kilojoules than before you began the Biggest Loser Eating Plan.

SHOPPING LIST

Before you begin this plan, make sure you have everything you need in the house. Shop the day before so that all you need to buy each week are some of the fresh ingredients. Photocopy the shopping list on these pages and take it with you. Some things you'll only have to buy once for the two weeks.

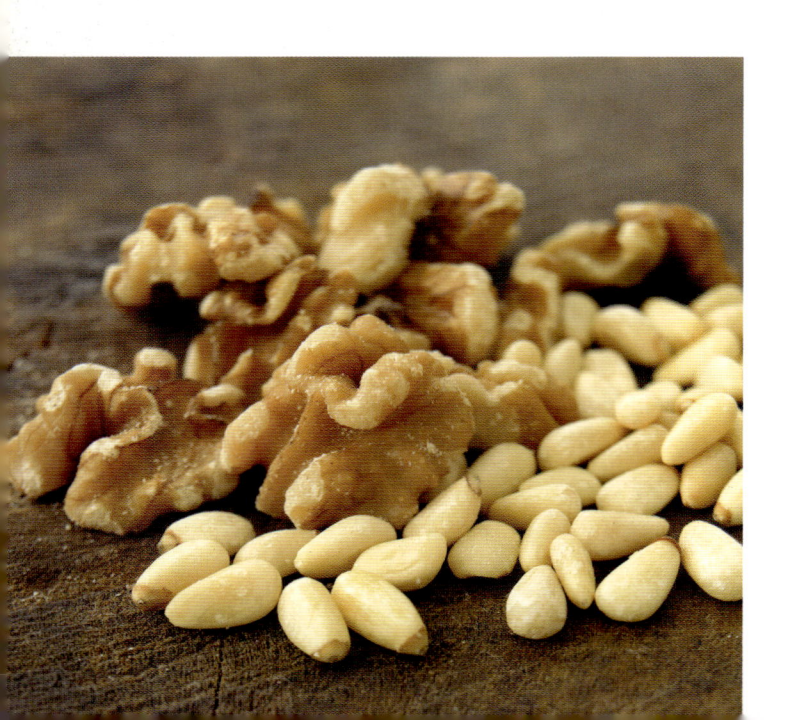

Week 1

Grocery
low-fat/light margarine
reduced-fat cheddar cheese
light soy sauce
low-fat mayonnaise
tahini
low-fat salad dressing
olive oil, in liquid form and as a spray for cooking
couscous
pearl barley
brown rice
rolled oats
wheatgerm
natural muesli
rice crackers
rye crackers
can of baked beans
cans of tuna in springwater
can of four-bean mix
eggs
instant miso soup
olives
LSA

Perishables
skim or low-fat milk
low-fat natural yoghurt
reduced-fat cottage cheese
wholegrain bread
wholegrain rolls

Meat and delicatessen
barramundi fillet
fish fillet such as whiting or flake
chicken breast fillet
chicken thigh fillets
steak
diced lamb
pork chop
slices of roast beef

Fruit and vegetables
fruit as snacks (2 pieces per day)
lemons
oranges
spinach
carrots
celery
cucumber
tomatoes
salad greens
spring onions
alfalfa sprouts
fennel
sweet potatoes
onions
eggplant
pumpkin
capsicum
zucchini
green beans
mushrooms
bok choy
broccoli
asparagus
snow peas
onions (red and brown)
garlic

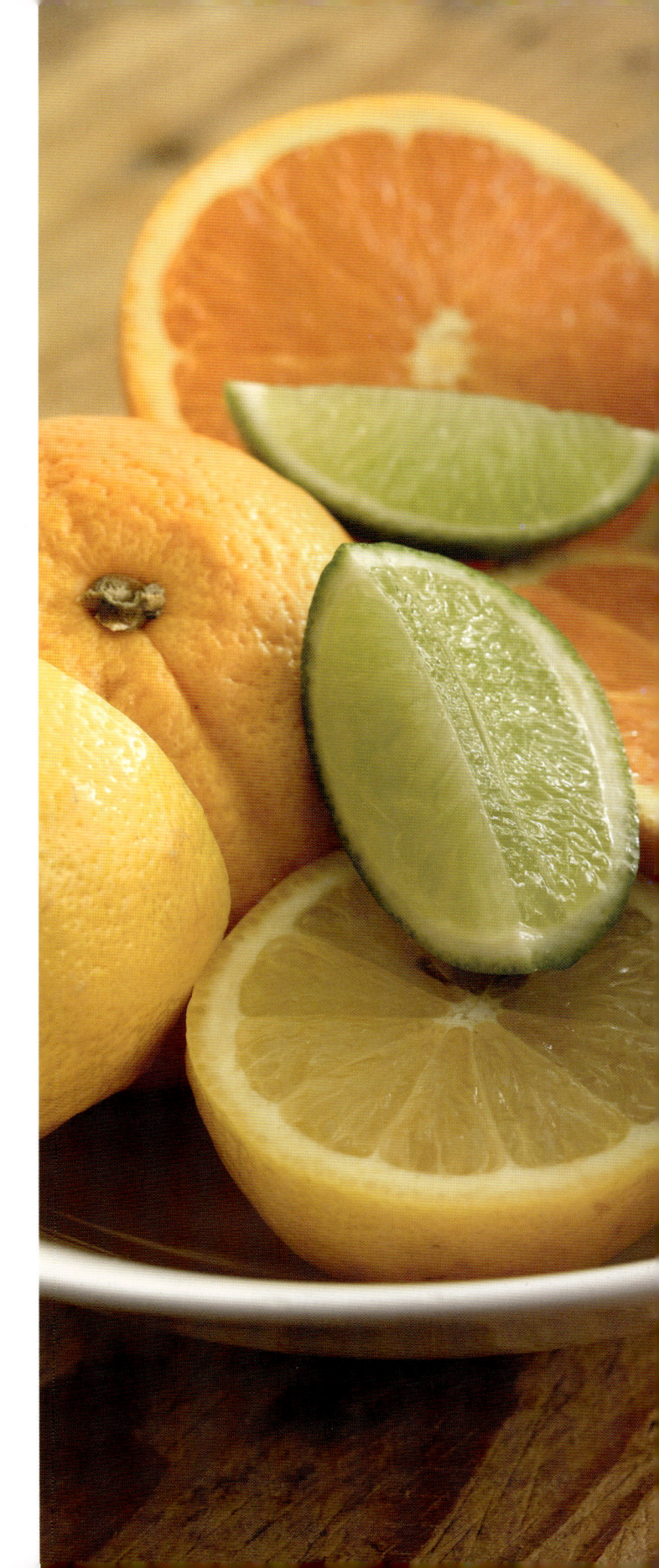

Week 2

Grocery
low-fat/light margarine
reduced-fat cheddar cheese
sweet chilli sauce
low-fat satay sauce
tahini
low-fat salad dressing
olive oil, in liquid form and as a spray for cooking
cellophane noodles
couscous
brown rice
rolled oats
wheatgerm
buckwheat
high-fibre cereal
rye crackers
can of baked beans
cans of low-salt tomatoes
cans of tuna in springwater
can of four-bean mix
eggs
chicken stock
instant miso soup
olives
brazil nuts

Perishables
skim or low-fat milk
low-fat natural yoghurt
reduced-fat cottage cheese
reduced-fat fetta cheese
hummus
wholegrain bread
sourdough bread
wholegrain rolls

Meat and delicatessen
barramundi fillet
snapper fillet
chicken breast fillets
minute steak
steak
pork chop
slices of roast beef
slices of lean ham

Fruit and vegetables
fruit as snacks (2 pieces per day)
lemons
spinach
carrots
celery
cucumber
cherry tomatoes
tomatoes
salad greens
alfalfa sprouts
dill
fennel
sweet potatoes
potatoes
onions
eggplant
pumpkin
capsicum
zucchini
corn
beetroot
broccoli
mushrooms
onions (red and brown)
garlic

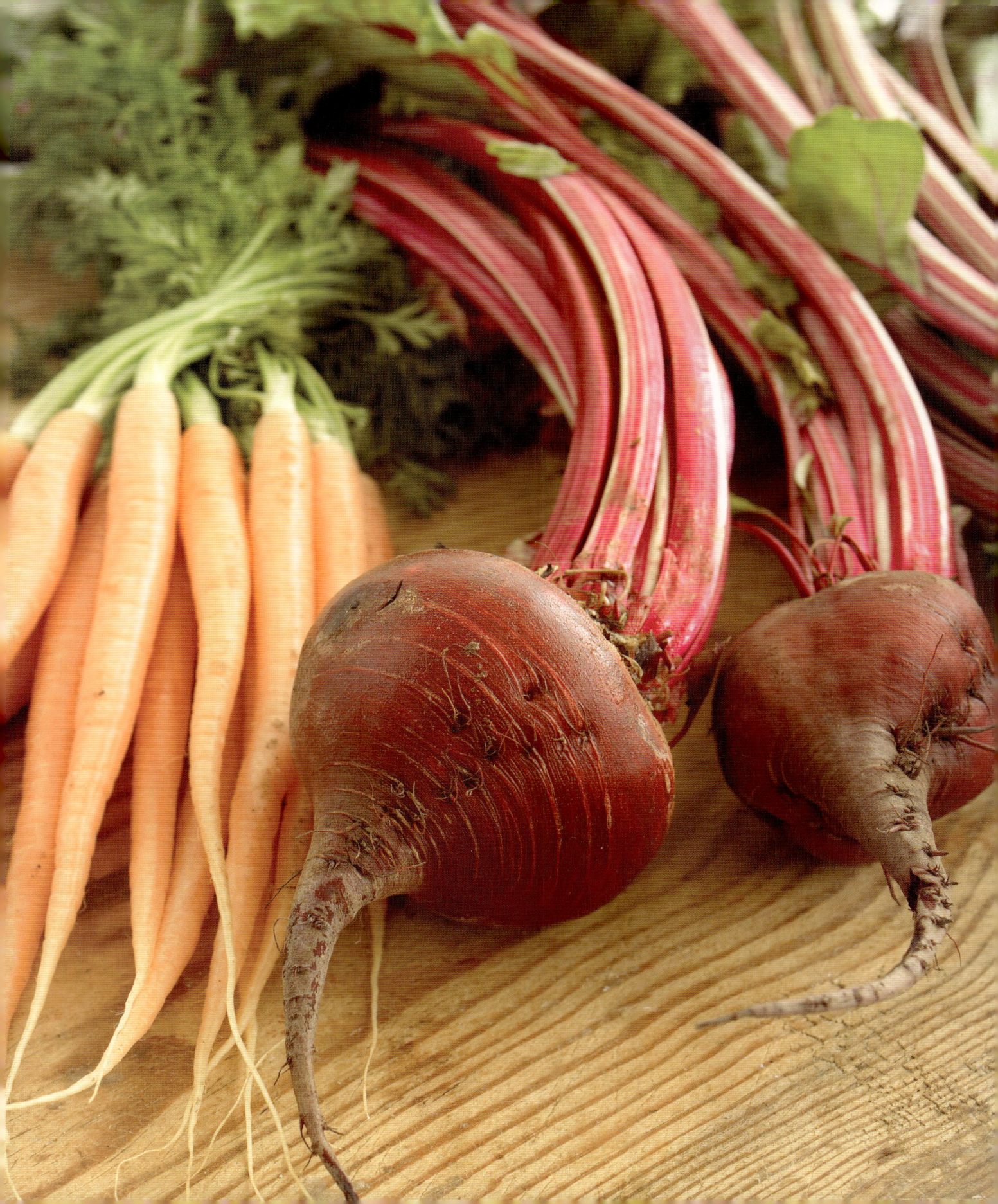

MENU PLANS

Follow these menu plans over the two weeks. Aim to prepare your food ahead so you're not tempted to pop into the local takeaway or café.

KICKSTART WEEK 1

	Day 1	Day 2	Day 3
Breakfast	1 cup Porridge (see p 154) with ½ cup skim milk, 1 piece fruit and 1 tablespoon wheatgerm	Omelette made with 3 egg whites, 1 cup chopped mushrooms and 1 tomato 1 slice wholegrain toast with light margarine	½ cup natural muesli with ½ cup skim milk and 1 piece fruit
Snack	200 g low-fat natural yoghurt 1 piece fruit	Fruit smoothie made with 200 ml skim milk, 1 piece fruit, dash of vanilla essence and a pinch of cinnamon	2 rye crackers with 30 g reduced-fat cottage cheese, 1 tomato and alfalfa sprouts
Lunch	1 small (130 g) can baked beans on 1 slice wholegrain toast with light margarine 1 cup dressed green salad leaves with ½ tomato, ¼ sliced cucumber and 1 tablespoon sliced onion	Chicken roll (1 wholemeal bread roll with light margarine, 80 g chicken breast and 1 cup dressed green salad leaves)	1 small (95 g) can tuna in springwater, 1 small (125 g) can four-bean mix, ¾ cup dressed green salad leaves, 1 spring onion and ¼ cucumber
Snack	1 cup raw vegetable pieces (carrot, celery and broccoli) with 1 tablespoon tahini	2 rice crackers with 30 g reduced-fat cheddar cheese 200 g low-fat natural yoghurt	200 g low-fat natural yoghurt with 1 piece fruit and 1 tablespoon LSA
Dinner	120 g white fish fillet baked in foil with juice of ¼ lemon, 1 tablespoon dill and 2 cloves garlic ½ cup cooked couscous ¾ cup steamed vegetables	160 g grilled steak ½ cup cooked rice ¾ cup steamed vegetables	Chicken Cacciatore (see p 195) ½ cup cooked rice 1 cup dressed green salad leaves

Day 4	Day 5	Day 6	Day 7
200 g low-fat natural yoghurt with 1 piece fruit	½ cup natural muesli with ½ cup skim milk and 1 piece fruit	1 cup Porridge (see p 154) with ½ cup skim milk, 1 piece fruit and 1 tablespoon LSA	Scrambled eggs made with 3 egg whites, 1 tomato and 1 cup baby spinach leaves served on 1 slice wholegrain toast with light margarine.
1 boiled egg mixed with ¼ cup reduced-fat cottage cheese and 1 cup of shredded lettuce with dressing on 2 rye crackers	2 rye crackers with 1 cup shredded lettuce leaves and 1 small (85 g) can tuna in spring-water mixed with low-fat mayonnaise	1 cup miso soup 1 wholegrain bread roll with light margarine	200 g low-fat natural yoghurt with 1 piece fruit and 1 tablespoon LSA
Lamb and Barley Hotpot (see p 172) 1 slice wholegrain bread with light margarine	Roast beef roll (1 wholegrain bread roll with light margarine, 2 slices roast beef, 1 medium tomato and 1 cup dressed green salad leaves)	Spiced Vegetable Ratatouille (see p 230) 1 cup cooked couscous	Tuna roll (1 wholegrain bread roll with light margarine, 1 small (95 g) can tuna in springwater, and 1 cup dressed green salad leaves)
1 cup raw vegetable pieces (carrot, celery and broccoli) with 1 tablespoon tahini	200 g low-fat natural yoghurt with 1 piece fruit	200 g low-fat natural yoghurt with 1 piece fruit	2 rye crackers with 30 g reduced-fat cheddar cheese and 1 tomato
120 g white fish fillet baked in foil with juice of ¼ lemon, 1 tablespoon dill and 2 cloves garlic 1½ cups Spiced Vegetable Ratatouille (see p 230)	Fried rice (½ cup cooked brown rice, 1 egg and 1½ cups cooked vegetables with soy sauce)	100 g Herb-crusted Grilled Pork (see p 212) Fennel and Orange Salad (see p 180) 1 cup steamed green vegetables	120 g grilled steak ¾ cup cooked couscous ½ cup steamed vegetables

KICKSTART WEK 2

	Day 1	Day 2	Day 3
Breakfast	1 cup Porridge (see p 154) with ⅔ cup skim milk 1 piece fruit	1⅓ cup high-fibre cereal with ½ cup skim milk 1 piece fruit	Omelette made with 3 egg whites, 1 slice lean ham and 50 g reduced-fat ricotta 1 slice wholegrain toast with light margarine
Snack	200 g low-fat natural yoghurt with 1 piece fruit and 4 brazil nuts, chopped	2 rye crackers with 30 g reduced-fat cottage cheese, 1 tomato and alfalfa sprouts	Fruit smoothie made with 200 ml skim milk, 1 piece fruit and 1 tablespoon wheatgerm
Lunch	1 small (130 g) can baked beans on 1 slice wholegrain toast with light margarine and 1 cup dressed green salad leaves	Chicken salad roll (1 mixed grain bread roll with light margarine, 65 g chicken, 1 cup torn lettuce leaves, capsicum and tomatoes)	Tuna and bean roll (mixed-grain bread roll with light margarine, 1 small (95 g) can tuna in springwater and ½ small (125 g) can four-bean mix with 1 cup green salad leaves)
Snack	1 cup raw vegetable pieces (carrot, celery and broccoli) with 2 tablespoons hummus	200 g low-fat natural yoghurt with 1 piece fruit	2 rye crackers with 30 g reduced-fat cheddar cheese and 1 medium tomato
Dinner	100 g Herb-crusted Grilled Pork (see p 212) ½ cup roast vegetables ¾ cup cooked couscous with 3 slices apple	100 g Snapper with (1 serve) Greek Salad (see p 222) ¼ cup cooked brown rice	Chicken Cacciatore (see p 195) ½ cup cooked brown rice 1 cup steamed green vegetables

Day 4	Day 5	Day 6	Day 7
1 cup high-fibre cereal with 200 ml skim milk 1 piece fruit	Fruit smoothie made with 200 ml skim milk, 1 piece fruit, 1 tablespoon wheatgerm and 100 g low-fat natural yoghurt	Scrambled eggs made with 3 egg whites, 1 cup cooked mushrooms and 1 cup baby spinach leaves 1 slice wholegrain toast with light margarine	2 Buckwheat Pancakes (see p 157) 100 g low-fat natural yoghurt with 1 piece fruit and 1 tablespoon wheatgerm
200 g low-fat natural yoghurt with 1 piece fruit and 1 tablespoon LSA	1 piece mixed-grain bread with light margarine, 30 g reduced-fat cheddar cheese and 1 medium tomato	Fruit smoothie made with 200 ml skim milk and 1 piece fruit	Fruit smoothie made with 200 ml skim milk, 1 piece fruit and 1 tablespoon wheatgerm
Vegetables Stuffed with Spiced Rice (see p 228) 1 cup dressed green salad leaves	Roasted Vegetable and Couscous Salad (see p 175) with 1½ cups rocket leaves	Roast beef roll (1 wholemeal bread roll with light margarine, 2 slices roast beef, 1 cup torn lettuce, slices of tomato and cucumber)	1 hard-boiled egg mashed with ½ tablespoon low-fat mayonnaise and 1 cup dressed green salad leaves on 1 slice mixed-grain toast
1 cup miso soup 1 mixed grain bread roll with light margarine	100 g low-fat natural yoghurt with 1 piece fruit and and 1 tablespoon LSA	1 cup raw vegetable pieces (carrot, celery and broccoli) with dip of 100 g low-fat natural yoghurt or reduced-fat ricotta, a squeeze of lemon juice and 1 tablespoon tahini	2 rye crackers with 1 small (95 g) can tuna in springwater, slices of tomato and onion, alfalfa and ¼ tablespoon chilli sauce
Steak Sandwich (see p 206) with 1 piece toasted sourdough 1 cup dressed green salad leaves	75 g grilled chicken breast with 30 g low-fat satay sauce ½ cup cooked rice 1½ cups steamed vegetables	120 g barramundi, baked in foil with juice of ¼ lemon, 1 tablespoon dill and 2 cloves of garlic 1 cup dressed green salad leaves and 75 g cellophane noodles OR 1 medium foil-baked jacket potato	70 g grilled steak ½ cup cooked brown rice 1½ cups steamed vegetables, tossed with 1½ teaspoons olive oil and a squeeze of lemon juice

Exercise

This two-week program is designed to get you out walking for 12 days with one rest day each week. Use these first two weeks to check out your local area and explore parts of your neighbourhood you've never been to. Change your route each day if you think you'll get bored. Look out for hills so that you can plan ahead, ready for the next day when you need to increase the intensity and work a little harder. Keep your eyes open for park benches and children's playgrounds as these can be used for some of the exercises in the following LifeStyle Plan.

The KickStart Plan focuses on cardiovascular training (cardio) rather than resistance training, although some resistance exercises are introduced in the second week. Walking and jogging are used but you can take on any kind of cardio exercise that you enjoy, such as cycling, cross-training, stair climbing or a combination of several cardio exercises, following the time periods set out in the plan.

The intensity levels vary in the plan and gradually increase over the second week. As with any exercise, listen to your body. Remember, you need to be moving out of your exercise comfort zone so you should be puffing and sweating. Take a water bottle with you and sip regularly during your workout. However, if you feel dizzy or faint, stop immediately and rest.

WARM UP AND COOL DOWN

Begin each session with a 5-minute warm-up: start walking at a normal pace, gradually increase your speed and start to swing your arms as you walk so that your heart-rate begins to rise and you are puffing. Remember to test the intensity at which you are working – ideally, you can still speak but you are breathing hard (try reciting your shopping list or singing a song – it shouldn't be too easy).

After each session, slow down to a relaxed walk and, once your breathing and heart-rate have returned to normal, spend 5–10 minutes doing the stretches on pages 130–133, first working your major muscle groups (your quadriceps, hamstrings, calves, chest, shoulders and back) and then moving on to other stretches. You will be using these stretches after all your workouts, so it's worth becoming familiar with them.

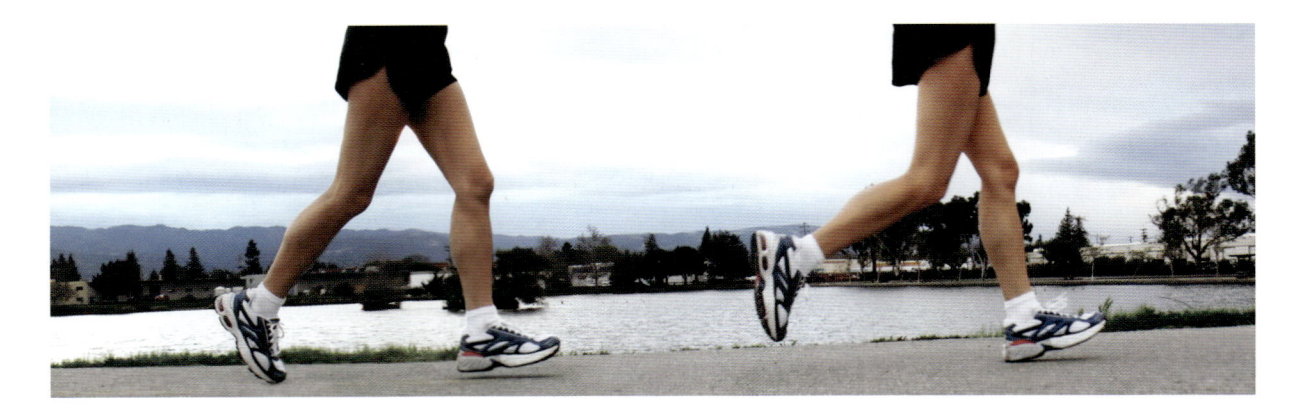

WEEK 1

Your first week on the plan will get your body moving and help you get used to setting aside time each day for activity. Read the Week 1 program so you have an idea of what you'll be doing each day, then write it in your training diary so you're organised and ready to go.

KICKSTART WEEK 1

DAY	BEGINNER	INTERMEDIATE	ADVANCED
1	Cardio – walk Stride along at a steady pace. **20–30 min**	Cardio – walk Stride along at a steady pace. **30–40 min**	Cardio – walk or jog Stride or jog along at a steady pace. **40–50 min**
2	Cardio – walk Stride along at a steady pace. **20–30 min**	Cardio – walk Stride along at a steady pace. **30–40 min**	Cardio – walk or jog Stride or jog along at a steady pace. **40–50 min**
3	Cardio – walk Stride along at a steady pace. **30–40 min**	Cardio – walk Stride along at a steady pace. **35–45 min**	Cardio – walk or jog Stride or jog along at a steady pace. **45–55 min**
4	Cardio – walk Add intensity by adding a hill. Keep a steady pace. **25–35 min**	Cardio – walk Add intensity by adding a hill – walk up and down twice. **30–40 min**	Cardio – walk or jog Add intensity by adding a hill – walk/jog up and down twice. **40–50 min**
5	Cardio – walk Stride along at a steady pace. **30–40 min**	Cardio – walk Stride along at a steady pace. **35–45 min**	Cardio – walk or jog Stride along at a steady pace. **45–55 min**
6	Cardio – walk Add intensity by adding a hill. Keep a steady pace. **30–40 min**	Cardio – walk Add intensity by adding a hill – walk up and down twice. **35–45 min**	Cardio – walk or jog Add intensity by adding a hill – walk/jog up and down twice. **40–50 min**
7	Rest day	Rest day	Rest day

WEEK 2

Now in your second week of the KickStart Plan, the intensity levels gradually increase. Resistance exercises are also included; see pages 134–142 for the correct technique for these exercises. If you feel uncomfortable doing step-ups or push-ups in public, finish your cardio and complete these at home.

KICKSTART WEEK 2

DAY	BEGINNER	INTERMEDIATE	ADVANCED
8	Cardio – walk Stride along at a steady pace for **30–40 min**. Find a curb or step and complete 30 step-ups on each leg.	Cardio – walk Stride along at a steady pace for **40–50 min**. Find a curb or step and complete 40 fast step-ups on each leg.	Cardio – walk or jog Stride along at a steady pace for **45–55 min**. Find a curb or step and complete 50 fast step-ups on each leg.
9	Cardio – walk Find an incline and incorporate this into your walk. If you're near the beach, walk through the sand for greater intensity. Keep up a steady pace for **30–40 min**.	Cardio – walk Find an incline and incorporate this into your walk, going up and down twice. If you're near the beach, walk through the sand for greater intensity. Keep up a steady pace for **40–50 min**.	Cardio – walk or jog Find an incline and incorporate this, walking or jogging up and down 2 or 3 times. If you're near the beach, walk through the sand for greater intensity. **45–55 min**
10	Cardio – walk Stride along at a steady pace. **30–40 min**	Cardio – walk Stride along at a steady pace. **35–45 min**	Cardio – walk or jog Stride along at a steady pace. **40–50 min**
11	Cardio – walk Stride along at a steady pace for **30–40 min**. Then, using a curb or step, complete 30 fast step-ups on each leg followed by a maximum of 10 push-ups on your knees. Add in 10 crunches to finish.	Cardio – walk Stride along at a steady pace for **40–50 min**. Find a curb or step and complete 40 fast step-ups on each leg.	Cardio – walk or jog Stride along at a steady pace for **45–55 min**. Find a curb or step and complete 50 fast step-ups on each leg.

Note how many step-ups, push-ups and crunches you completed in your training diary.

KICKSTART WEEK 2

DAY	BEGINNER	INTERMEDIATE	ADVANCED
12	**Cardio – walk** Stride along at a steady pace. **30–40 min**	**Cardio – walk** Stride along at a steady pace. **35–45 min**	**Cardio – walk or jog** Stride along at a steady pace. **45–55 min**
13	**Cardio – walk** Stride along at a steady pace for **20–30 min**. Then, using a curb or step, complete 30 fast step-ups on each leg followed by 10 push-ups on your knees. Add in 10 crunches to finish.	**Cardio – walk** Stride along at a steady pace for **30–40 min**. Then, using a curb or step, complete 40 fast step-ups on each leg followed by 15 push-ups on your knees. Add in 20 crunches to finish.	**Cardio – walk or jog** Stride along at a steady pace for **35–40 min**. Then, using a curb or step, complete 50 fast step-ups on each leg followed by 20 push-ups on your toes. Add in 30 crunches to finish.
	Note how many step-ups, push-ups and crunches you completed in your training diary.		
14	*Rest day*	*Rest day*	*Rest day*

'I was overweight simply because I ate more than I used. I chose the easy option of being fat and made excuses that I was happy to be fat – yeah, well, I was lying.' **'Big Wal' Milberg, Series One**

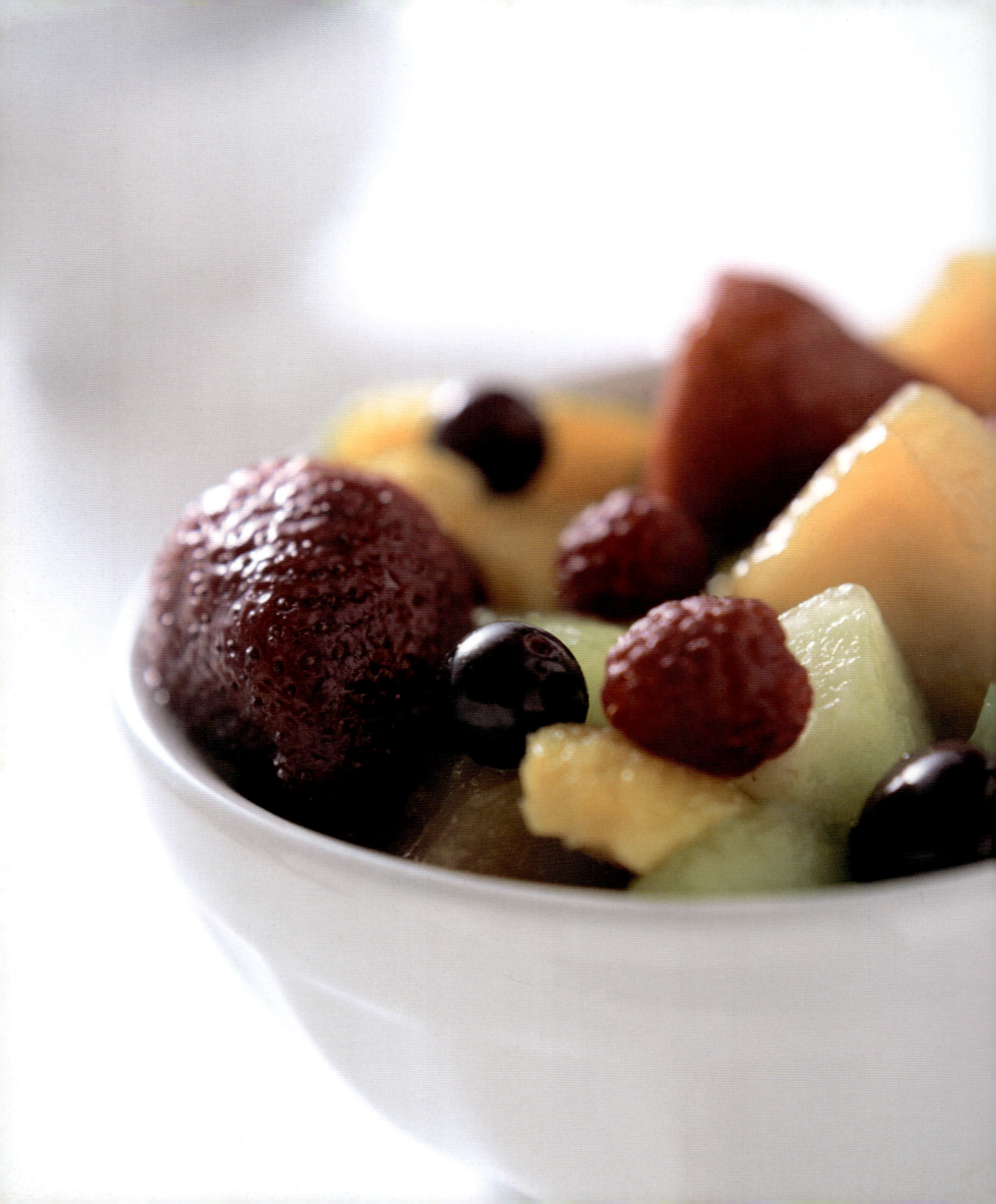

The LifeStyle Plan

You've spent two weeks on the KickStart Plan, exercising six days a week and following a healthy, portion-controlled eating plan. How do you feel? Good? You're now ready to move on to the LifeStyle Plan, challenging yourself with new exercise programs and enjoying more delicious recipes that will help you continue to eat healthily and lose weight. This three-month plan helps you turn your behavioural changes into lifelong good habits, from choosing healthy food, limiting portion sizes and planning your meals, to increasing your incidental activity and exercising six days a week.

Eating

The LifeStyle Plan includes three sample-week menu plans, one for each of the following daily kilojoule limits: 6000 kilojoules, 8000 kilojoules and 10,000 kilojoules. The menu plans ensure you receive all the necessary nutrients, fibre, vitamins and minerals at the recommended daily intake for good nutrition, and include three meals and two snacks each day. Use the menu plan for your kilojoule level for the first week and then adapt it using the recipes in Recipes for Life (page 147) and what you have learnt in Part Two.

If you find that you're just getting too hungry on your chosen plan, move to a menu plan for one of the higher daily kilojoule limits. That way you're still eating healthy, nutritious food and probably still consuming fewer kilojoules than before you began the Biggest Loser Eating Plan. Even if you have the occasional lapse, remember that it's not all-or-nothing. Little changes can make a difference, and they're better than doing nothing at all.

In the long term as you lose weight, you may need to reduce your kilojoule intake to keep losing weight or to maintain your weight. Try out one of the lower kilojoule intake menu plans to get a feel for how much food that amounts to – for example, if you lose weight on the 10,000-kilojoule plan, make the 8000-kilojoule plan your maintenance plan.

COOKING FOR HEALTH

Healthy eating is delicious when you know some of the tricks of the trade. It doesn't mean that you can't treat yourself occasionally, or still enjoy your favourite recipes. By changing an ingredient or the cooking technique, you can update recipes and create healthy versions of your favourite foods.

Try some of these ideas for modifying recipes:

- Reduce the amount of oil, butter or margarine a recipe requires. If a recipe calls for ½ cup, using ⅓ generally won't affect the result. For a cake, replace some of the butter or margarine with apple purée to keep it moist.
- Use skim milk or low-fat milk instead of full-cream milk.
- Replace any butter or oil needed for frying or stir-frying by using a non-stick pan or a cooking (oil) spray, or line the pan with baking paper and spray with the oil spray.
- Use reduced-fat cheese, ricotta and mayonnaise to replace full-fat versions.
- Use low-fat natural yoghurt or evaporated skim milk to replace cream.
- Choose fish canned in water instead of oil.
- Use herbs and spices to enhance flavour rather than salt, reduce the amount of salt, or don't use it at all (unless it's needed to help plain flour rise).
- Reduce sugar in baking. Try adding cinnamon, nutmeg, allspice, vanilla or almond essence for sweetness.
- Use wholegrains such as whole-wheat flour, wholegrain pasta and brown rice instead of the white refined varieties.

A HEALTHY KITCHEN

You may already have a well-stocked kitchen, but here are a few items that will help you cook healthy meals:

- measuring cups and spoons
- measuring scale
- measuring jug
- colander
- steamer
- non-porous chopping boards
- wok
- non-stick frypan (reducing the amount of oil needed)
- baking dish
- wooden spoons
- baking paper
- oil spray
- herbs and spices
- plastic containers with airtight lids for storage and taking lunch to work
- sharp knifes including a cook's knife and a smaller paring knife (these can be bought relatively cheaply so replace any old knives)
- microwave.

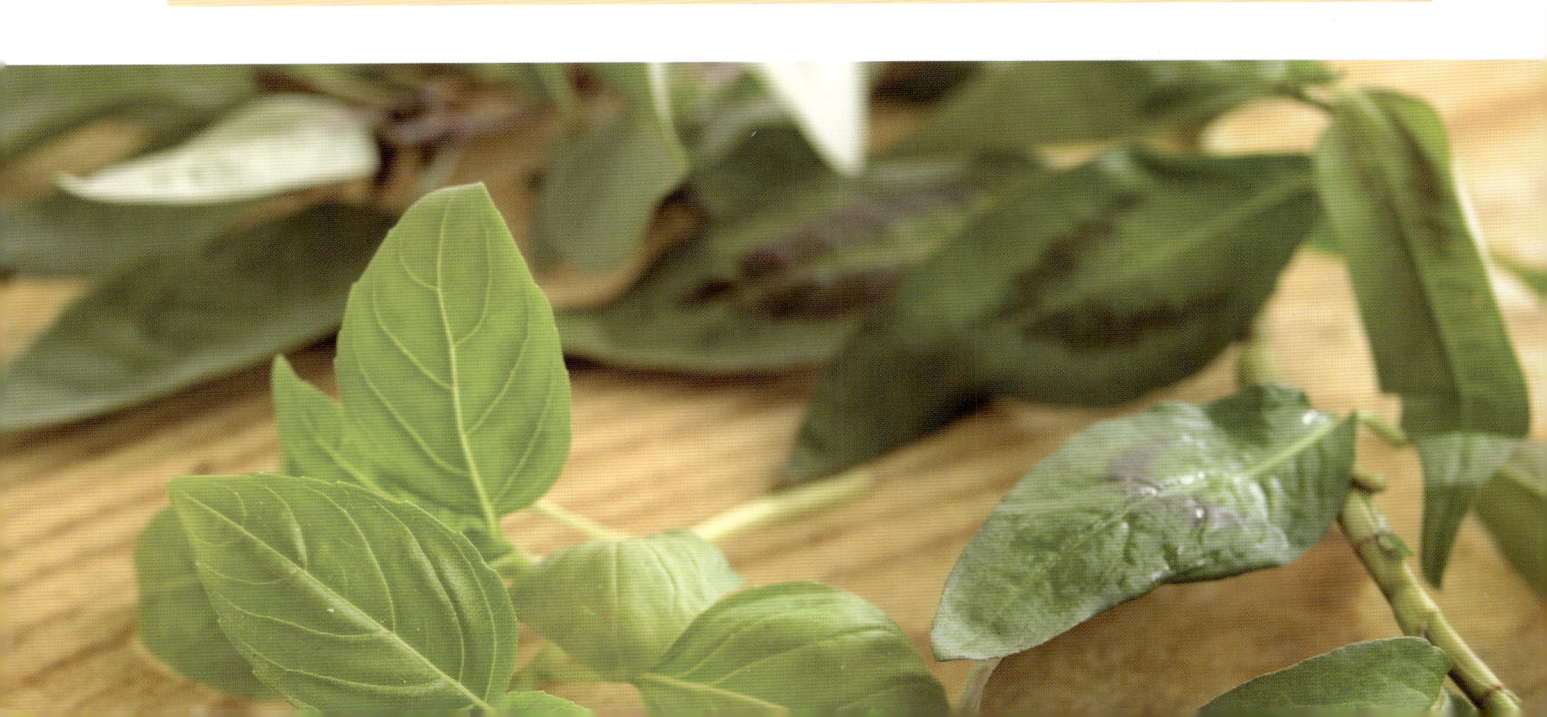

- Substitute up to half of the white flour required with whole-wheat flour.
- Add vegetables, such as baby spinach, canned low-salt tomatoes, grated carrot or zucchini, to meat dishes.
- Dilute bottled Asian, Indian and pasta sauces with either a can of diced low-salt tomatoes or skim evaporated milk.
- Add baby spinach or other dark green salad leaves to stir-fries and salads.
- Don't peel fruit and vegetables, even if the recipe says to.
- Choose raisins instead of choc-chips when making cookies.
- Use marinades to flavour meats rather than sauces and gravies.
- Substitute full-fat sour cream with light sour cream, or use cottage cheese mixed with lemon juice instead.
- Replace up to 40 per cent of mince in recipes with beans, red lentils, tofu, brown rice or couscous.
- Use two egg whites to replace one whole egg.
- Replace breadcrumbs with wholemeal or wholegrain crumbs.
- Find a similar recipe that has a lower fat content.

You can improve your health and reduce your fat and salt intake by using healthy cooking methods and making healthy choices when shopping:

- Select lean cuts of meat and trim all visible fat from meat before cooking. When cooking stews, simmer then cool and skim any fat from the surface.
- Use a rack when roasting to allow the fat to run off.
- Cook stews and sauces a day before you need them. Not only will they taste better, but also the fat can be scraped off the top.
- Remove the skin from chicken, no matter how good it looks!
- Reduce the amount of meat served by having a moderate portion size and increasing the amount of vegetables on your plate.
- Use cooking methods such as steaming, roasting, stir-frying, microwaving and poaching instead of frying.
- Don't put salt on the table.
- Reduce your salt intake by limiting canned foods; condiments such as tomato sauce, olives and pickles; and processed meats such as ham, salami and bacon.
- Use reduced-salt varieties of canned food where possible.
- Enjoy frozen yoghurt instead of ice-cream, or choose the low-fat varieties.
- Add extra salad items or cooked vegetable to lunches and dinners.
- Increase the amount of fruit, vegetables and wholegrains you eat.
- Eat smaller portions; use smaller plates, smaller glasses and cups and smaller cutlery.
- Eat regular meals.
- Don't eliminate foods, just reduce the amount.

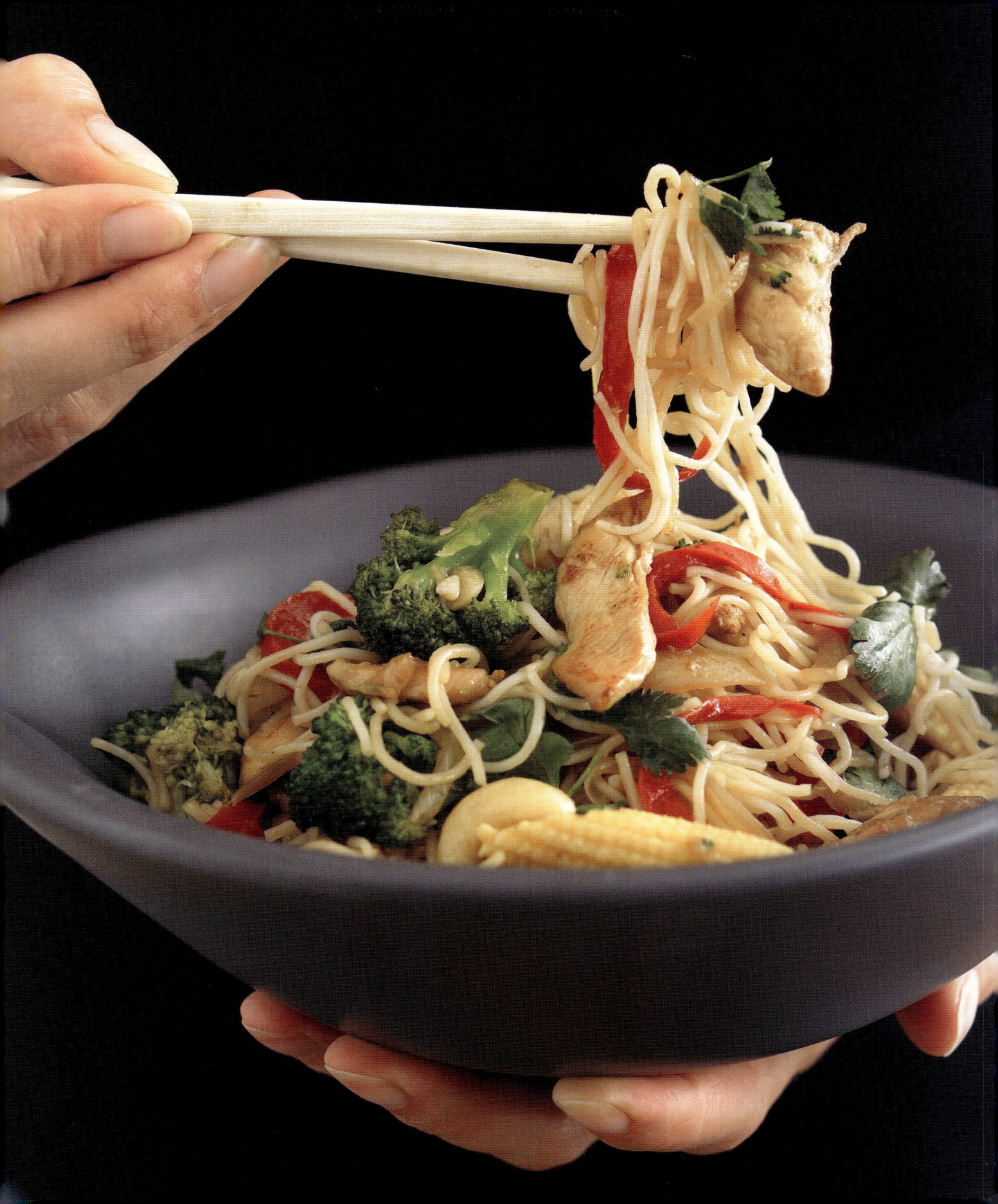

SAMPLE MENU PLAN — 6000 KJ INTAKE

	Day 1	Day 2	Day 3
Breakfast	½ cup natural muesli with ½ cup skim milk and 1 tablespoon LSA 1 piece fruit	1 cup high-fibre cereal with ½ cup skim milk, 1 tablespoon LSA and 1 medium banana	1 cup Bircher Muesli (see p 152)
Snack	2 rice crackers with 30 g reduced-fat cottage cheese, 1 tomato and alfalfa sprouts	200 g low-fat natural yoghurt with 1 piece fruit	60 g reduced-fat cottage cheese mixed with 2 tablespoons chopped sun-dried tomatoes on 4 rye crackers
Lunch	1 slice wholegrain toast with light margarine, ½ cup baked beans, 1 poached egg and 1 cup cooked spinach	Open chicken sandwich (1 slice wholegrain bread with light margarine, 1 teaspoon mustard, grilled skinless chicken breast fillet and 1 cup of dressed salad greens, slices of cucumber and capsicum)	Ham roll (1 wholegrain bread roll with light margarine, 1 teaspoon mustard, 1 slice lean ham, 1 medium tomato and 1 cup dressed green salad leaves)
Snack	200 g low-fat natural yoghurt with 1 piece fruit, 1 tablespoon LSA and 2 teaspoons honey	4 rye crackers with 2 slices lean ham and 1 tomato	Fruit smoothie made with 200 ml skim milk, 1 piece fruit and 1 tablespoon wheatgerm, dash of vanilla essence and a pinch of cinnamon
Dinner	Snapper with Greek Salad (see p 222)	Spiced Vegetable Ratatouille with Couscous (see p 230)	Chicken and Spinach Lasagne (see p 200) 1 cup dressed green salad leaves

Day 4	Day 5	Day 6	Day 7
½ cup natural muesli with ½ cup skim milk and 1 tablespoon LSA 1 piece fruit	200 g low-fat natural yoghurt with 2 pieces fruit, 1 tablespoon LSA and 1 tablespoon wheatgerm	Scrambled Eggs with Smoked Salmon (see p 162) on sourdough toast with light margarine	Buckwheat Pancakes (see p 157) with 1 piece fruit and 1 tablespoon low-fat natural yoghurt
2 rye crackers with 1½ hard-boiled eggs, 1 cup dressed green salad leaves and alfalfa sprouts	1 cup raw vegetable pieces (carrot, celery and broccoli) with 2 tablespoons hummus and 1 tablespoon tahini	Fruit smoothie made with 200 ml skim milk, 1 piece fruit, 1 tablespoon wheatgerm, dash of vanilla essence and a pinch of cinnamon	Fruit smoothie made with 200 ml skim milk, 1 piece fruit and 1 tablespoon wheatgerm
Roasted Vegetable and Couscous Salad (see p 175)	Steak Sandwich (see p 206)	Tuna and bean roll (wholemeal bread roll with light margarine, 1 small (95 g) can tuna in springwater, 1 small (125 g) can four-bean mix and 1 cup dressed green salad leaves)	Open salmon sandwich (1 piece wholegrain bread with light margarine, 3 slices smoked salmon, 1 cup watercress, ¼ sliced onion and 1 tablespoon reduced-fat cream cheese)
125 g frozen yoghurt 1 piece fruit	Fruit smoothie made with 200 ml skim milk, 1 piece fruit, 1 tablespoon wheatgerm, dash of vanilla essence and a pinch of cinnamon	Apple and Rhubarb Crumble (see p 232) with 3 tablespoons low-fat natural yoghurt	1 cup raw vegetable pieces (carrot, celery and broccoli) with 2 tablespoons hummus and 1 tablespoon tahini
Chicken and Cashew Stir-fry (see p 198)	Swordfish with Roast Tomato and Rocket Salad (see p 224) 1½ cups cooked vegetables ¾ cup oven chips	Braised Lamb Shanks with Lentil and Onion Stew (see p 210) 1 cup dressed green salad leaves	Grilled Eye Fillet with Mustard Polenta (see p 203) 1 cup dressed green salad leaves

SAMPLE MENU PLAN — 8000 KJ INTAKE

	Day 1	Day 2	Day 3
Breakfast	1½ cups high-fibre cereal with ½ cup skim milk 1 piece fruit	1 cup Porridge (see p 154) with ½ cup skim milk, 1 piece fruit, 1 tablespoon LSA and 1 tablespoon honey	¾ cup Bircher Muesli (see p 152)
Snack	Cheese sandwich (2 slices wholemeal bread with 30 g reduced-fat cheddar cheese and 1 cup dressed green salad leaves)	2 slices wholemeal fruit bread with 60 g reduced-fat cottage cheese 1 piece fruit	1 cup Bacon, Lentil and Tomato Soup (see p 168) 1 slice wholegrain toast with light margarine
Lunch	1½ cups Lamb and Barley Hotpot (see p 172) 1 wholegrain bread roll with light margarine	100 g grilled skinless chicken breast ½ cup Spiced Vegetable Ratatouille with (1 serve) Couscous (see p 230)	Roast beef roll (1 wholegrain bread roll with light margarine, 1 teaspoon mustard, 2 slices roast beef, 1 cup dressed green salad leaves, slices of cucumber and tomato)
Snack	Fruit smoothie made with 200 ml skim milk, 1 piece fruit, 2 tablespoons wheatgerm, dash of vanilla essence and a pinch of cinnamon 2 rye crackers with 1 small (95 g) can tuna in springwater, 1 spring onion and 1 tablespoon low-fat mayonnaise	1 cup raw vegetable pieces (carrot, celery and broccoli) with 2 tablespoons hummus and 1 tablespoon tahini	Fruit smoothie made with 200 ml skim milk, 1 piece fruit, dash of vanilla essence and a pinch of cinnamon Rye crackers with 30 g reduced-fat cheddar cheese, tomato and alfalfa on rye crackers
Dinner	Grilled Eye Fillet with Mustard Polenta (see p 203) ¾ cup steamed vegetables	Swordfish with Roast Tomato and Rocket Salad (see p 224) 1 cup steamed vegetables ¾ cup cooked brown rice or oven chips	Chicken and Spinach Lasagne (see p 200) 1 cup dressed green salad leaves

Day 4	Day 5	Day 6	Day 7
1⅓ cups high-fibre cereal with ½ cup skim milk 1 piece fruit	Scrambled eggs made with 3 egg whites, 1 grilled tomato on 2 slices wholegrain toast spread with 1½ tablespoons avocado	1 cup Porridge (see p 154) with ½ cup skim milk, 1 piece fruit, 1 tablespoon LSA and 1 tablespoon honey	Spanish-style Baked Eggs (see p 164) 1 slice wholegrain toast with light margarine
2 boiled eggs mashed with 1 tablespoon low-fat mayonnaise and 1 cup dressed green salad leaves on 4 rye crackers	1 cup Lamb and Barley Hotpot (see p 172) 1 slice wholegrain toast with light margarine	Fruit smoothie made with 200 ml skim milk, 1 piece fruit, 1 tablespoon honey, 2 tablespoons wheatgerm, dash of vanilla essence and a pinch of cinnamon	200 g low-fat natural yoghurt with 2 pieces fruit, 1 tablespoon honey and 1 tablespoon LSA
Tuna and bean roll (1 wholegrain bread roll with light margarine, 1 small (95 g) can tuna in springwater, 1 small (125 g) can four-bean mix, 1 cup dressed green salad leaves and slices of cucumber and tomato)	Corn Fritters with Smoked Salmon and Coriander Dressing (see p 189) 1 piece fruit	Spiced Lamb Pockets (see p 187)	Ocean Trout Panzanella Salad (see p 216)
200 g low-fat natural yoghurt with 2 pieces fruit, 1 tablespoon honey and 1 tablespoon LSA	4 rye crackers with light margarine, 60 g reduced-fat cheddar cheese and 2 slices lean ham 1 piece fruit	1 cup raw vegetable pieces (carrot, celery and broccoli) with 2 tablespoons hummus and 1 tablespoon tahini	Ham and cheese sandwich (2 slices wholegrain bread, with 30 g low-fat cottage cheese, 2 slices lean ham and 1 tablespoon chopped sun-dried tomatoes)
Yoghurt-marinated Lamb Cutlets (see p 209) 1 cup cooked couscous 100 g Tabouleh (see p 179)	Beef Stir-fry with Hokkien Noodles (see p 201) 1½ cups steamed vegetables	Fried rice (1 cup cooked brown rice, 1 cup steamed vegetables and 100 g grilled skinless chicken breast with soy sauce)	1 cup cooked wholemeal pasta with 1 small (95 g) can tuna in springwater, 2 tablespoons chopped olives and 2 tablespoons pesto 1 cup dressed green salad leaves

SAMPLE MENU PLAN — 10,000 KJ INTAKE

	Day 1	Day 2	Day 3
Breakfast	1½ cups high-fibre cereal with ½ cup skim milk 1 piece fruit	¾ cup Bircher Muesli (see p 152) with 1 piece fruit	Scrambled eggs made with 4 egg whites and 1 yolk with 1 cup baby spinach laeves, ½ cup sliced mushrooms and 2 slices wholegrain toast with light margarine
Snack	Cheese and tomato sandwich (2 slices wholegrain bread with light margarine, 2 slices lean ham, 30 g reduced-fat cheddar cheese, 1 tomato and 1 cup dressed greens)	Grilled mushrooms, 30 g reduced-fat fetta and 1 cup rocket leaves on 1 slice wholemeal toast with light margarine	2 rye crackers with 30 g reduced-fat cheddar cheese 1 cup raw vegetable pieces (carrot, celery and broccoli) with 2 tablespoons hummus and 1 tablespoon tahini
Lunch	1 large baked potato with 1 small can baked beans and 30 g reduced-fat cottage cheese 1 cup dressed green salad leaves	Spiced Lamb Pockets (see p 187)	Tuna sandwich (2 slices wholemeal bread with 1 small (95 g) can tuna in springwater, 1 small (125 g) can four-bean mix, 2 tablespoons corn kernels, 1 spring onion and low-fat mayonnaise)
Snack	4 rye crackers with 185 g can tuna in springwater and 80 g corn kernels Fruit smoothie made with 200 ml skim milk, 1 piece fruit, 1 tablespoon honey, 2 tablespoons wheatgerm, 1 tablespoon LSA, dash of vanilla essence and a pinch of cinnamon	Fruit smoothie made with 200 ml skim milk, 1 piece fruit, 1 tablespoon wheatgerm, and 1 tablespoon honey Carrot, Sultana and Walnut Muffin (see p 240)	200 g low-fat natural yoghurt, with 1 piece fruit, 1 teaspoon honey and 1 tablespoon LSA
Dinner	Chicken and Cashew Stir-fry (see p 198)	Beef Stir-fry with Hokkien Noodles (see p 201)	Chicken and Spinach Lasagne (see p 200) ½ cup cooked wholemeal pasta 1 cup dressed green salad leaves

Day 4	Day 5	Day 6	Day 7
1 cup Porridge (see p 154) with ½ cup skim milk, 1 piece fruit, 1 tablespoon LSA and 1 tablespoon honey	1⅓ cups high-fibre cereal, ½ cup skim milk and 2 tablespoons LSA	Italian Omelette (see p 160) and 2 slices wholegrain toast with light margarine	1 cup Porridge (see p 154) with ½ cup skim milk and 1 piece fruit
Lamb and Barley Hotpot (see p 172) 1 slice wholegrain toast with light margarine	Bacon, Lentil and Tomato Soup (see p 168) 2 slices wholegrain toast with light margarine	200 g low-fat natural yoghurt with 2 pieces fruit, 1 tablespoon honey and 1 tablespoon LSA	Roasted Vegetable and Couscous Salad (see p 175) 2 slices wholegrain toast with light margarine
Roast beef rolls (2 medium wholegrain bread rolls with light margarine, 1 teaspoon mustard, 4 slices roast beef, 2 medium tomatoes and 2 cups dressed green salad leaves)	Steak Sandwich (see p 206)	Fried rice (1 cup brown rice, 120 g grilled skinless chicken breast and 1 cup cooked vegetables with soy sauce and sesame oil)	2 taco shells with Nacho sauce (see p 207), 1 tomato and 1 cup shredded lettuce topped with 1 tablespoon light sour cream
Apple and Rhubarb Crumble (see p 210)	Cheese sandwich (2 slices wholegrain bread with light margarine, 1 teaspoon mustard, 30 g reduced-fat cheddar cheese and 1 cup dressed green salad leaves)	4 rye crackers with 30 g reduced-fat cheddar cheese 1 cup raw vegetable pieces (carrot, celery and broccoli) with 2 tablespoons hummus and 1 tablespoon tahini	4 rye crackers with 1 small (95 g) can tuna in springwater Fruit smoothie made with 200 ml skim milk, 1 piece fruit, dash of vanilla essence and a pinch of cinnamon
Braised Lamb Shank with Lentil and Onion Stew (see p 210) 1 cup dressed green salad leaves	150 g white fish fillet baked in foil with juice of ¼ lemon, 1 tablespoon dill leaves and 2 cloves garlic 1½ cups Spiced Vegetable Ratatouille with Couscous (see p 230) 1 cup dressed green salad leaves Pear and Coconut Spring Rolls (see p 235)	Grilled Eye Fillet with Mustard Polenta (see p 203) 1 cup steamed green vegetables	Herb-crusted Grilled Pork (see p 212) 1 cup Orange and Fennel Salad (see p 180) 1 cup steamed vegetables

Exercise – Program 1

Program 1 is a great way for you to build on your achievements from the KickStart Plan. Consisting of 50 per cent cardio and 50 per cent resistance (circuit) training, you can choose to exercise outdoors, at home or in a gym.

You'll be exercising six days a week, alternating between cardio and resistance training (the resistance training will be done in a circuit format). You don't need to go to a gym to do the resistance circuit training in this program, but an optional gym resistance-training program has been included in case you belong to a gym or are thinking of joining one. The gym program can replace the resistance circuit on days 2 and 6.

WHAT'S YOUR INTENSITY?

Intensity is the amount of effort you use to exercise. The intensity you train at plays a vital role in how good your results are. In some of the Biggest Loser exercise programs you'll need to be able to gauge your intensity so you know to work harder or slow down as needed. Use a heart-rate monitor to rate your intensity (see pages 78–79) or use the scale below.

- Levels 1–3   your resting heart rate (when you are sitting still or just slightly moving)
- Level 4   slow walking pace, or moving around the house
- Level 5   your heart-rate is slightly elevated but you can still hold a conversation
- Level 6   your body is warm, your heart-rate is up and you are puffing
- Level 7   you can still talk but your focus is more on the body working
- Level 8   your heart-rate is definitely elevated, body working hard
- Level 9   your heart is pounding as if you've just done a 10-second sprint
- Level 10   you're purple in the face, heart-rate through the roof, can't speak!

Before starting your cardio workouts, warm up for a good 5–7 minutes, gradually building up to an intensity level of 5 or 6. For the actual workout, lift your intensity to level 7 or 8 and maintain this as outlined in the relevant workout program. For the cool-down, spend 5 minutes gradually reducing the intensity down to a level 4. Then spend 5–10 minutes stretching all major muscle groups (see pages 130–133 for the stretches).

Use these intensity guidelines for any cardio exercise you do (for example, cycling, running or walking).

The key with these workouts is to keep going and be consistent. If you feel a little bored or stale, mix the activities up. If you're a gym member, take an aerobics class instead of your usual cardio training, or try a piece of equipment you don't normally use. If you don't have access to gym facilities, try going for a swim or a bike ride to keep things interesting.

First read through the entire program and make notes in your training diary about which level is right for you for both the cardio and resistance sessions and what that involves (the time, the exercises and the intensity levels). This way you can personalise the program for yourself.

The table below shows the overall plan for the six-weeks of program 1 – that is, which days you'll be doing cardio training (and whether it will be interval or endurance cardio) and which days you'll be doing resistance training (and don't forget to enjoy your rest day too!).

PROGRAM 1 – SIX-WEEK SUMMARY: BEGINNER

DAY	WEEK 1	WEEK 2	WEEK 3	WEEK 4	WEEK 5	WEEK 6
1	Endurance cardio	Endurance cardio	Endurance cardio	Endurance cardio	Interval cardio	Interval cardio
2	Circuit or gym resistance	Circuit or gym resistance	Circuit or gym resistance	Circuit or gym resistance	Circuit or gym resistance	Circuit or gym resistance
3	Endurance cardio	Endurance cardio	Interval cardio	Interval cardio	Endurance cardio	Endurance cardio
4	Circuit	Circuit	Circuit	Circuit	Circuit	Circuit
5	Endurance cardio	Endurance cardio	Endurance cardio	Endurance cardio	Interval cardio	Interval cardio
6	Circuit or gym resistance	Circuit or gym resistance	Circuit or gym resistance	Circuit or gym resistance	Circuit or gym resistance	Circuit or gym resistance
7	Rest	Rest	Rest	Rest	Rest	Rest

PROGRAM 1 – SIX-WEEK SUMMARY: INTERMEDIATE

DAY	WEEK 1	WEEK 2	WEEK 3	WEEK 4	WEEK 5	WEEK 6
1	Endurance cardio	Endurance cardio	Endurance cardio	Interval cardio	Interval cardio	Interval cardio
2	Circuit or gym resistance	Circuit or gym resistance	Circuit or gym resistance	Circuit or gym resistance	Circuit or gym resistance	Circuit or gym resistance
3	Endurance cardio	Endurance cardio	Interval cardio	Endurance cardio	Endurance cardio	Endurance cardio
4	Circuit	Circuit	Circuit	Circuit	Circuit	Circuit
5	Endurance cardio	Endurance cardio	Endurance cardio	Interval cardio	Interval cardio	Interval cardio
6	Circuit or gym resistance	Circuit or gym resistance	Circuit or gym resistance	Circuit or gym resistance	Circuit or gym resistance	Circuit or gym resistance
7	*Rest*	*Rest*	*Rest*	*Rest*	*Rest*	*Rest*

PROGRAM 1 – SIX-WEEK SUMMARY: ADVANCED

DAY	WEEK 1	WEEK 2	WEEK 3	WEEK 4	WEEK 5	WEEK 6
1	Endurance cardio	Endurance cardio	Endurance cardio	Interval cardio	Interval cardio	Interval cardio
2	Circuit or gym resistance	Circuit or gym resistance	Circuit or gym resistance	Circuit or gym resistance	Circuit or gym resistance	Circuit or gym resistance
3	Endurance cardio	Interval cardio	Interval cardio	Endurance cardio	Endurance cardio	Endurance cardio
4	Circuit	Circuit	Circuit	Circuit	Circuit	Circuit
5	Endurance cardio	Endurance cardio	Endurance cardio	Interval cardio	Interval cardio	Interval cardio
6	Circuit or gym resistance	Circuit or gym resistance	Circuit or gym resistance	Circuit or gym resistance	Circuit or gym resistance	Circuit or gym resistance
7	*Rest*	*Rest*	*Rest*	*Rest*	*Rest*	*Rest*

WARM UP AND COOL DOWN

As with the KickStart Plan, begin each session with a 5-minute warm-up: start walking at a normal pace, gradually increase your speed and start to swing your arms as you walk so that your heart-rate begins to rise and you are puffing. Cool down after each session by spending 5–10 minutes doing the stretches on pages 130–133. When you're doing your cardio training, slow down the intensity so that your heart-rate returns to normal, then do the stretches.

PROGRAM 1 CARDIO TRAINING

Your body taps into different energy systems depending on the type of exercise you do. For example, your body burns fuel differently for a quick burst of energy such as a sprint, which can only be maintained for a few minutes, than it does for a steady paced 10-kilometre run. To maximise your fat-burning potential and to effectively increase your fitness levels, vary the exercise types and intensities you do. In your Biggest Loser cardio workout, you'll do both endurance and interval cardio. They are described on the following pages, with your weekly Program 1 Cardio Workout.

Endurance cardio

Endurance cardio refers to a steady, continuous state of exercising. Your heart-rate is reasonably elevated, to level 7 or 8, and you can maintain a consistent speed for around 30–40 minutes at a time. Choose your endurance cardio session time based on the exercising levels below. This is the time your endurance cardio session will run for in Program 1.

YOUR ENDURANCE CARDIO LEVEL

BEGINNER	INTERMEDIATE	ADVANCED
Endurance cardio 25–35 min Work at a steady rate throughout, maintaining an intensity level of around 7 or 8.	**Endurance cardio** 35–45 min Work at a steady rate throughout, maintaining an intensity level of around 7 or 8.	**Endurance cardio** 45–55 min Work at a steady rate throughout, maintaining an intensity level of around 7 or 8.

Interval cardio

Interval cardio refers to shorter bursts (intervals) of more intense exercising, interspersed with more moderate cardio. Your heart-rate will rise to level 8 or 9 for a couple of minutes as you speed up or add in a hill, and then you return to endurance cardio with your intensity at level 7 for 10 minutes, then you add the interval intensity again. This challenges your body, burns fat and increases your cardiovascular capacity. Try interval training by jogging, running or sprinting the distance between electricity poles. See if you can build up to jogging one span then sprinting two or three spans before jogging one again. Always use a watch or timer when performing intervals; if you just try to guess the time, you'll pull up early. Remember, be disciplined and stick exactly to the pre-set interval periods, even when it gets really tough. Stay focused, dig deep and completely finish each one. Choose your interval cardio session times based on the exercising levels below and note the breakdown of the time by intensity level.

YOUR INTERVAL CARDIO LEVEL

BEGINNER	INTERMEDIATE	ADVANCED
Interval cardio 20–30 min/session. Keep a steady rate of cardio for 8 minutes, then add intensity by including a hill or moving faster for 2 minutes. Return to a steady lower intensity.	Interval cardio 25–35 min/session. Keep a steady rate, then every 8–10 minutes increase the intensity by including a hill or moving faster for 2 minutes. Return to a steady lower intensity.	Interval cardio 35–45 min/session. Keep a steady rate, then every 8–10 minutes increase the intensity by including a hill or moving faster for 4 minutes. Return to a steady lower intensity.
Warm-up 7–8 min, level 7 2 min, level 9 6 min, level 7 2 min, level 9 5 min, level 7 2 min, level 9 Cool-down	Warm-up 7 min, level 7 2 min, level 9 6 min, level 7 2 min, level 9 5 min, level 7 3 min, level 9 3 min, level 8 1 min, level 9.5 Cool-down	Warm-up 7 min, level 7 3 min, level 9 7 min, level 7 3 min, level 9 6 min, level 7 4 min, level 9 5 min, level 7 3 min, level 9 1 min, level 9.5 Cool-down

Cardio training overview

The table below shows you how long your three weekly cardio sessions should be, based on your exercise level, and how many of those will be endurance and interval cardio.

CARDIO: SIX-WEEK SUMMARY

WEEK	BEGINNER	INTERMEDIATE	ADVANCED
1	Endurance cardio x 3 20–30 min/session Keep a steady rate throughout.	Endurance cardio x 3 30–40 min/session Keep a steady rate throughout.	Endurance cardio x 3 40–50 min/session Keep a steady rate throughout.
2	Endurance cardio x 3 30–40 min/session Keep a steady rate throughout.	Endurance cardio x 3 40–50 min/session	Endurance cardio x 2 Interval cardio x 1 45–55 min/session
3	Endurance cardio x 2 Interval cardio x 1 30–40 min/session	Endurance cardio x 2 Interval cardio x 1 40–50 min/session	Endurance cardio x 2 Interval cardio x 1 50–55 min/session
4	Endurance cardio x 2 Interval cardio x 1 30–40 min/session	Endurance cardio x 1 Interval cardio x 2 40–50 min/session	Endurance cardio x 1 Interval cardio x 2 45–55 min/session
5	Endurance cardio x 1 Interval cardio x 2 40–50 min/session	Endurance cardio x 1 Interval cardio x 2 45–55 min/session	Endurance cardio x 1 Interval cardio x 2 50–55 min/session
6	Endurance cardio x 1 Interval cardio x 2 45–55 min/session	Endurance cardio x 1 Interval cardio x 2 45–55 min/session	Endurance cardio x 1 Interval cardio x 2 50–55 min/session

'Now that I've lost weight, I have so much more energy, a real zest for life. I feel absolutely amazing compared with how I used to feel. These days I often wear a Superman t-shirt, because that's how I feel – I know that if I set my mind to it, I can achieve anything.'

Shane Giles, Series One

PROGRAM 1 RESISTANCE TRAINING

The Biggest Loser Exercise Plan includes resistance training – using this in your workouts will really make the difference with your weight-loss and muscle tone. In resistance training, your body has to push against a load, forcing your muscles to work harder and therefore become stronger. The load can be weights or your own body weight – for example, push-ups are hard because you are trying to push your full weight upwards. Whereas cardio training burns fat and improves your cardiovascular health, resistance training raises your metabolic rate, builds lean muscle tissue, and strengthens and tones your muscles. The increased activity of your muscles rebuilding and repairing after resistance training will keep your body's fat-burning rate up all day (even while you're asleep, your body will burn fat at an accelerated rate as a result of weight training). This enhances the fat-burning results from your cardio workouts. Together, resistance and cardio training are the real weight-loss deal!

The key to performing resistance training is to think about moving and working the muscle you are targeting rather than focusing on the weight itself. Technique is absolutely vital – perform an exercise incorrectly and, at best, you will not be appropriately training the target muscles you are aiming for. At worst, you could injure yourself. Concentration is everything in resistance training. It's not a time for chat – focus on the muscle and feel its movement as you perform each perfect rep.

Your resistance training will be done in a circuit, meaning you'll move through a series of exercises involving high repetitions (reps), each targeting a different body part or muscle group, with minimal rest between exercises. The exercise sequence allows each muscle group time to recover while you are working another muscle area. Once you've completed the full circuit, take a brief rest before beginning the second round. Circuit training not only improves your fat-burning ability, it also introduces you to the use of resistance (in this case, your own body weight).

Choose from the following three programs based on your exercise level – beginner, intermediate or advanced. The programs show the intensity you should work at, the exercise sequence, the number of repetitions you need to perform for each exercise, the rest you should have between each exercise type, and the number of times you should perform the complete circuit (these change depending on which level you're working at and which week it is). Take your time to study the program so you really understand what you need to do. It might look a little overwhelming or strange at first, but it's worth following – this program has been created for optimum weight-loss and muscle tone.

Before beginning your program, read the description of each exercise and look at the photographs (see page 130 onwards), so you fully understand what each exercise is and how it should be performed correctly.

Equipment needed

There are three exercises in the Biggest Loser circuit training that require a resistance band. If you don't have one, you can skip these exercises or use light hand-weights for two of them (not the upper back row), but it's a good idea to buy a resistance band. A great tool for doing resistance training at home or outside, it's a length of stretchy rubber tube with handles on the end. You can buy one for about $15 from most sports shops.

RESISTANCE CIRCUIT: BEGINNER

	WEEK 1	WEEK 2	WEEK 3	WEEK 4	WEEK 5	WEEK 6
INTENSITY						
EXERCISE	REPS	REPS	REPS	REPS	REPS	REPS
Bodyweight squats	12–15	15–18	16–20	12–15	15–18	16–20
Push-ups on knees	12–15	15–18	16–20	12–15	15–18	16–20
Upper back row	12–15	15–18	16–20	12–15	15–18	16–20
Static lunges	12–15	15–18	16–20	12–15	15–18	16–20
Shuttle runs	1 min	2 min	3 min	1 min	2 min	3 min
Bench dips	12–15	15–18	16–20	12–15	15–18	16–20
Bicep curls	12–15	15–18	16–20	12–15	15–18	16–20
Calf raises	12–15	15–18	16–20	12–15	15–18	16–20
Shoulder presses	12–15	15–18	16–20	12–15	15–18	16–20
Ricochets	12–15	15–18	16–20	12–15	15–18	16–20
Crunches	12–15	15–18	16–20	12–15	15–18	16–20
Rest between stations	60 sec	60 sec	60 sec	45 sec	45 sec	30 sec
Rest between circuits	3 min	3 min	3 min	3 min	3 min	3 min
No. of circuits	2	2	2	2	3	3

RESISTANCE CIRCUIT: INTERMEDIATE

	WEEK 1	WEEK 2	WEEK 3	WEEK 4	WEEK 5	WEEK 6
INTENSITY						
EXERCISE	REPS	REPS	REPS	REPS	REPS	REPS
Bodyweight squats	15–18	16–20	20–25	15–18	16–20	20–25
Push-ups on knees or toes	15–18	16–20	20–25	15–18	16–20	20–25
Upper back row	15–18	16–20	20–25	15–18	16–20	20–25
Static lunges	15–18	16–20	20–25	15–18	16–20	20–25
Shuttle runs	1 min	2 min	3 min	1 min	2 min	3 min
Bench dips	15–18	16–20	20–25	15–18	16–20	20–25
Bicep curls	15–18	16–20	20–25	15–18	16–20	20–25
Calf raises	15–18	16–20	20–25	15–18	16–20	20–25
Shoulder presses	15–18	16–20	20–25	15–18	16–20	20–25
Ricochets	15–18	16–20	20–25	15–18	16–20	20–25
Crunches	15–18	16–20	20–25	15–18	16–20	20–25
Rest between exercises	60 sec	60 sec	45 sec	45 sec	30 sec	30 sec
Rest between circuits	3 min	3 min	3 min	3 min	3 min	3 min
No. of circuits	2	2	2	2	3	3

RESISTANCE CIRCUIT: ADVANCED

EXERCISE	WEEK 1 REPS	WEEK 2 REPS	WEEK 3 REPS	WEEK 4 REPS	WEEK 5 REPS	WEEK 6 REPS
Bodyweight squats	15–20	20–25	25–30	15–20	20–25	25–30
Push-ups on toes until you need to move to knees	15–20	20–25	25–30	15–20	20–25	25–30
Upper back row	15–20	20–25	25–30	15–20	20–25	25–30
Static lunges	15–20	20–25	25–30	15–20	20–25	25–30
Shuttle runs	2 min	3 min	4 min	2 min	3 min	4 min
Bench dips	15–20	20–25	25–30	15–20	20–25	25–30
Bicep curls	15–20	20–25	25–30	15–20	20–25	25–30
Calf raises	15–20	20–25	25–30	15–20	20–25	25–30
Shoulder presses	15–20	20–25	25–30	15–20	20–25	25–30
Ricochets	15–20	20–25	25–30	15–20	20–25	25–30
Crunches	15–20	20–25	25–30	15–20	20–25	25–30
Rest between exercises	60 sec	60 sec	45 sec	45 sec	30 sec	25 sec
Rest between circuits	3 min	3 min	3 min	3 min	3 min	3 min
No. of circuits	2	2	2	2	3	3

OPTIONAL PROGRAM 1
GYM-BASED RESISTANCE TRAINING

If you belong to a gym and want an incredibly effective resistance-training program, replace your resistance circuit sessions with this twice a week on days 2 and 6 (stick with the resistance circuit on day 4). Photocopy the program below and take it with you to the gym. It's suitable for beginners and more advanced exercisers, but you should be guided by a trainer until you are competent and confident with the technique. It's a great way to start resistance training and, before you know it, you'll be comfortable using the machines and you'll be noticing great changes in your body and strength.

This program isn't a circuit, so just perform the complete sequence once. Make sure you warm up with 5 minutes of cardio before you start and do the cool-down stretches on pages 130–133 once you've finished your session.

Weeks 1 and 2

Perform four sets of each exercise – 12 reps first set, 10 second set, then 8, then 6. Rest for 30 seconds between each set and 60 seconds between each exercise. Choose a weight that is heavy enough so you can just finish each set. The weight should increase slightly for each set. Ask a trainer to check your form and ensure each rep is performed perfectly.

Weeks 3 to 6

Perform four sets of each exercise – 12 reps first set, 10 second set, then 8, then 6. Rest for 30 seconds between each set and 60 seconds between each exercise. Choose a weight that is heavy enough so you can just finish each set. After your fourth set, rest for 30 seconds, return the weight to your 10 or 8 rep weight and then do 1 full-on set to muscle failure (approximately 12–15 reps). Then rest for 60 seconds and move to your next exercise.

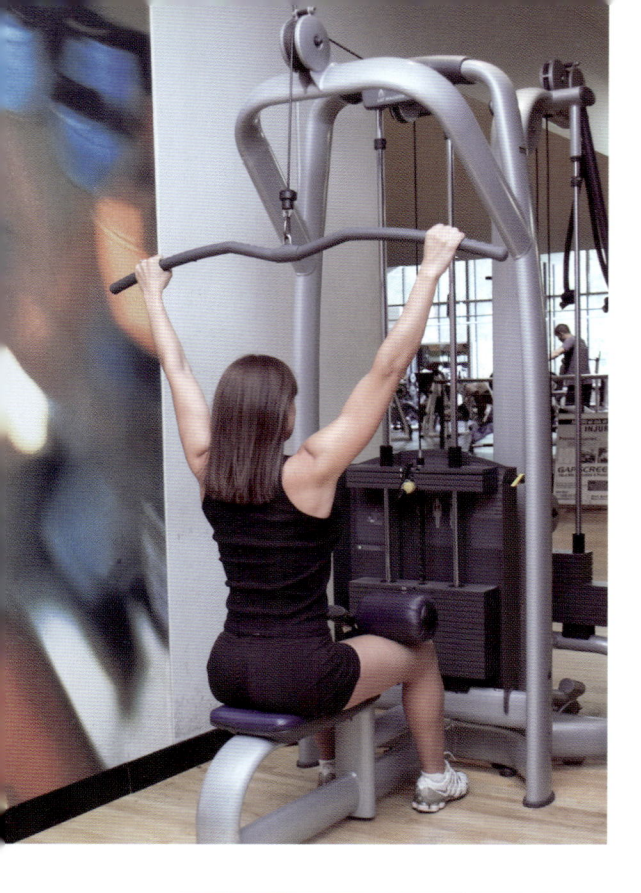

GYM TRAINING

EXCERCISE	REPS
Machine chest press	12, 10, 8, 6
Lat pull-down	12, 10, 8, 6
Machine shoulder press	12, 10, 8, 6
Leg press	12, 10, 8, 6
Lying leg curl	12, 10, 8, 6
Bicep curl	12, 10, 8, 6
Lying bar extension	12, 10, 8, 6
Rest between exercises	60 sec

Exercise – Program 2

By now you are feeling and looking great – and after two weeks on the KickStart Plan and six-weeks on Program 1 you're now ready for Program 2. You'll have improved your fitness and may now even consider joining a gym. Working out at a gym isn't essential, but it will push your fitness to the next level where you'll see amazing results. For example, the cardio machines such as the treadmill, cross trainer and bike all have pre-set interval programs so you simply pick your level and go for it.

Program 2 has a new weekly plan for your cardio and resistance workouts. It uses the same gym resistance training workout as in Program 1, so if you've been including it in your training, keep going but increase the weights for all exercises and do the workout three times a week rather than two. If you didn't do the gym resistance training in Program 1 but would like to begin now, see the previous page for the details. If you're sticking with the resistance circuit, you'll still be challenged – there's a whole new higher intensity resistance circuit and you're ready for it!

PROGRAM 2 – SIX-WEEK SUMMARY: BEGINNER

DAY	WEEK 1	WEEK 2	WEEK 3	WEEK 4	WEEK 5	WEEK 6
1	Circuit or gym resistance	gym resistance	Endurance cardio	Endurance cardio	Circuit or gym resistance	Endurance cardio
2	Endurance cardio	Interval cardio	Circuit or gym resistance	Endurance cardio	Interval cardio	Circuit or gym resistance
3	Circuit or gym resistance	Circuit or gym resistance	Interval cardio	Circuit or gym resistance	Circuit or gym resistance	Interval cardio
4	Interval cardio	Endurance cardio	Circuit or gym resistance	Interval cardio	Endurance cardio	Circuit or gym resistance
5	Circuit or gym resistance	Circuit or gym resistance	Endurance cardio	Circuit or gym resistance	Circuit or gym resistance	Endurance cardio
6	Endurance cardio	Interval cardio	Circuit or gym resistance	Endurance cardio	Interval cardio	Circuit or gym resistance
7	Rest	Rest	Rest	Rest	Rest	Rest

PROGRAM 2 – SIX-WEEK SUMMARY: INTERMEDIATE

DAY	WEEK 1	WEEK 2	WEEK 3	WEEK 4	WEEK 5	WEEK 6
1	Circuit or gym resistance	Endurance cardio	Endurance cardio	Circuit or gym resistance	Endurance cardio	Endurance cardio
2	Endurance cardio	Interval cardio	Circuit or gym resistance	Endurance cardio	Interval cardio	Circuit or gym resistance
3	Circuit or gym resistance	Circuit or gym resistance	Interval cardio	Circuit or gym resistance	Circuit or gym resistance	Interval cardio
4	Interval cardio	Endurance cardio	Circuit or gym resistance	Interval cardio	Endurance cardio	Circuit or gym resistance
5	Circuit or gym resistance	Circuit or gym resistance	Endurance cardio	Circuit or gym resistance	Circuit or gym resistance	Endurance cardio
6	Endurance cardio	Interval cardio	Circuit or gym resistance	Endurance cardio	Interval cardio	Circuit or gym resistance
7	Rest	Rest	Rest	Rest	Rest	Rest

As with Program 1, read through all the programs first and personalise the program in your training diary. Read the descriptions of the new exercises (see pages 134–145) so you feel comfortable performing them. The table below shows you the overall plan for the six-weeks of Program 2 – and you'll see it's been mixed up a little from Program 1, just to keep things interesting. Check which days you'll be doing cardio training (and whether it will be interval or endurance cardio) and which days you'll be doing resistance training. Feel free to mix things up – there are options and, as long as you maintain balance and allow your body time to recover between similar sessions, you can swap an interval workout for an additional circuit. Enjoy!

WARM UP AND COOL DOWN

As with the KickStart Plan and Program 1, it's essential to begin each session with a 5-minute warm-up: start walking at a normal pace, gradually increase your speed and start to swing your arms as you walk so that your heart-rate begins to rise and you are puffing. Cool down after each session by spending 5–10 minutes doing the stretches on pages 130–133. When you're doing your cardio training, slow down the intensity so that your heart-rate returns to normal, then do the stretches.

PROGRAM 2 – SIX-WEEK SUMMARY: ADVANCED

DAY	WEEK 1	WEEK 2	WEEK 3	WEEK 4	WEEK 5	WEEK 6
1	Circuit or gym resistance	Endurance cardio	Endurance cardio	Circuit or gym resistance	Endurance cardio	Endurance cardio
2	Interval cardio	Interval cardio	Circuit or gym resistance	Interval cardio	Interval cardio	Circuit or gym resistance
3	Circuit or gym resistance	Circuit or gym resistance	Interval cardio	Circuit or gym resistance	Circuit or gym resistance	Interval cardio
4	Endurance cardio	Endurance cardio	Circuit or gym resistance	Endurance cardio	Endurance cardio	Circuit or gym resistance
5	Circuit or gym resistance	Circuit or gym resistance	Endurance cardio	Circuit or gym resistance	Circuit or gym resistance	Endurance cardio
6	Interval cardio	Interval cardio	Circuit or gym resistance	Interval cardio	Interval cardio	Circuit or gym resistance
7	Rest	Rest	Rest	Rest	Rest	Rest

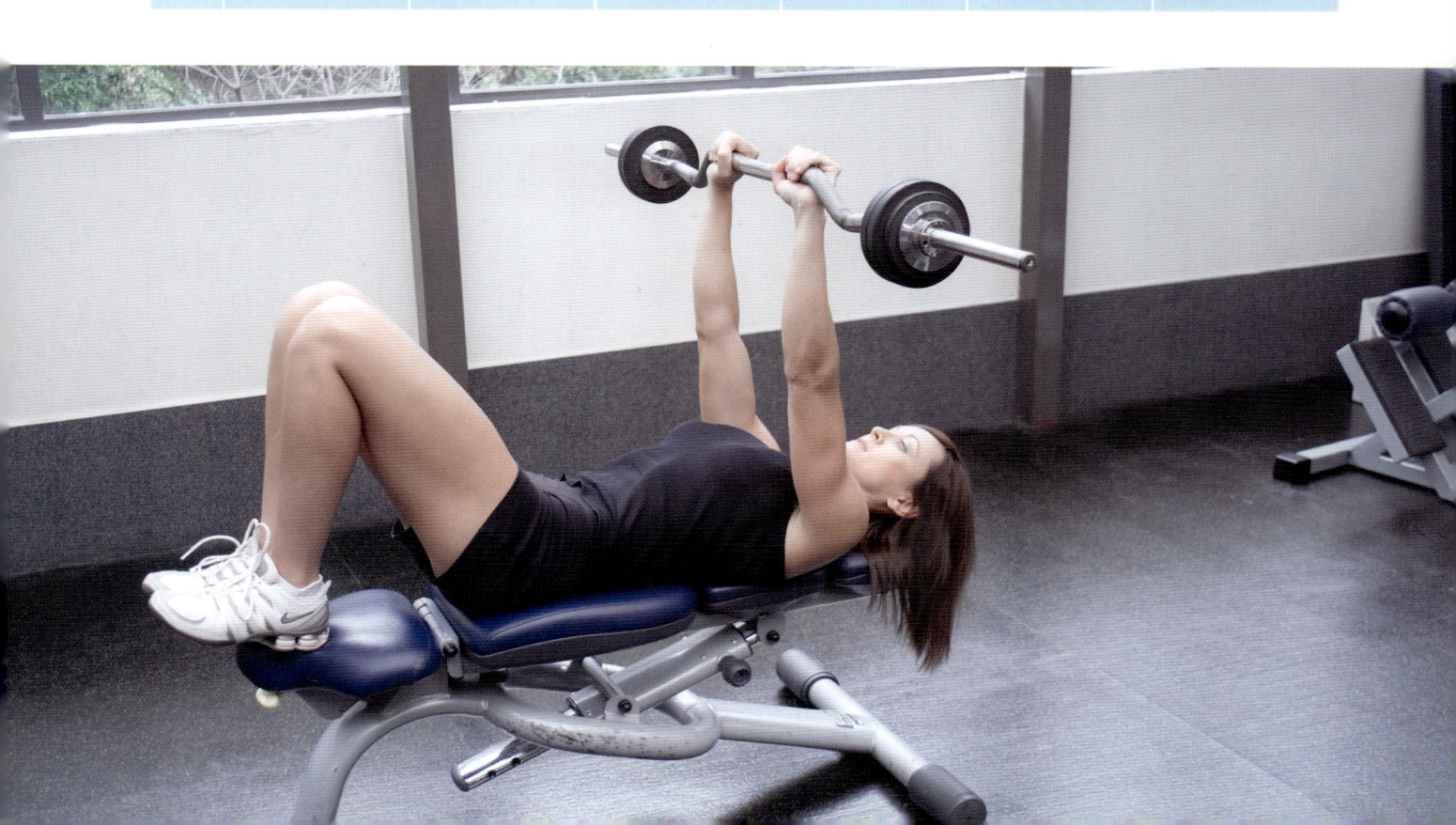

PROGRAM 2 CARDIO TRAINING

In Program 2, the endurance cardio time/levels remain the same. If you've been exercising at the beginner level, now is a good time to move up to the intermediate level (see page 111 in Program 1 for the endurance cardio levels). The interval cardio levels have changed, so check the table below for your new timing pattern (see page 108 in Program 1 for the intensity levels).

Interval cardio

Choose your interval cardio session times based on the exercising levels below and note the breakdown of the time by intensity level.

YOUR INTERVAL CARDIO LEVEL

BEGINNER	INTERMEDIATE	ADVANCED
Interval cardio 30–40 min/session Steady rate of cardio for 7 minutes, then add intensity (up to a level 8 or 9) by including a hill or moving faster for 2–3 minutes. Return to a slightly slower steady intensity (level 7) then pick up the pace again. The time difference between intervals gradually reduces throughout the session.	Interval cardio 30–40 min/session Keep a steady rate, then every 6 or so minutes, increase the intensity (up to a level 8 or 9) by including a hill or moving faster for 2–3 minutes. Return to a slightly slower steady intensity (level 7) then pick up the pace again. The time difference between intervals gradually reduces throughout the session.	Interval cardio 35–45 min session Keep a steady rate, then every 5–6 minutes, increase the intensity (up to a level 8 or 9) by including a hill or moving faster for 2–3 minutes. Return to a slightly slower steady intensity (level 7) then pick up the pace again. The time difference between intervals gradually reduces throughout the session.
Warm-up 7 min, level 7 2 min, level 9 7 min, level 7 3 min, level 9 6 min, level 7 2 min, level 9 6 min, level 7 3 min, level 9 Cool-down	Warm-up 6 min, level 7 2 min, level 9 6 min, level 7 3 min, level 9 5 min, level 7 3 min, level 8 4 min, level 7 2 min, level 9 2 min, level 8 1 min, level 9.5 Cool-down	Warm-up 6 min, level 7 2 min, level 9 6 min, level 7 3 min, level 9 5 min, level 7 2 min, level 9 5 min, level 7 3 min, level 9 4 min, level 7 2 min, level 9 1 min, level 9.5 Cool-down

Cardio training overview

The table below shows you how long your three weekly cardio sessions should be, based on your exercise level, and how many of those will be endurance and interval cardio.

CARDIO: SIX-WEEK SUMMARY

WEEK	BEGINNER	INTERMEDIATE	ADVANCED
1	Endurance cardio x 2 Interval cardio x 1	Endurance cardio x 2 Interval cardio x 1	Endurance cardio x 1 Interval cardio x 2
2	Endurance cardio x 2 Interval cardio x 2	Endurance cardio x 2 Interval cardio x 2	Endurance cardio x 2 Interval cardio x 2
3	Endurance cardio x 2 Interval cardio x 1	Endurance cardio x 2 Interval cardio x 1	Endurance cardio x 2 Interval cardio x 1
4	Endurance cardio x 2 Interval cardio x 1	Endurance cardio x 2 Interval cardio x 1	Endurance cardio x 1 Interval cardio x 2
5	Endurance cardio x 2 Interval cardio x 2	Endurance cardio x 2 Interval cardio x 2	Endurance cardio x 2 Interval cardio x 2
6	Endurance cardio x 2 Interval cardio x 1	Endurance cardio x 2 Interval cardio x 1	Endurance cardio x 2 Interval cardio x 1

PROGRAM 2 RESISTANCE TRAINING

As with Program 1, choose from the following three programs based on your exercise level – beginner, intermediate or advanced. The programs show the intensity you should work at, the exercise sequence, the number of repetitions you need to perform for each exercise, the rest you should have between each exercise type, and the number of times you should perform the complete circuit (these change depending on which level you're working at and which week it is).

Before beginning your program, thoroughly read the descriptions of each exercise and look at the photographs (see pages 134–145), so you full understand what each exercise is and how it should be performed correctly.

RESISTANCE CIRCUIT: BEGINNER

EXERCISE	WEEK 1 REPS	WEEK 2 REPS	WEEK 3 REPS	WEEK 4 REPS	WEEK 5 REPS	WEEK 6 REPS
Step-ups	12–15	15–18	16–20	12–15	15–18	16–20
Push-ups on toes or knees	12–15	15–18	16–20	12–15	15–18	16–20
Walking lunges	12–15	15–18	16–20	12–15	15–18	16–20
Supermen	12–15	15–18	16–20	12–15	15–18	16–20
Shuttle runs	1 min	2 min	3 min	1 min	2 min	3 min
Bicep curls	12–15	15–18	16–20	12–15	15–18	16–20
Reverse crunches	12–15	15–18	16–20	12–15	15–18	16–20
Close-grip push-ups	12–15	15–18	16–20	12–15	15–18	16–20
Pulsing squats	12–15	15–18	16–20	12–15	15–18	16–20
Shoulder presses	12–15	15–18	16–20	12–15	15–18	16–20
Bicycle crunches	12–15	15–18	16–20	12–15	15–18	16–20
Rest between stations	1 min	45 sec	30 sec	45 sec	30 sec	20 sec
Rest between circuits	3 min	3 min	2 min	3 min	2 min	1 min, 30 sec
No. of circuits	2	2	2	2	3	3

RESISTANCE CIRCUIT: INTERMEDIATE

EXERCISE	WEEK 1 REPS	WEEK 2 REPS	WEEK 3 REPS	WEEK 4 REPS	WEEK 5 REPS	WEEK 6 REPS
Step-ups	15–18	16–20	20–25	15–18	16–20	20–25
Push-ups on toes	15–18	16–20	20–25	15–18	16–20	20–25
Walking lunges	15–18	16–20	20–25	15–18	16–20	20–25
Supermen	15–18	16–20	20–25	15–18	16–20	20–25
Shuttle runs	1 min	2 min	3 min	1 min	2 min	3 min
Bicep curls	15–18	16–20	20–25	15–18	16–20	20–25
Reverse crunches	15–18	16–20	20–25	15–18	16–20	20–25
Close-grip push-ups	15–18	16–20	20–25	15–18	16–20	20–25
Pulsing squats	15–18	16–20	20–25	15–18	16–20	20–25
Shoulder presses	15–18	16–20	20–25	15–18	16–20	20–25
Bicycle crunches	15–18	16–20	20–25	15–18	16–20	20–25
Rest between stations	45 sec	30 sec	20 sec	30 sec	20 sec	10 sec
Rest between circuits	2 min	2 min	1 min, 30 sec	2 min	1 min, 30 sec	1 min
No. of circuits	2	2	2	2	3	3

RESISTANCE CIRCUIT: ADVANCED

	WEEK 1	WEEK 2	WEEK 3	WEEK 4	WEEK 5	WEEK 6
INTENSITY						
EXERCISE	REPS	REPS	REPS	REPS	REPS	REPS
Step-ups	15–20	20–25	25–30	15–20	20–25	25–30
Normal or wide push-ups	15–20	20–25	25–30	15–20	20–25	25–30
Walking lunges	15–20	20–25	25–30	15–20	20–25	25–30
Supermen	15–20	20–25	25–30	15–20	20–25	25–30
Shuttle runs	2 min	3 min	4 min	2 min	3 min	4 min
Bicep curls	15–20	20–25	25–30	15–20	20–25	25–30
Reverse crunches	15–20	20–25	25–30	15–20	20–25	25–30
Close-grip push-ups	15–20	20–25	25–30	15–20	20–25	25–30
Pulsing squats	15–20	20–25	25–30	15–20	20–25	25–30
Shoulder presses	15–20	20–25	25–30	15–20	20–25	25–30
Bicycle crunches	15–20	20–25	25–30	15–20	20–25	25–30
Rest between stations	30 sec	20 sec	10 sec	20 sec	10 sec	no rest
Rest between circuits	1 min	1 min	1 min	45 sec	30 sec	20 sec
No. of circuits	2	2	2	2	3	3

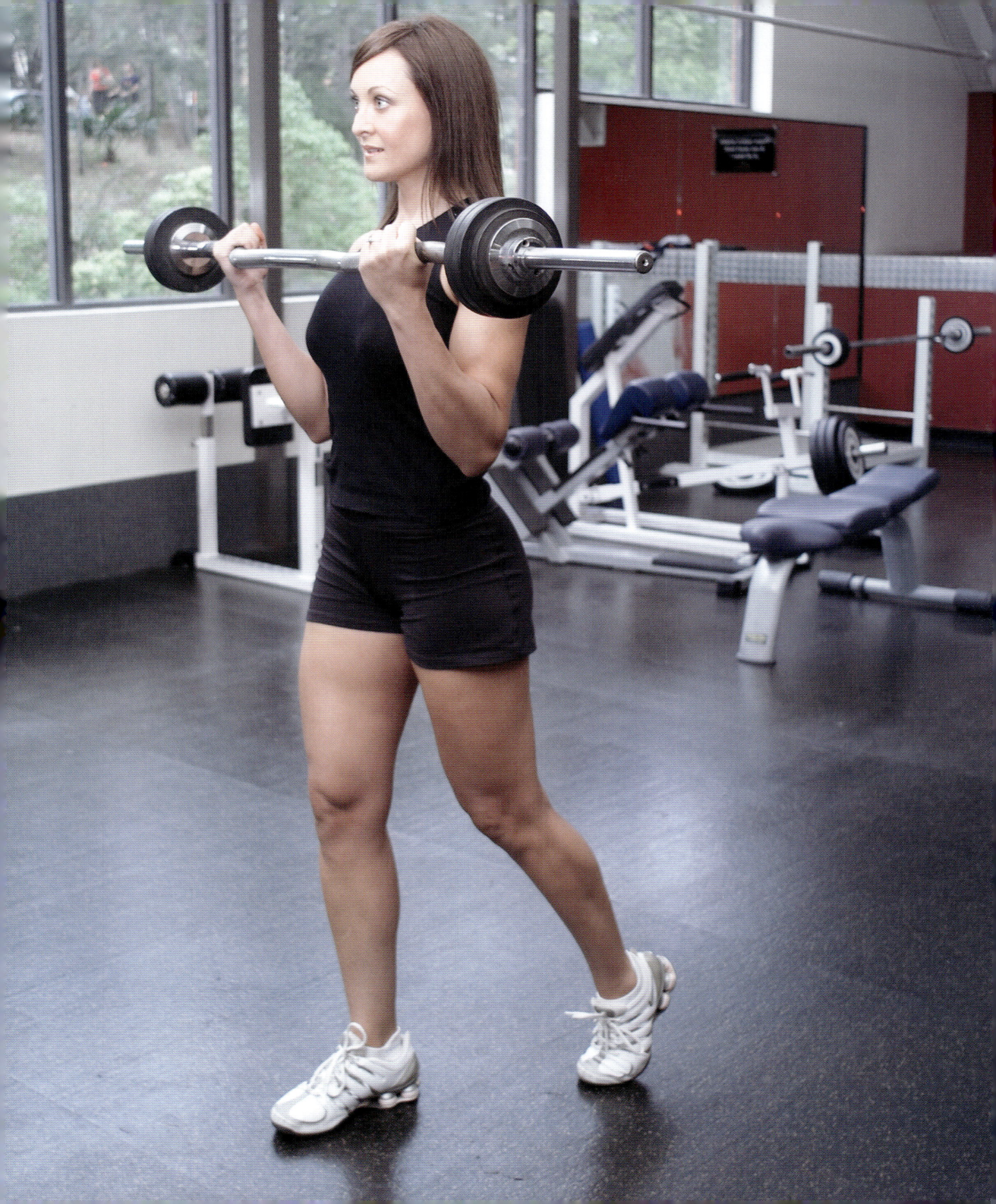

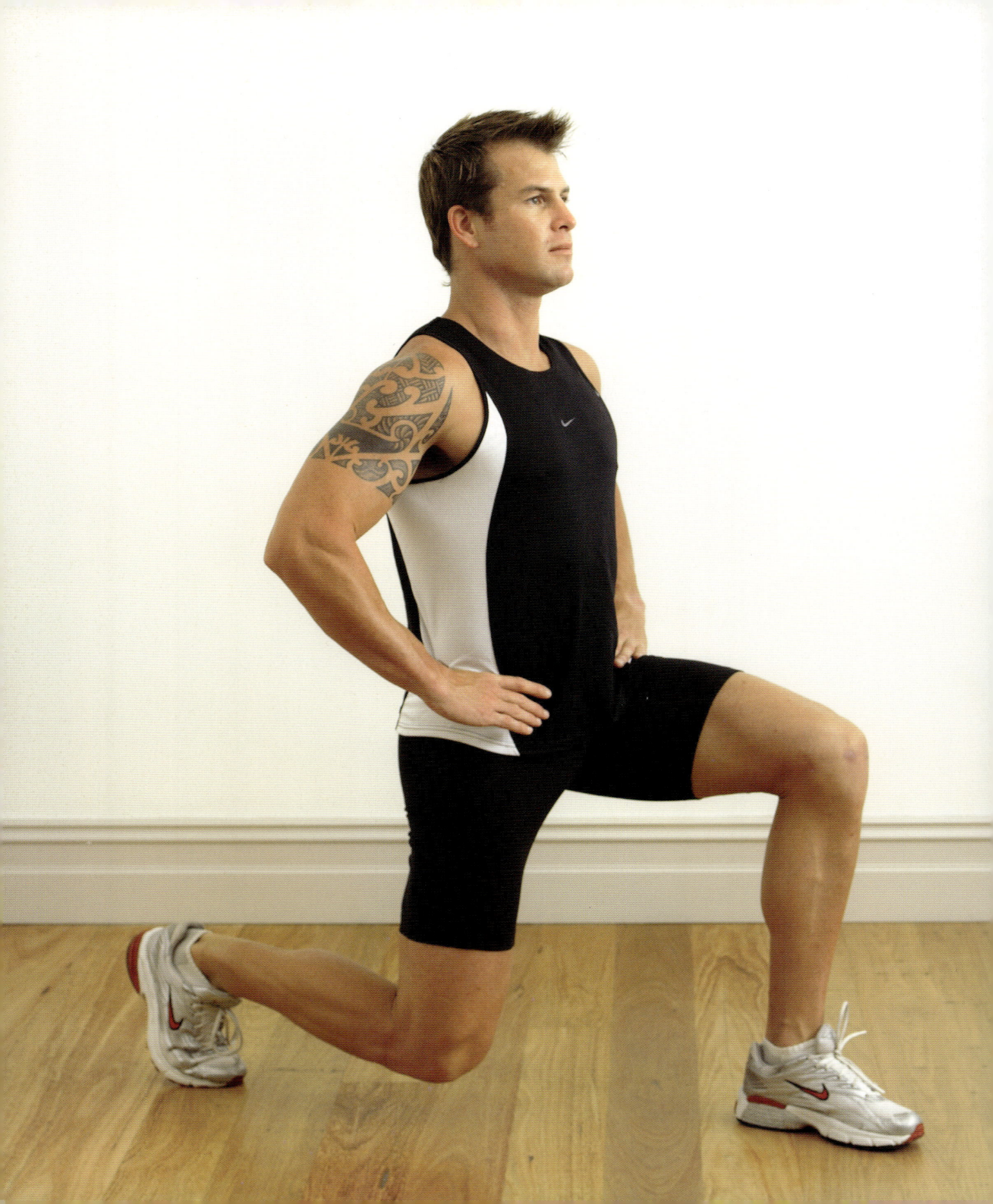

The Exercises

You've read through your programs, now learn how to do the exercises. The Australian Biggest Loser trainers Shannan Ponton and Michelle Bridges take you through all the stretches and exercises, showing you how to do them properly. Good form and correct technique are vital, so take your time with each exercise until you have it mastered.

Stretches

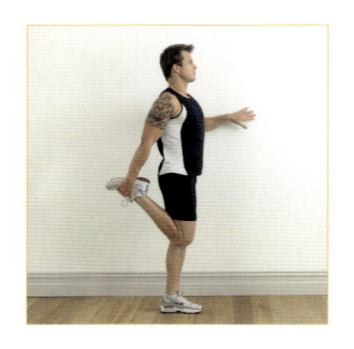

Quads
Hold on to a chair or wall to balance with your left hand and shift your weight onto your left foot. Lift your right foot behind into your right hand and gently draw it up and back to your backside until you feel a good stretch through the front of the thigh. Try to keep your knees together. Hold for 15–30 seconds, then change legs.

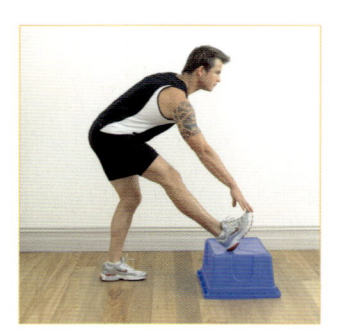

Hamstrings
Lift one heel up onto a step, tilt forwards pushing your hips backwards, gently drawing the toe of the foot towards you until you feel a good stretch through the back of the leg. Hold for 15–30 seconds, then change legs.

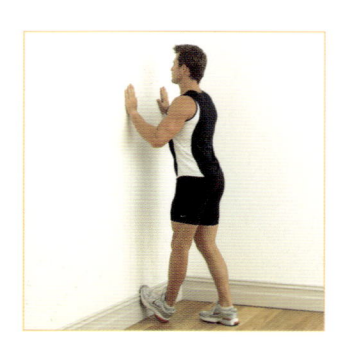

Calves
Face a wall and place the ball of your foot against the wall keeping the heel on the ground. Gently bring your weight forward so that your nose is to the wall. Try to keep the front leg straight or until you feel a decent stretch through the calf muscle. Hold for 15–30 seconds, then change legs.

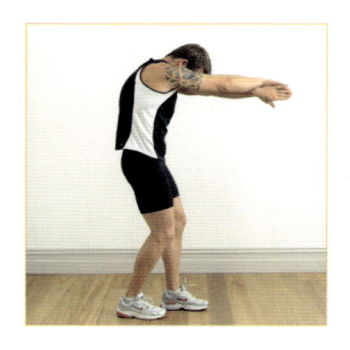

Upper back
Stand with your arms straight out in front of you with your thumbs pointing downwards. Cross your arms placing the palms together. Apply a little pressure between the hands and gently draw your arms forward, curling the upper back and dropping the head. Hold for 15–30 seconds.

Chest and shoulders

Link your hands behind your back, drop your shoulders and gently lift your hands up. Hold for 15–30 seconds.

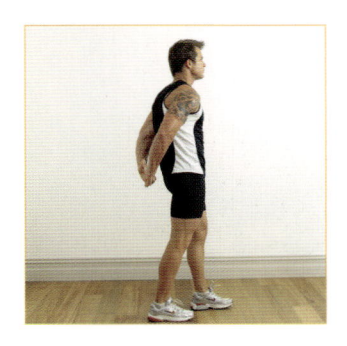

Hip flexor

Kneel on one knee with your front leg bent at 90 degrees. Gently shift your weight forward and place your hands behind your head. You should feel a stretch running vertically down the front of your hip, from your hip bone to the top of your thigh.

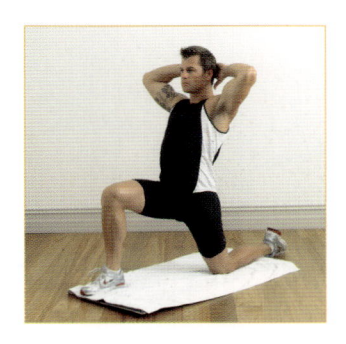

Triceps

Lift one arm directly above your head, bend the elbow taking the hand down towards your spine. Rest the other forearm on your head and take hold of the bent elbow gently drawing it back until you feel the stretch through the back of the arm. Change sides.

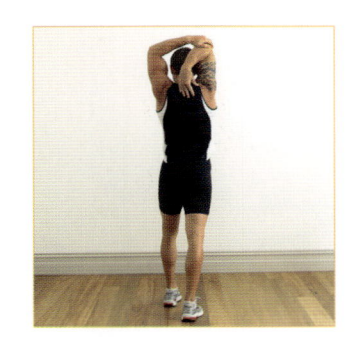

Biceps

Stand side-on and an arm's length away from a wall. Place the hand closest to the wall straight out to the side and slightly behind your body. Turn your fingers backwards pointing away from your body and push your hand flat against the wall. Gently turn your head away from the wall. Hold the stretch for 30 seconds and repeat on the other side.

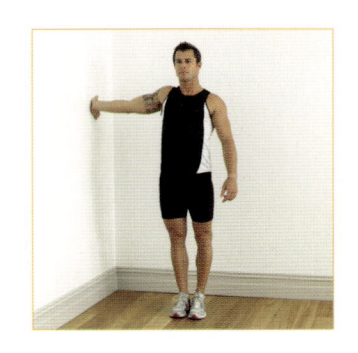

Glutes
Lie on your back and cross your right ankle over your left bent knee. Lift your left foot off the ground and take your hands around the front of, or under, your left knee. Draw the knee towards you, keeping your head and shoulders on the ground. Hold for 15–30 seconds and repeat on the other side.

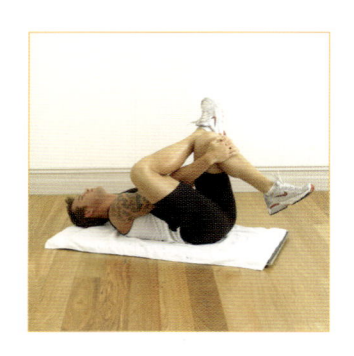

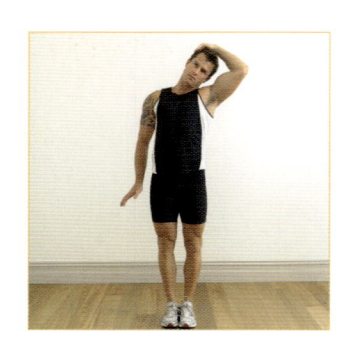

Neck
Place your hand on your head and gently tilt it towards one side without applying much pressure at all. Hold. Release your hand, take your head back to the neutral position and repeat on the other side. Finally, draw your chin into your chest and place both hands on your head, very gently applying a small amount of pressure. Hold for 15–30 seconds.

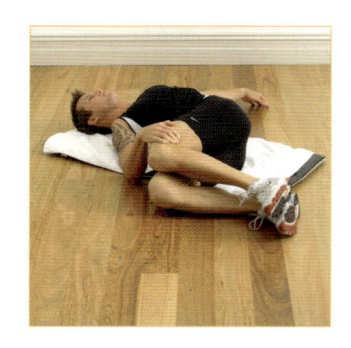

Lower back twist
Lie flat on your back with your arms straight out to your sides, palms facing down. Slide your feet up towards your backside, keeping them flat on the floor. Gently roll your legs across your body so that the bottom leg rests on the ground and your top knee sits directly on the bottom leg. To add some intensity to this stretch place your hand, on the side that your legs are positioned, on top of your top leg and gently pull towards the floor. Hold for 30 seconds and return to the start position before repeating on the other side.

Back stretch

Start in a kneeling position, on all fours. Gently lower your stomach towards the ground; at the same time gently raise your head and look towards the sky, being careful not to strain your neck. Hold this position for 10 seconds. Gently reverse the movement by pulling your stomach up and in, belly button to spine, making your back arch skyward as high as you can. At the same time lower your head and look towards the floor, pulling your chin as close as possible to your chest. Hold this position for 10 seconds. This sometimes called the cat stretch.

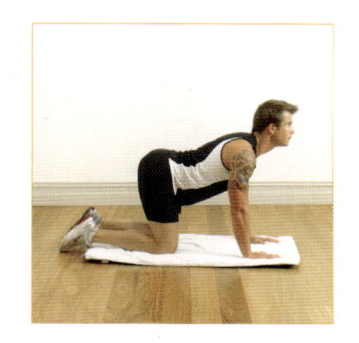

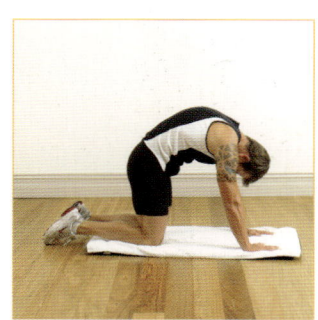

Advanced back stretch

Only do this stretch if your back is in good health. Standing up, bend over taking your hands behind your knees (keep your knees slightly bent). Hug your chest to your knees and gently arch your back upwards, relaxing the muscles along your spine all the way up to your neck. Hold for 15–30 seconds. Gently release, keeping your knees bent as you stand up.

Resistance circuit exercises

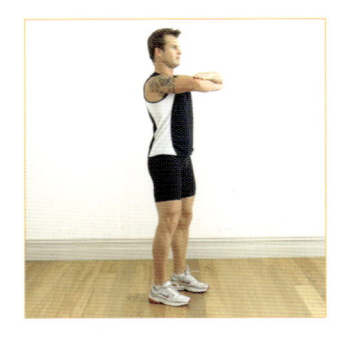

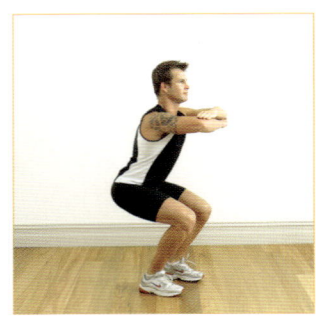

Bodyweight squat

This exercise targets your thighs, hips and backside. Stand with your feet hip-width apart and toes pointing forwards. Cross your hands over your chest lifting your elbows out in front. Brace your abdominals and, keeping your back straight, squat down until your thighs are roughly parallel to the floor. Push up through your heels as you rise.

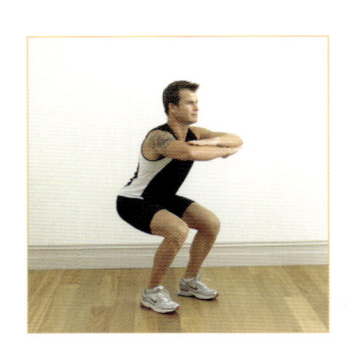

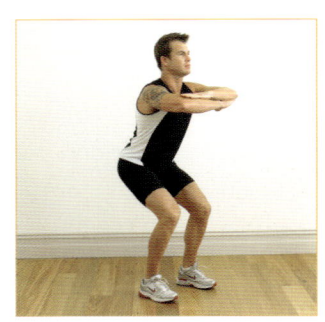

Pulsing squat

You can turn the squat intensity up a notch by holding the squat low and adding a small pulse at the bottom of the range. Squat down until your thighs are parallel to the floor and then try doing 10 small pulses, keeping your back straight and abdominals strong before you rise.

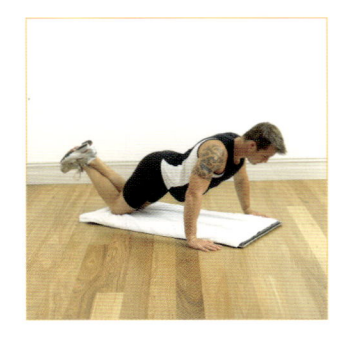

Push-up on knees

A great upper body strength-builder, this exercise works the chest and shoulders. Begin on your knees with your hands shoulder-width apart in front of you and your ankles crossed behind you. Bring your weight forward between your hands so that they are level with your chest. Brace your abdominals and keeping your back in its natural curve and your head up, lower your upper body almost to the ground. Push up through the heels of the hands to return to your starting position.

Push-up on toes

If you are exercising at the advanced level, increase the difficulty by performing your push-ups on your toes.

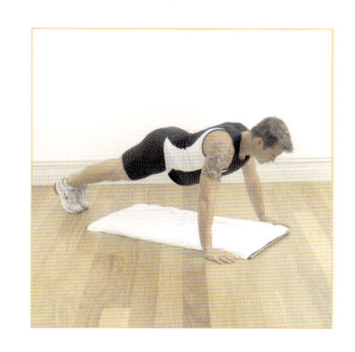

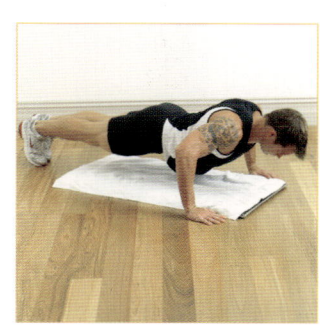

Close-grip push-up

An alternative to the push-up, this time focusing on the back of the upper arms – the triceps. Begin on your knees but place your hands just chest-width apart with your fingers pointing forwards. Draw your elbows towards each other and bring your weight forward so that your hands are directly beneath your chest. Keeping your back in its natural curve, head up and tummy tight, bend at the elbows bringing your chest close to the ground. As you push up ensure your elbows brush your ribs at the sides. Need an additional challenge? Take it to your toes!

Wide push-up

For an additional challenge with your push-ups, choose a wide push-up. You begin as you would a normal push-up except you move your hands further apart, at least another hand-span out from normal push-ups.

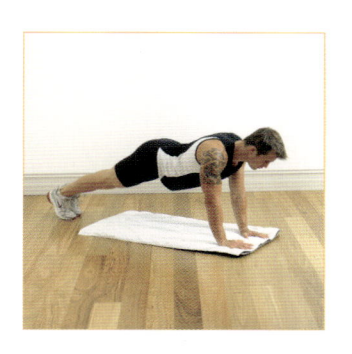

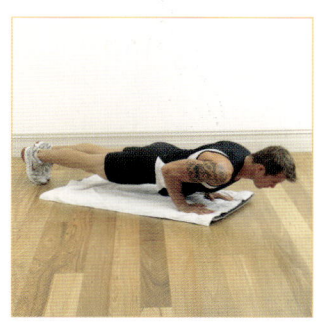

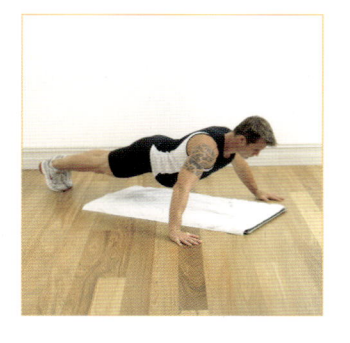

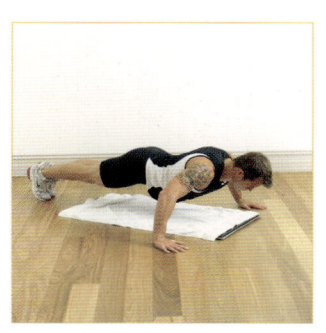

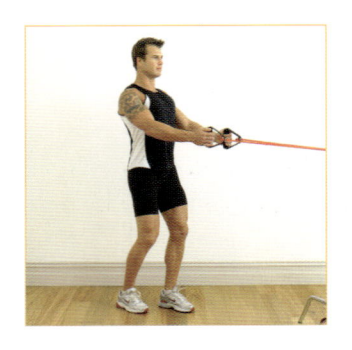

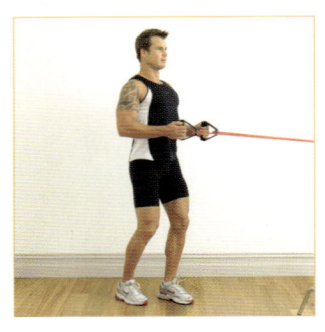

Upper back row

This exercise strengthens your back and biceps. You need a resistance band for this one. Wrap the band around a tree, signpost or seat. Grasp the two handles (vertically, with one in each hand), standing facing the band's anchor point. Starting with your arms extended, squeeze your elbows back in a rowing motion and try to bring your shoulder blades together. Hold for a second, then slowly release the contraction returning to the start position.

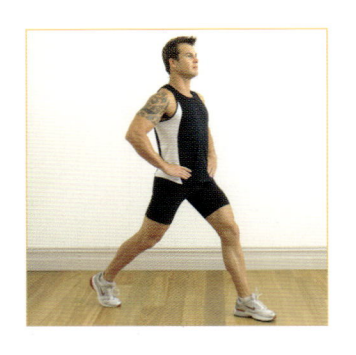

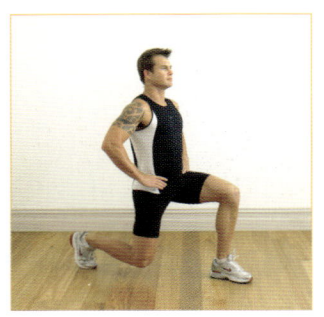

Static lunge

This is one of the best exercises for toning and strengthening your thighs and buttocks. Stand with feet hip-width apart as if each foot is on a train track. Take a long step forwards so that your front knee is behind your front toe (not beyond it) and the thigh is roughly parallel to the floor. Brace your abdominals, keeping your torso upright, bend the back knee down towards the floor. Push up off front heel to rise up and then drop the back knee again. Repeat the same leg for the number of required repetitions and then change legs.

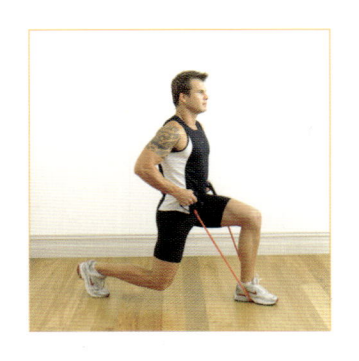

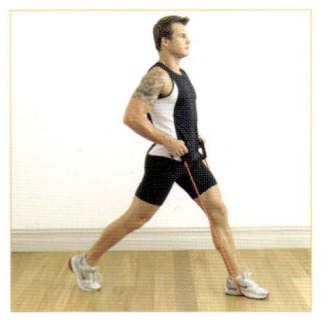

To take this exercise to the next level, try staying at the lowest part of the lunge with your back knee close to the floor and lifting only halfway back up. To increase the intensity, place the resistance band under your front foot and hold the handles at your hips or shoulders.

Walking lunge

This style of lunge requires a little more balance and coordination. Begin as you would for a static lunge with your feet hip-width apart and your hands on your hips. Take a long stride forwards, dropping the back knee down towards the floor. Push off the front heel and bring the back foot level with the front one. Lead off with the opposite foot, drop the other knee down and drive forwards. To increase the intensity, hold hand-weights by your sides.

Shuttle run

This is good to get your heart-rate up and test your agility and speed. Choose two points that are approximately 10 metres apart. Run back and forth between the two points, touching the ground for an added exertion.

Bench dips

Designed to target the triceps at the back of the upper arms, dips can be performed on a sturdy bench, step or chair. Sit upright on the edge of the bench, step or chair and place your hands hip-width apart, palms down, fingers pointing forward and gripping the edge. Walk your heels forward keeping your knees at 90 degrees and slide your bottom off the bench with elbows slightly bent. Lower your body by bending your elbows until they are at a 90-degree angle. Push up off your hands to return to start position.

For an intermediate version, walk your feet further out in front of you. Ensure you still keep your bottom close to the bench or chair as you perform the dips.

For the advanced version, rest your feet on another chair or bench in front of you, keeping your bottom close to the bench as you complete the exercise.

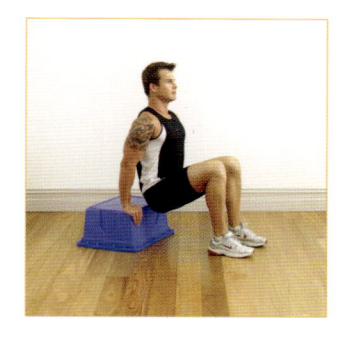

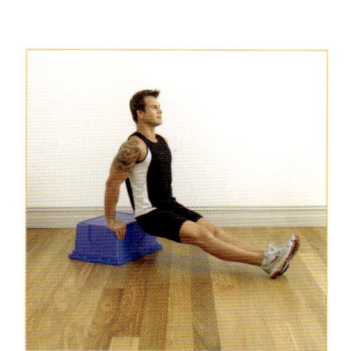

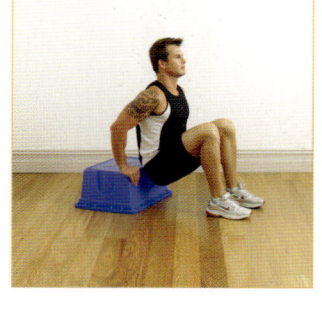

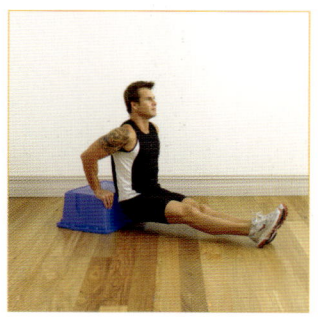

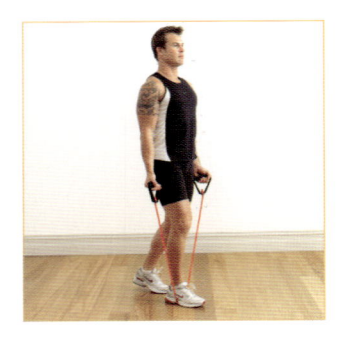

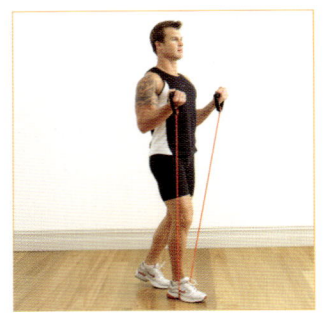

Resistance-band bicep curl

Stand on the band, keeping your elbows by (but not touching) your side. Slowly curl your hands towards your shoulders. The elbow joint should be the only joint moving. Once you reach the top, squeeze for a second then return to the start position.

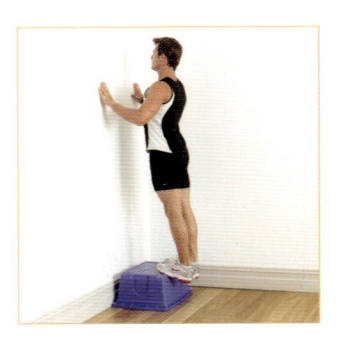

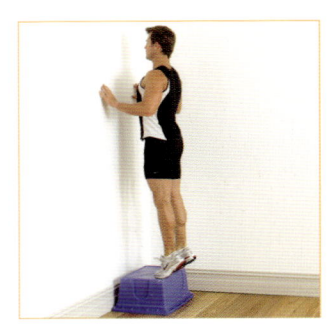

Calf raises

Often neglected, the calves have their own exercise right here. Stand on a step with your heels lowered, balancing on the balls of your feet. For added stability hold on to the wall or banister. Slowly lift your heels as high as you can until you feel a little pinch through the back of the calf muscle. Gently lower back to the starting position and repeat.

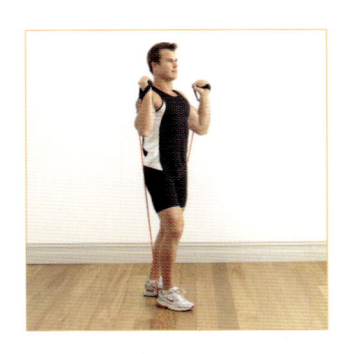

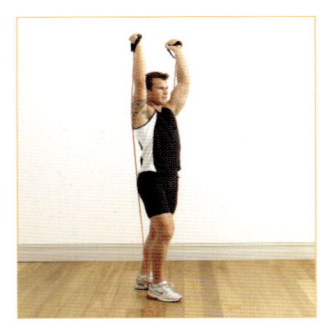

Resistance-band shoulder press

Stand on the band and keep your abdominals braced. Holding one handle in each hand, bring your hands up next to your shoulders, then press your hands straight up above your head so that your elbows are next to your ears. Hold for a second and return to start position at your shoulders.

Ricochets

This exercise will lift your heart-rate and test your agility. Because it can be hard on weak joints and shins, only do this exercise if you are working at the intermediate or advanced level. Stand with your feet together and arms by your sides. Keeping your feet together, jump forward 30 centimetres or so. Jump back to the starting position. Jump to your left, back to the start, then to the right, back to the start, and then behind you. Repeat this sequence, keeping your ground contact time minimal and your feet together.

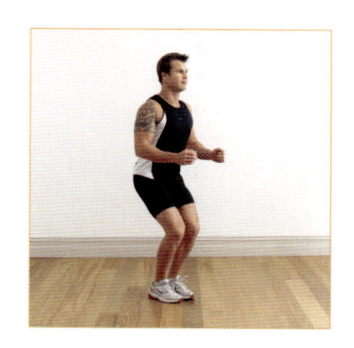

Standard crunch

Lie on your back with your knees bent and feet flat on the ground pulled towards your buttocks. Place your hands on your thighs and gently slide your hands up towards your knees. Don't pull with your neck. Concentrate on curling your chest towards your hips, not sitting straight up.

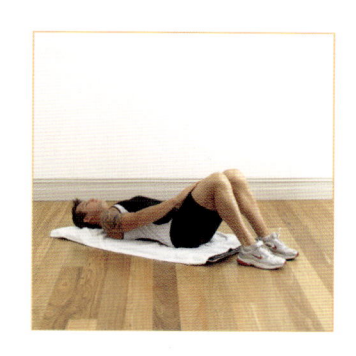

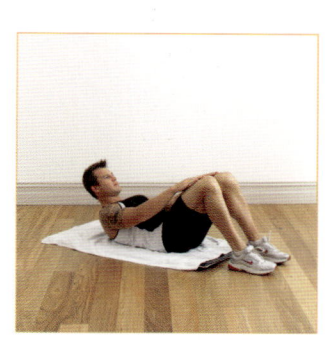

Oblique crunch

Lying on your back, place your left hand behind your head and your right hand at 45 degrees down from your shoulder flat on the ground. Crunch the left side of your torso, diagonally across your body, bringing your left shoulder off the ground and heading towards your right hip. Squeeze at the top and return to start position. Repeat on the other side.

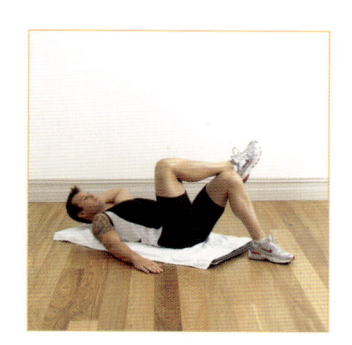

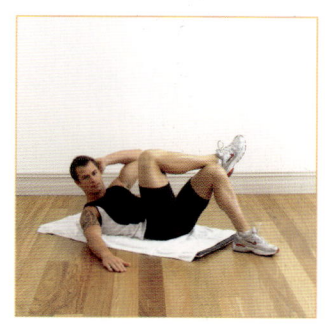

Bicycle crunch

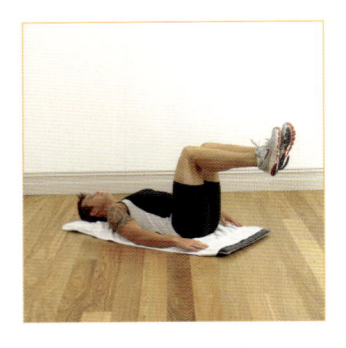

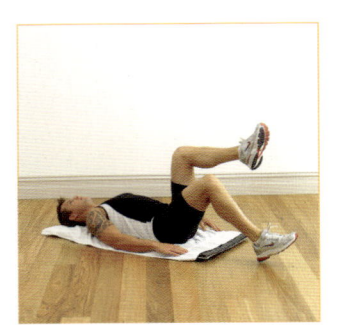

The bicycle crunch works all your abdominal muscles and it's no ride in the park. Lie on your back with your knees bent at 90 degrees (into your chest) and your arms by your sides. Alternately lower each foot to the ground, keeping the angle of your knee fixed. Be careful to keep your abdominals braced throughout and maintain the natural curve in your spine (don't over-arch or flatten it). To reduce the intensity of the exercise, do not extend your legs as low to the ground.

An advanced variation includes your upper body. Place your arms directly over your head so that they are resting on the ground. As one leg extends, bring the same arm over your head and towards your leg in an arc as if following that leg. As the knee bends and you withdraw the leg, the arm returns over your head again.

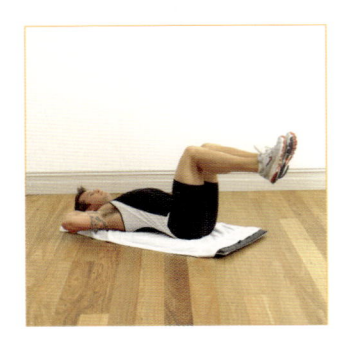

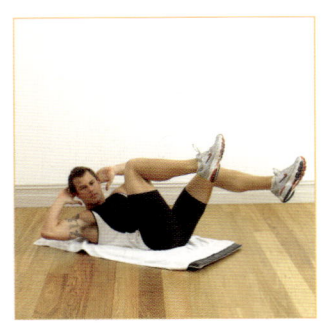

Take the exercise to a different level by adding a twist to really work your abdominals. Bring your fingers to your ears, bending your elbows out wide. As each knee comes into your chest, draw the opposite shoulder across to meet it. Rather than taking each foot to the ground, straighten the leg off the ground. Alternate sides.

Reverse crunch

Lie flat on your back with your knees bent and feet either on the ground or just off. Have your hands by your sides, palms down. Keeping your head down and your hands flat (not under your backside), roll the lower half of your body upwards, bringing your knees in towards your chest. Don't lift, just crunch or roll the lower half of your body inwards towards your chest. Slowly return to the starting position.

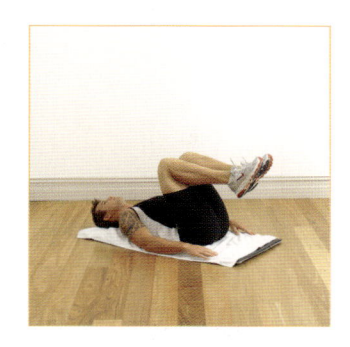

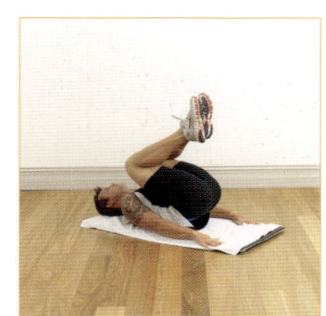

Advanced crunch

Choose this exercise if you are working at the advanced level only. Lie on your back with your knees bent, your elbows out wide and your fingers by your ears. Draw your belly button down towards the floor as you lift your shoulders forwards and up. Hold at the top for a second and then ease back down.

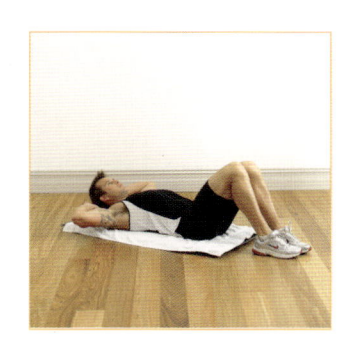

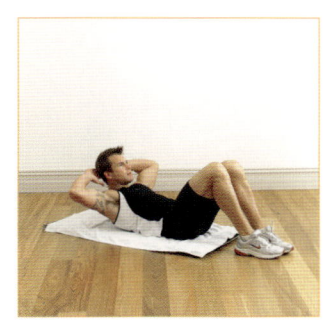

Step-ups

Lean, toned legs could be yours with this exercise. Find a step that is ideally between 20 and 50 centimetres high. Maintaining good posture, step one leg up and then the other and step down with the first then the second leg. Repeat half your set on one leg and then change lead legs to keep it balanced. Increase the intensity by jogging up and down and gradually performing the exercise more quickly.

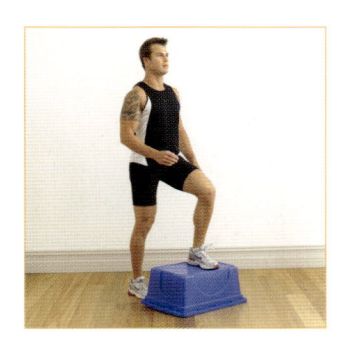

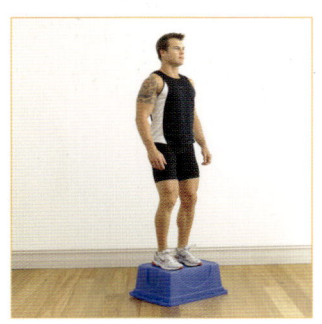

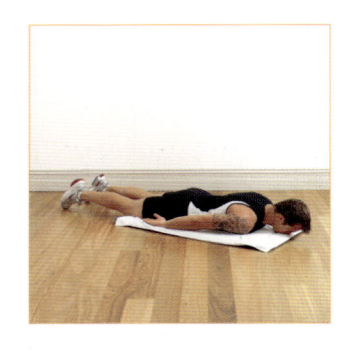

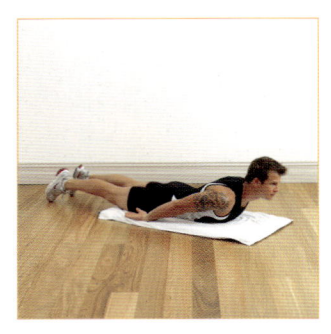

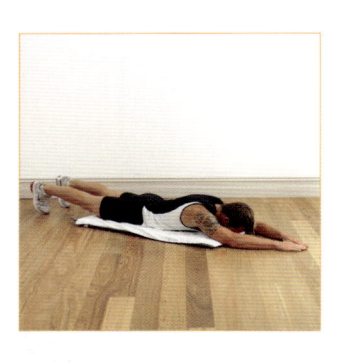

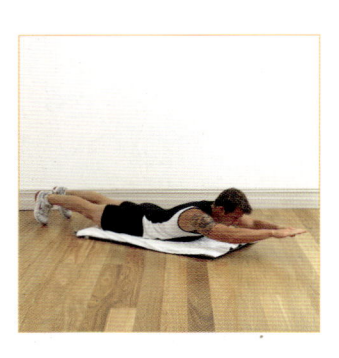

Superman

This exercise is very effective for strengthening your back. Lie face down on the floor with your hands down at your sides, palms up. (Place a rolled towel under your forehead if you feel more comfortable with your face clear of the floor.) Raise your chest and head off the floor, keeping your feet in contact with the floor. You don't need to lift very high to get the benefit of this exercise; instead, perform each repetition in a slow and controlled manner.

For an advanced version, lift alternate legs or both legs at the same time. To increase resistance, extend your arms out in front like Superman.

Gym resistance exercises

Machine chest press
Targets your chest and triceps. Sit in the machine with the handles level with the middle of your chest. Grasp the handles and push forward until your elbows are nearly straight (don't lock your elbows), keeping your chin up and the natural curve in your back (don't completely flatten your back on the back support). Hold for a second and return to the start.

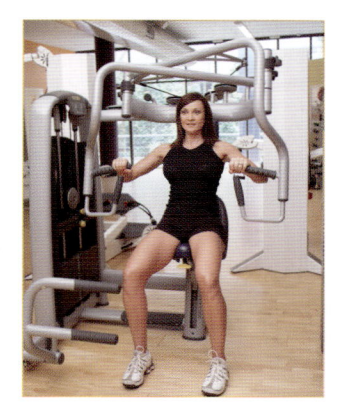

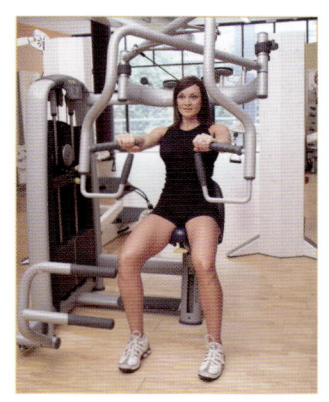

Lat pull-down
Targets your back and biceps. Sit facing the machine and grasp the handles just wider than shoulder width. Starting with your arms fully extended, squeeze the bar down slowly, stopping just under your chin. Make sure you sit up tall, chin up and keep a natural curve in your spine. Don't hunch forward.

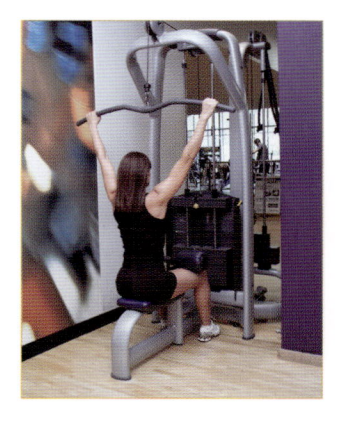

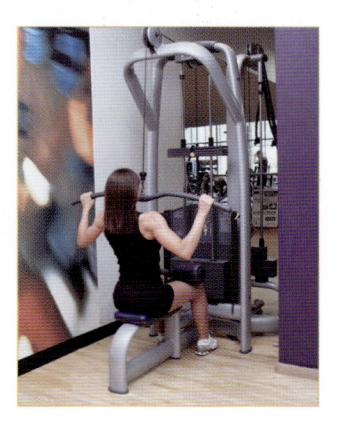

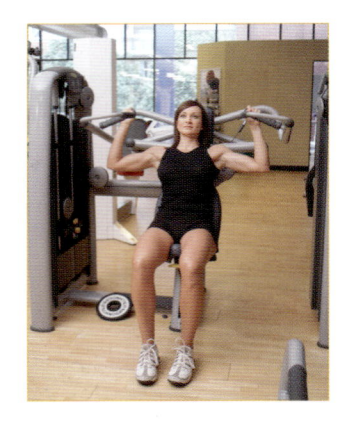

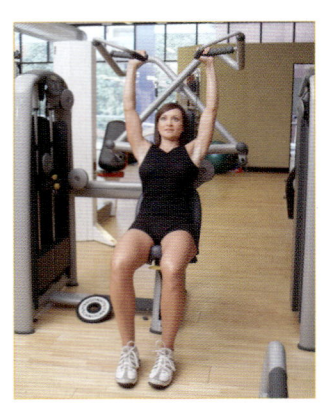

Machine shoulder press

Targets your shoulders and triceps. Sit facing away from the machine with your back against the back support and your hands underneath the handles. Grasp the handles and push up until your elbows are nearly straight (don't lock them), keeping your chin up and the natural curve in your back (it should not be dead flat on the back support). Hold for a second and return to the start.

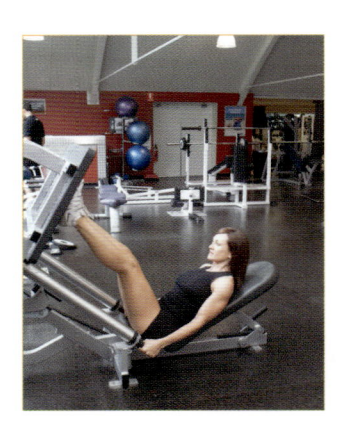

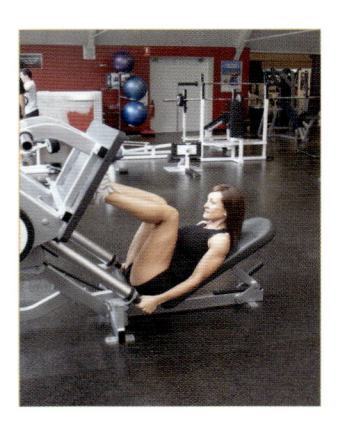

Leg press

Targets your backside, thighs and calves. Sit in the machine with your feet placed shoulder-width apart and your back and backside firmly supported by the seat. Remember to brace your core (your abdominals) and maintain a natural curve in your spine. Push the plate away and unlatch it. Slowly lower the plate towards your torso, making sure that your knees don't roll in (they should travel directly in the same line that your toes are pointed). Once your knees reach a 45-degree angle, push the plate away, trying to keep the weight on your heels.

Lying leg curl

Targets your hamstrings and calves. Lie face down on the machine. Adjust the leg pad so that it sits just on your Achilles tendon. Curl the pad up until it touches your backside, squeezing through your hamstrings and then lower slowly back to the start position.

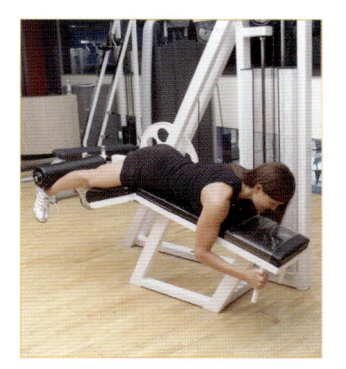

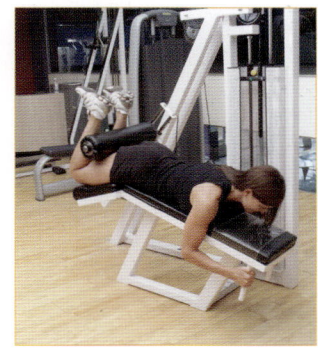

Bicep curl

Targets your biceps and forearms. Holding the bar, stand feet shoulder-width apart with one foot forward and one foot behind. Keeping your elbows by your side (but not touching) curl the bar upwards. The only joint moving should be your elbow. Once the bar is at the top, squeeze your bicep, hold for a second and then lower slowly to the start position.

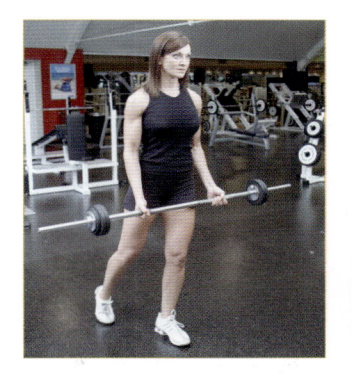

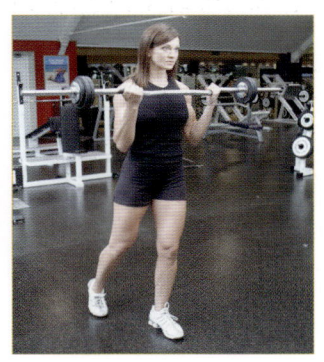

Lying bar extension

Targets your triceps. Lie flat on a bench holding a bar shoulder-width apart, with your arms held vertically from your torso. Slowly lower the bar towards your forehead, the only joint moving should be your elbow (upper arms stay vertical). Stop just before touching your forehead. Return the bar, through the same arc, to the start position.

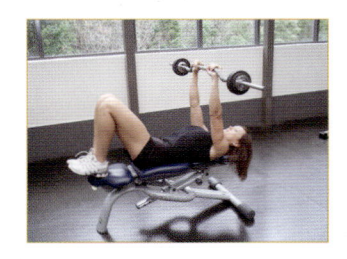

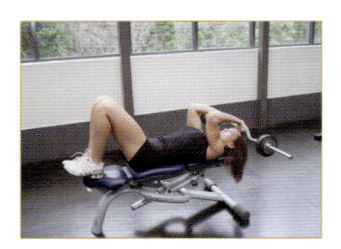

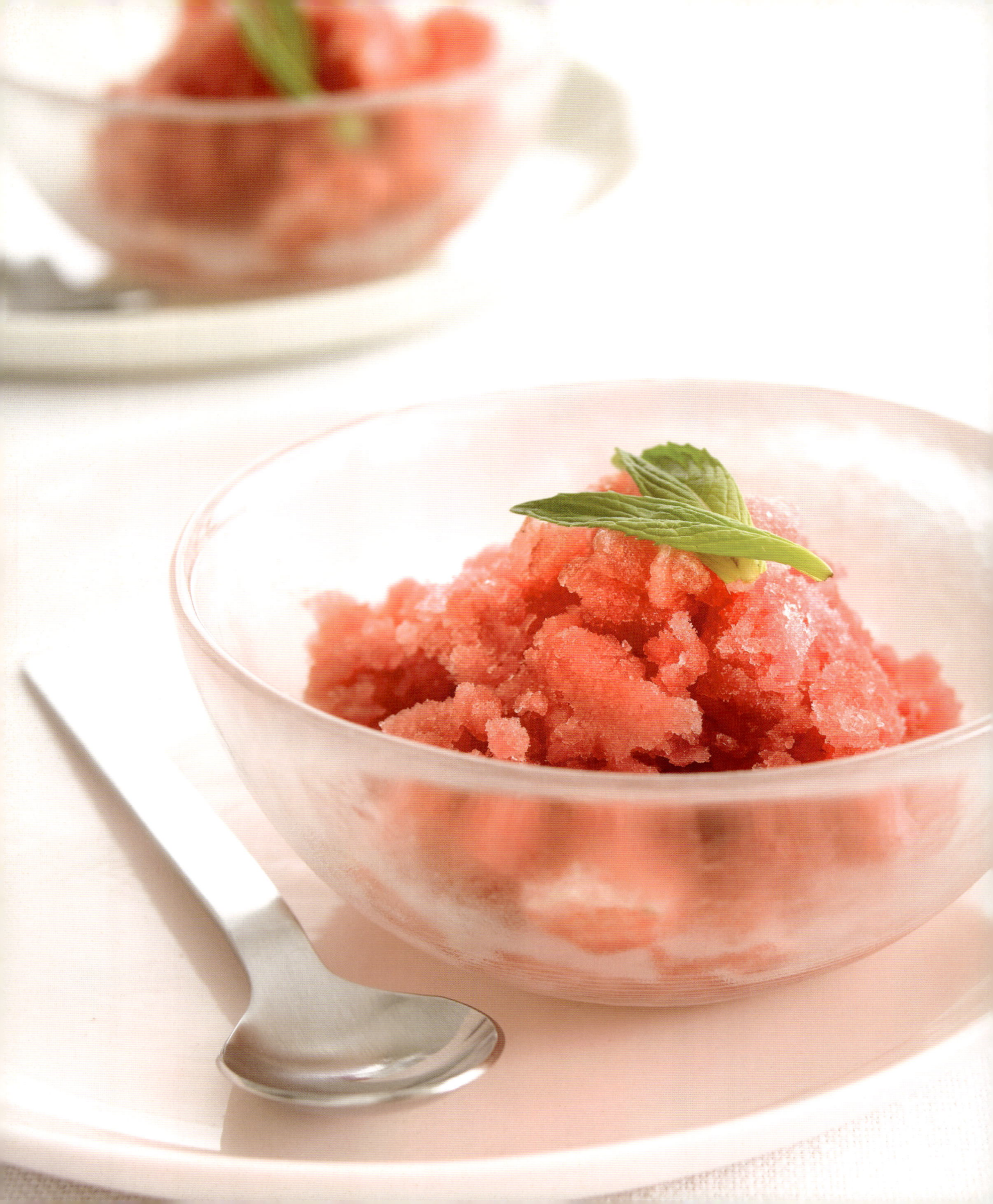

Recipes for Life

Losing weight doesn't mean you have to eat bland and boring food. Here are more than 60 simple and delicious recipes including breakfasts, light meals and dinners as well as desserts and sweet treats. The Biggest Loser recipes have been carefully devised and tested by experts, and offer a large range of fresh and mouth-watering meal options. A full nutrition analysis at the bottom of each recipe makes it easy to plan healthy eating.

Breakfasts

Banana smoothie

A quick all-in-one breakfast or instant energy lift for any time of day.

1 ripe banana, roughly chopped
1 tablespoon wheatgerm
¼ teaspoon ground cinnamon
3 tablespoons low-fat natural yoghurt
½ teaspoon honey
¾ cup low-fat milk

Place all ingredients in a blender and mix until smooth. Drink immediately.

Serves 1

NUTRITION ANALYSIS
PER SERVE
Total kJ: 979 kJ
Carbohydrates: 39.7 g
Fat: 1.7 g
Saturated fat: 0.9 g
Protein: 13.0 g
Fibre: 3.3 g

Tropical muesli

This is a light, sweet mix that will keep in an airtight container for up to two weeks. Serve topped with yoghurt and fruit.

olive oil spray
1 cup rolled oats
2 tablespoons honey
¼ cup shredded coconut
2 tablespoons flaked almonds
¼ teaspoon ground cinnamon
15 dried apricots, cut into 1 cm strips
1 tablespoon pepitas (pumpkin seed kernels)

Spray a large frying pan lightly with oil and add the oats. Toast gently over a low heat for 2–3 minutes until warmed through. Add honey and cook for 3–4 minutes, tossing well to coat.

Remove from heat and allow to cool. Meanwhile, lightly toast coconut and almonds in the frying pan for 1–2 minutes until golden. Remove from heat and add to the oats. Add cinnamon, apricots and pepitas and mix well to combine.

Serves 4

NUTRITION ANALYSIS
PER SERVE
Total kJ: 963 kJ
Carbohydrates: 31 g
Fat: 9.1 g
Saturated fat: 3.3 g
Protein: 4.9 g
Fibre: 3.8 g

Apple and carrot buzz

A great blast of energy to get you going in the morning.

1 green apple, cored and quartered
2 stalks celery, trimmed
2 carrots
2.5 cm piece fresh ginger, peeled

Pass all ingredients through a juicer and drink immediately.

Serves 1

Berry–mint smoothie

A wonderful refresher on hot summer days.

¼ cup frozen mixed berries
¾ cup strawberries, hulled
½ teaspoon honey
2 tablespoons low-fat natural yoghurt
½ cup unsweetened apple juice
¼ cup roughly chopped mint leaves
3 tablespoons rolled oats
5 ice cubes
mint leaves to garnish (optional)

Place all ingredients in a blender and mix until smooth. Drink immediately.

Serves 1

NUTRITION ANALYSIS

PER SERVE
Total kJ: 394 kJ
Carbohydrates: 20.9 g
Fat: 0.2 g
Saturated fat: 0.0 g
Protein: 1.7 g
Fibre: 1.1 g

NUTRITION ANALYSIS

PER SERVE
Total kJ: 869 kJ
Carbohydrates: 34.3 g
Fat: 2.9 g
Saturated fat: 0.8 g
Protein: 7.5 g
Fibre: 5.9 g

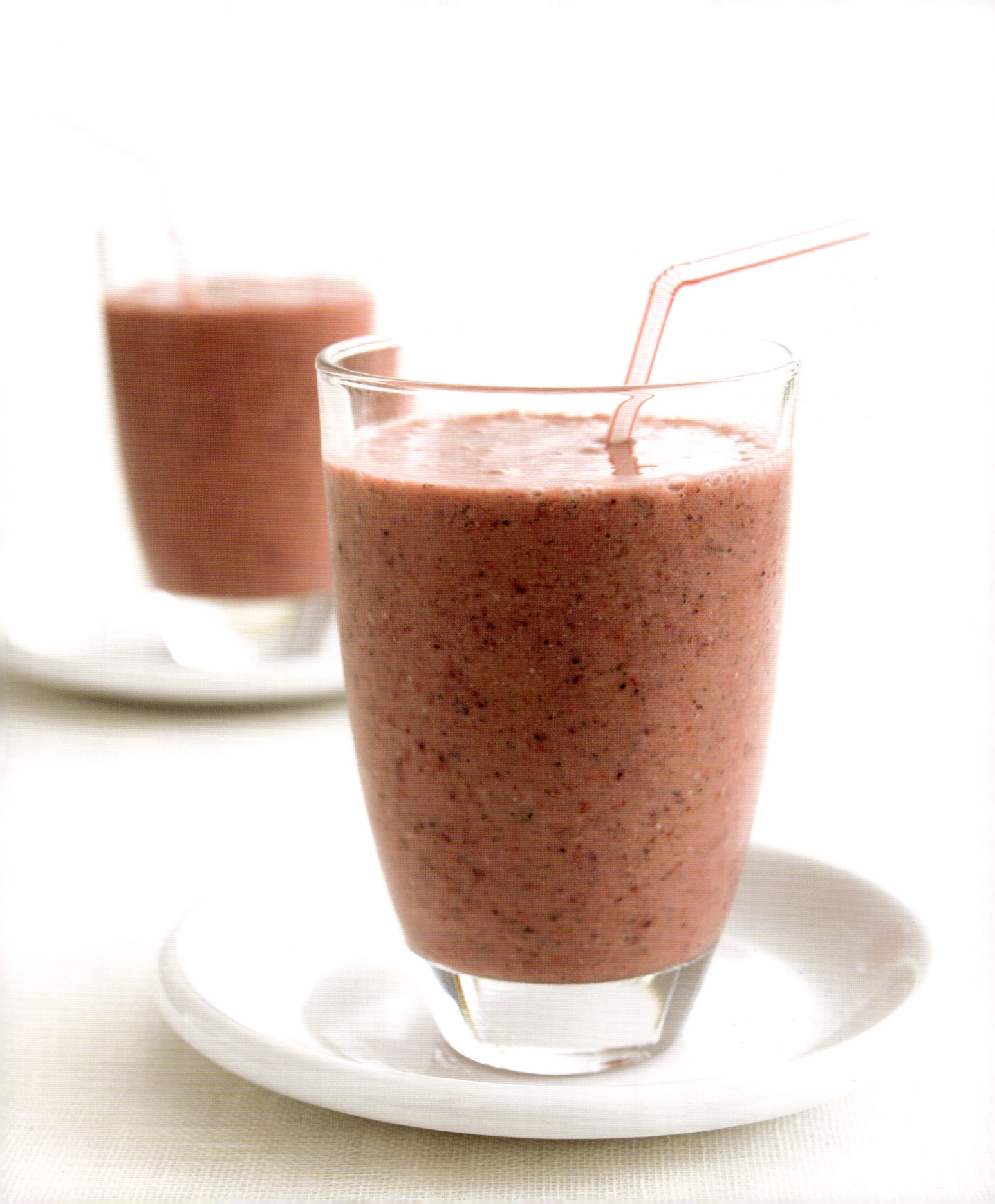

Winter fruit compote

Dried fruit is a great way to add sweetness and fibre without using sugar.

2 cups water
1 cup caster sugar
rind of 1 orange
2 cinnamon sticks
15 dried apricots, halved
10 pieces dried apple, halved
5 pieces dried pear, halved
5 pieces dried peach, halved
5 dried figs, halved
¼ cup raisins
¼ cup prunes, de-pitted and halved

Place water, sugar, orange rind, cinnamon sticks, apricots, apples, pears, peaches and figs in a large saucepan. Cook over a low heat for 7–10 minutes or until the fruit is tender. Remove from heat and add raisins and prunes. Can be served hot or cold.

Serves 8

NUTRITION ANALYSIS
PER SERVE
Total kJ: 205 kJ
Carbohydrates: 11.3 g
Fat: 0.1 g
Saturated fat: 0.0 g
Protein: 0.4 g
Fibre: 1.5 g

Bircher muesli

A light and colourful breakfast. Add any combination of nuts and seeds.

1½ cups rolled oats
1½ cups water
1 apple, grated
¾ cup low-fat natural yoghurt
¼ cup roughly chopped walnuts
2 tablespoons honey
1 teaspoon ground cinnamon
2 tablespoons pepitas (pumpkin seed kernels)

Soak the oats in the water overnight. Add remaining ingredients and mix well. Serve topped with seasonal fruit (or Stewed Apple and Rhubarb, see page 155).

Serves 4

NUTRITION ANALYSIS
PER SERVE
Total kJ: 1356 kJ
Carbohydrates: 42.0 g
Fat: 12.0 g
Saturated fat: 1.8 g
Protein: 9.0 g
Fibre: 4.3 g

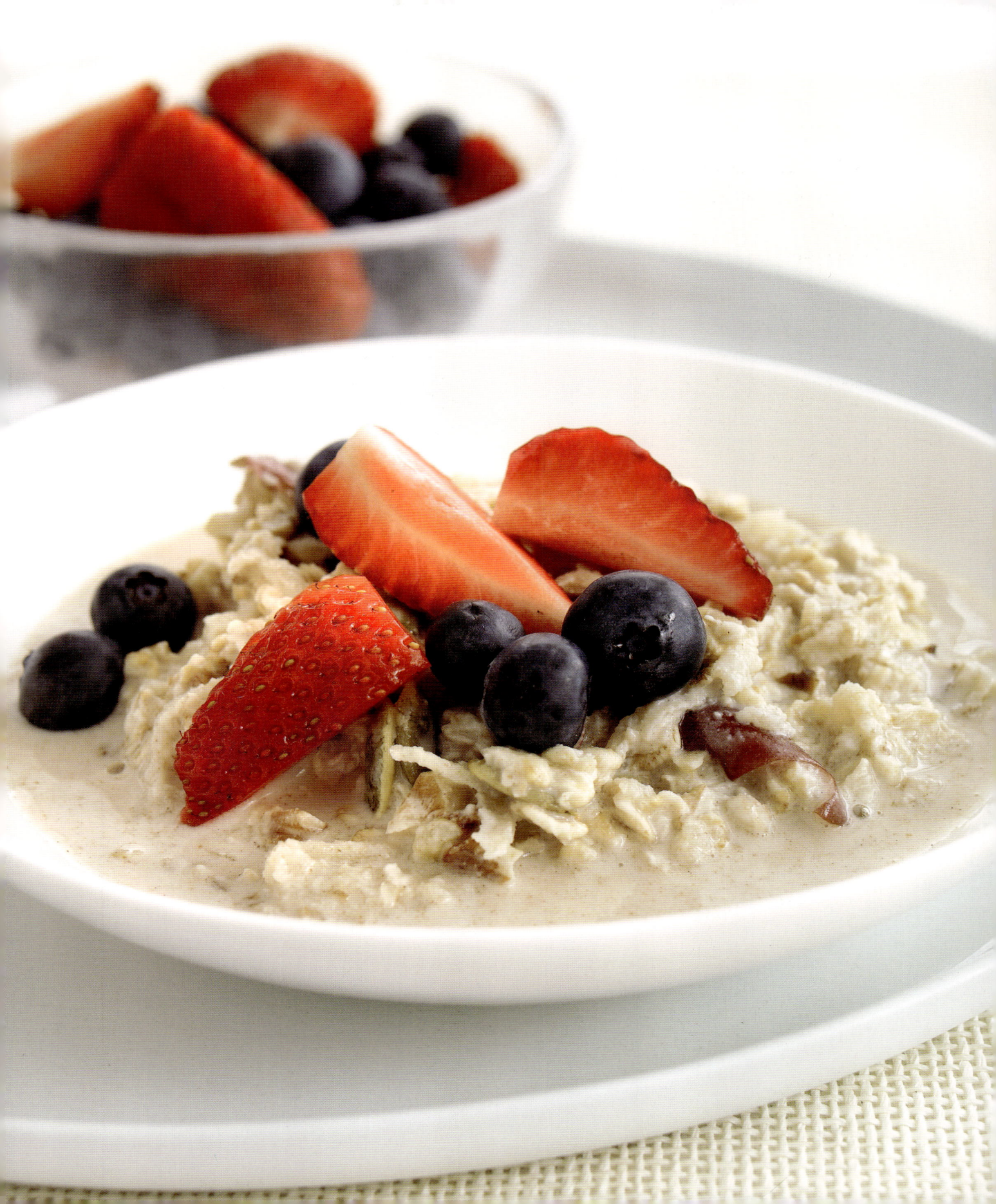

Porridge

Porridge is a delicious and satisfying breakfast, especially in winter. It is low-GI and provides energy to get you through the morning. Serve with Spiced Poached Pears (see opposite).

2 cups rolled oats
3 cups water
½ cup low-fat milk
4 tablespoons LSA*
2 teaspoons ground cinnamon

* LSA is a mixture of ground linseeds, sunflower seeds and almonds, and provides essential fatty acids, protein and fibre.

Soak oats in 2 cups of the water for a minimum of 30 minutes.

Cook oats in a large saucepan over a medium heat for 3–5 minutes. Add small amounts of the remaining water, stirring each time until absorbed. Stirring continuously will result in a creamier porridge. Add milk, stirring, until desired consistency is reached.

Remove from the heat and serve sprinkled with LSA and cinnamon.

Serves 4

NUTRITION ANALYSIS
PER SERVE
Total kJ: 1180 kJ
Carbohydrates: 29.2 g
Fat: 13.2 g
Saturated fat: 1.3 g
Protein: 9.5 g
Fibre: 4.5 g

Spiced poached pears

The rosewater here adds sweetness and a hint of the exotic. For a simple dessert serve pears with honey, low-fat natural yoghurt and walnuts.

6 ripe pears, peeled, cored and sliced lengthwise
4 cloves
1 cinnamon stick
rind of 1 orange
½ cup caster sugar
4 tablespoons rosewater (optional)

Place all ingredients in a snug-fitting saucepan and add enough water to just cover the pears. Place a saucer on top of the pears to keep them submerged, or give them a stir every now and again to ensure they cook evenly. Cook over a very low heat for 40 minutes until the pears are soft but retain their shape. Remove from the heat and serve, or store in an airtight container in the poaching liquid once cooled.

Serves 4

NUTRITION ANALYSIS
PER SERVE
Total kJ: 1043 kJ
Carbohydrates: 60.0 g
Fat: 0.2 g
Saturated fat: 0.0 g
Protein: 0.7 g
Fibre: 6.2 g

Stewed apple and rhubarb

Rhubarb is available all year round but is best in winter when the stalks are thicker and have a more intense colour. Wonderful served on porridge.

2 bunches (1.5 kg) rhubarb, washed, trimmed and de-stringed, then cut into 4 cm lengths
3 apples, peeled, cored and diced
1 cinnamon stick
2 star anise
1 vanilla bean, split lengthwise
½ cup caster sugar
3 tablespoons water

Place all ingredients in a large saucepan. Cover and cook over a medium heat, stirring occasionally, for 5–7 minutes or until the fruit is tender. Serve hot or refrigerate once cooled.

Serves 4

NUTRITION ANALYSIS
PER SERVE
Total kJ: 807 kJ
Carbohydrates: 46.8 g
Fat: 0.2 g
Saturated fat: 0.0 g
Protein: 1.0 g
Fibre: 3.0 g

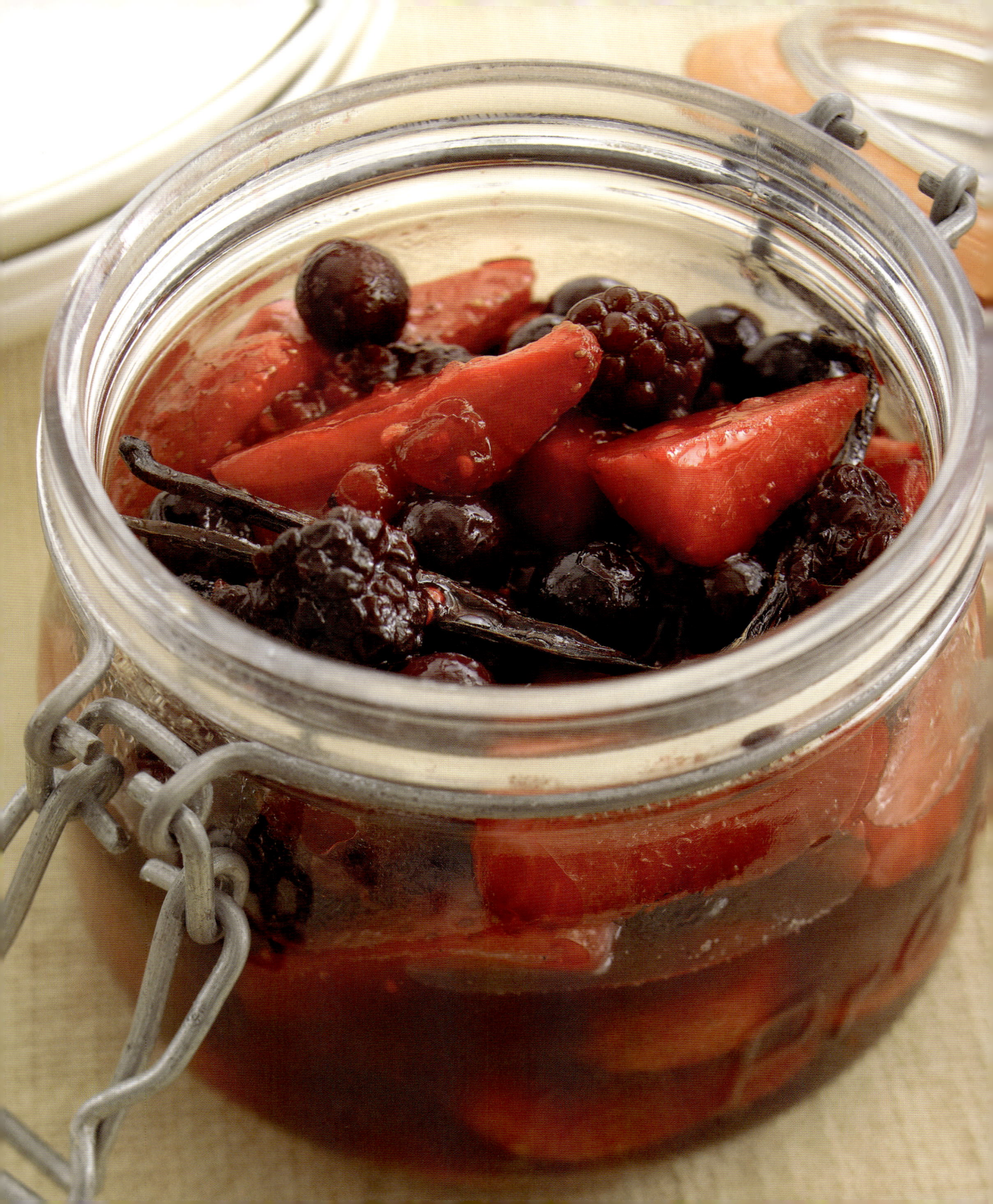

Berry compote

Very quick to make, this fruity mix is delicious with porridge or on pancakes.

- 1 cup frozen mixed berries
- ¾ cup strawberries, hulled and quartered
- ¼ cup caster sugar
- 1 vanilla bean, split lengthwise
- 1 tablespoon water

Place all ingredients in a small saucepan. Cook gently over a low heat for 10 minutes or until strawberries are tender. Serve hot or refrigerate once cooled.

Serves 8

NUTRITION ANALYSIS
PER SERVE
Total kJ: 198 kJ
Carbohydrates: 9.1 g
Fat: 0.1 g
Saturated fat: 0.0 g
Protein: 1.6 g
Fibre: 2.1 g

Buckwheat pancakes

Buckwheat actually contains no wheat or gluten, so is great for coeliacs.

- ¾ cup buckwheat flour
- ¼ cup caster sugar
- ¼ teaspoon ground nutmeg
- ½ teaspoon baking powder
- 3 tablespoons low-fat milk
- 1 egg yolk
- 3 egg whites
- olive oil spray

Combine flour, sugar, nutmeg and baking powder in a large mixing bowl. Add milk and egg yolk and mix thoroughly.

Whisk egg whites until fluffy and gently fold into the flour mixture, forming a smooth batter.

Heat a frying pan over medium heat and spray lightly with oil. Pour the batter into a jug and pour enough batter into the pan to coat the bottom. Cook until small bubbles form on the surface, then flip over and cook for a further couple of minutes or until golden. Serve warm topped with fresh or stewed fruits (or Berry Compote, see opposite).

Serves 4

NUTRITION ANALYSIS
PER SERVE
Total kJ: 731 kJ
Carbohydrates: 28.9 g
Fat: 1.7 g
Saturated fat: 0.6 g
Protein: 11.5 g
Fibre: 0.3 g

Slow-roasted garlic mushrooms

Mushrooms are a valuable source of protein and B vitamins. This recipe uses flat mushrooms but any type will do.

600 g flat mushrooms, wiped and stalks removed
4 cloves garlic, thinly sliced
light olive oil spray
4 sprigs thyme
75 g rocket leaves, washed
4 slices sourdough bread

Preheat oven to 180°C (350°F).

Place mushrooms and garlic in a baking dish. Spray lightly with oil and toss to coat. Add thyme sprigs and cover with a lid or foil. Bake for 1 hour, tossing occasionally.

Remove thyme and serve atop rocket leaves on unbuttered slices of toasted sourdough.

Serves 4

NUTRITION ANALYSIS
PER SERVE
Total kJ: 489 kJ
Carbohydrates: 11.2 g
Fat: 3.4 g
Saturated fat: 0.7 g
Protein: 9.5 g
Fibre: 6.4 g

Avocado and fetta salsa

Delicious on toast as a quick breakfast. The salsa can also be added to egg whites to make a tasty omelette.

olive oil spray
2 red onions, finely diced
2 cloves garlic, finely sliced
2 ripe roma tomatoes, diced
1½ ripe avocados, cut into 2 cm pieces
2 tablespoons chopped oregano leaves
80 g low-fat fetta, crumbled
freshly ground black pepper

Heat a large frying pan over a low heat and spray lightly with oil. Cook the onions and garlic gently for a few minutes until soft. Add the tomato, avocado and oregano and stir gently until warmed through. Add the fetta and allow to melt slightly. Season and serve warm.

Serves 4

NUTRITION ANALYSIS
PER SERVE
Total kJ: 1121 kJ
Carbohydrates: 4.5 g
Fat: 23 g
Saturated fat: 6.3 g
Protein: 8.4 g
Fibre: 3.2 g

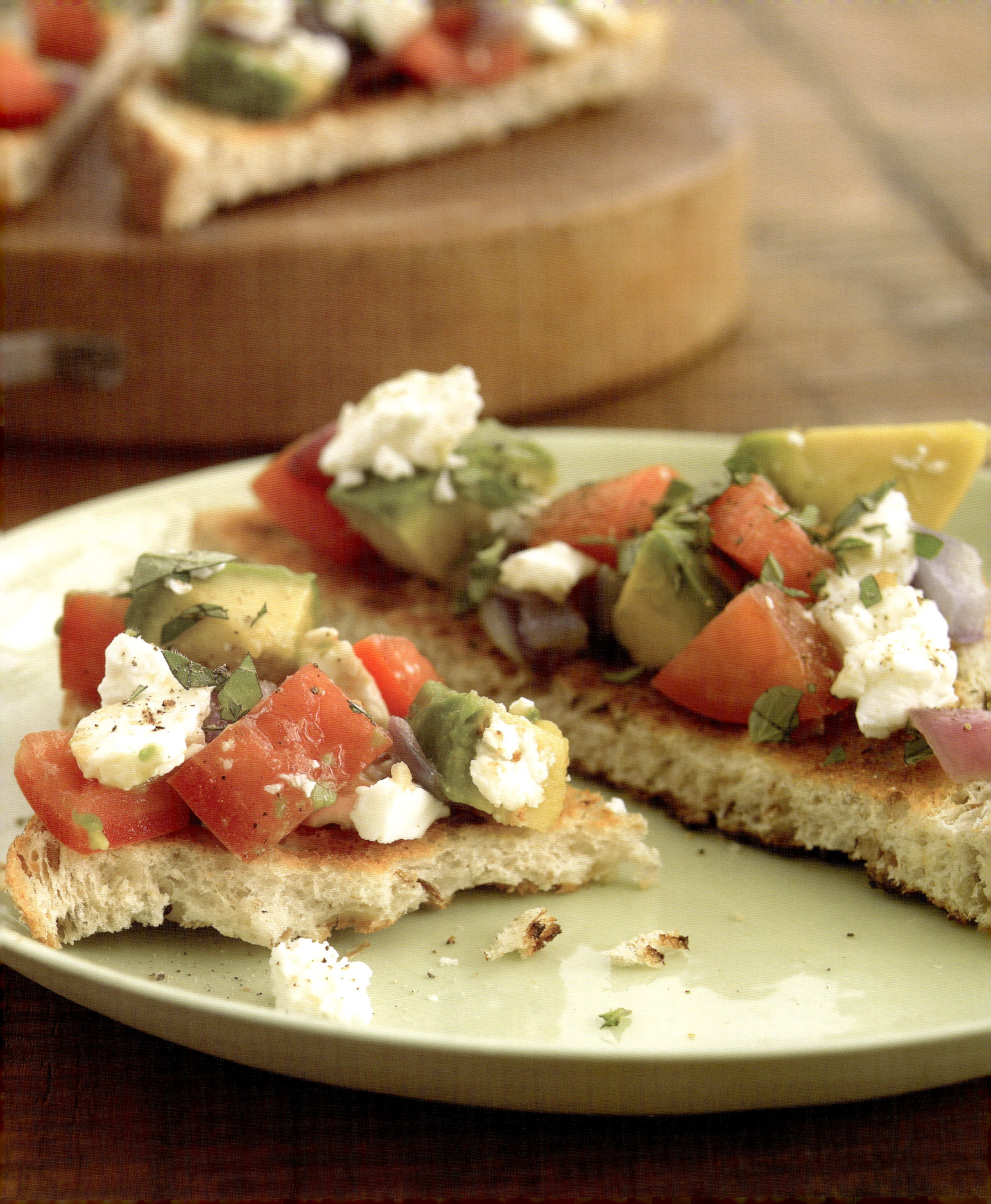

Italian omelette

A hearty and satisfying breakfast. For a vegetarian version, substitute a handful of chopped mushrooms for the ham.

olive oil spray
2 red onions, finely diced
2 cloves garlic, crushed
4 slices fat-free leg ham, chopped
4 eggs, lightly beaten
8 egg whites, lightly beaten
¼ cup skim milk
1 tablespoon grated reduced-fat cheddar cheese
1 tablespoon chopped oregano leaves
200 g reduced-fat ricotta

Heat a small frying pan over a low heat and spray lightly with oil. Gently cook the onions, garlic and ham for a few minutes until onions soften.

Combine eggs, egg whites, milk, cheese and oregano in a mixing bowl. Remove the onion mixture from the heat, allow to cool slightly, and fold into the eggs.

Spray the frying pan lightly with a little more oil and pour a quarter of the mixture into the pan. Cook over a medium heat until it begins to set. Sprinkle 50 g of the ricotta over one half of the omelette and use a spatula to fold the other side over to cover. Cook for a further 5 minutes. Loosen the base and sides and gently slide out of the pan. Repeat with remaining mixture.

Serves 4

NUTRITION ANALYSIS
PER SERVE
Total kJ: 973 kJ
Carbohydrates: 4.4 g
Fat: 12.7 g
Saturated fat: 5.8 g
Protein: 25.4 g
Fibre: 0.4 g

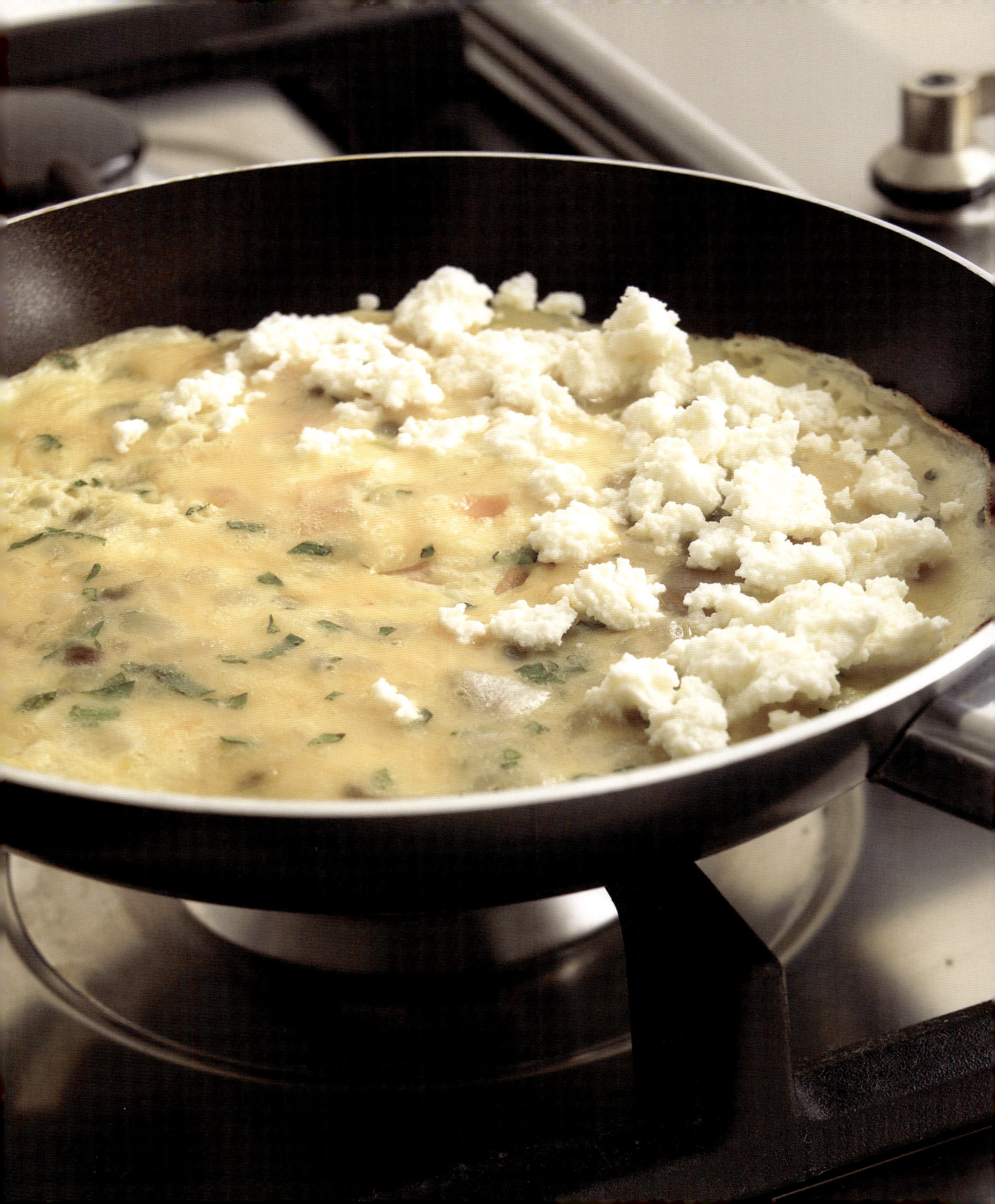

Scrambled eggs with smoked salmon

Salmon is a valuable source of essential fatty acids. This delicious breakfast takes just minutes to prepare.

olive oil spray
1 onion, finely diced
4 eggs
8 egg whites
8 slices smoked salmon, cut into 1 cm strips
2 tablespoons chopped chives
4 slices sourdough bread

Heat a large frying pan over a low–medium heat and spray lightly with oil. Add the onion and cook gently until soft.

Beat the eggs and egg whites together and pour into the pan. Stir continuously for 3–5 minutes until cooked.

Remove from heat and combine with the salmon and chives. Serve immediately on unbuttered slices of toasted sourdough.

Serves 4

NUTRITION ANALYSIS
PER SERVE
Total kJ: 998 kJ
Carbohydrates: 12.8 g
Fat: 8.4 g
Saturated fat: 2.2 g
Protein: 27 g
Fibre: 1.9 g

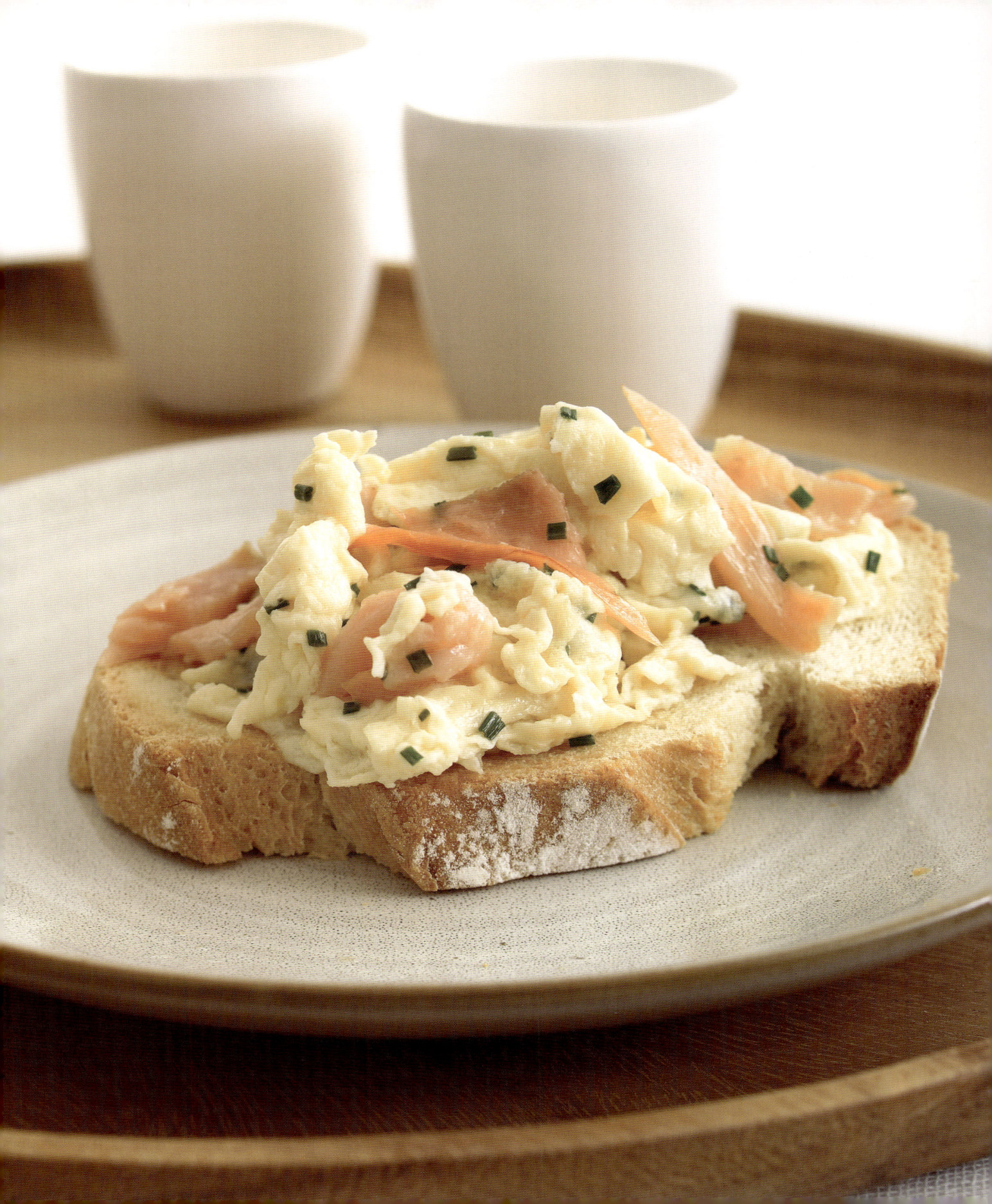

Spanish-style baked eggs

This is an interesting twist on eggs for breakfast, with robust flavours.

2 red capsicums
olive oil spray
1 onion, finely sliced
2 cloves garlic, finely sliced
100 g baby spinach leaves
2 cups tomato passata or
　Napoli Sauce (see page 182)
2 tablespoons capers, roughly chopped
10 pitted black olives, roughly chopped
⅓ cup torn basil leaves
8 eggs
extra basil leaves to garnish
freshly ground black pepper

Preheat oven to 160°C (320°F).

Lightly spray the capsicums with oil and hold over an open flame or place under a grill, until the skin blisters and blackens. Allow to cool then peel, remove stem and seeds and slice into 1 cm strips.

Heat a large, ovenproof pan over a medium heat and spray lightly with oil. Cook the onion and garlic gently for a few minutes until soft. Add the spinach leaves and allow to wilt. Add the capsicum, napoli sauce, capers, olives and basil and cook for a few minutes, stirring gently until warmed through.

Divide mixture between 4 individual ramekins (1½-cup capacity) and crack 2 eggs on top of each. Bake in the oven for 5–7 minutes or until egg whites are cooked but the yolks still soft. Sprinkle torn basil leaves on top, season and serve.

Serves 4

NUTRITION ANALYSIS
PER SERVE
Total kJ: 922 kJ
Carbohydrates: 11.9 g
Fat: 11.3 g
Saturated fat: 3.3 g
Protein: 15.6 g
Fibre: 4.0 g

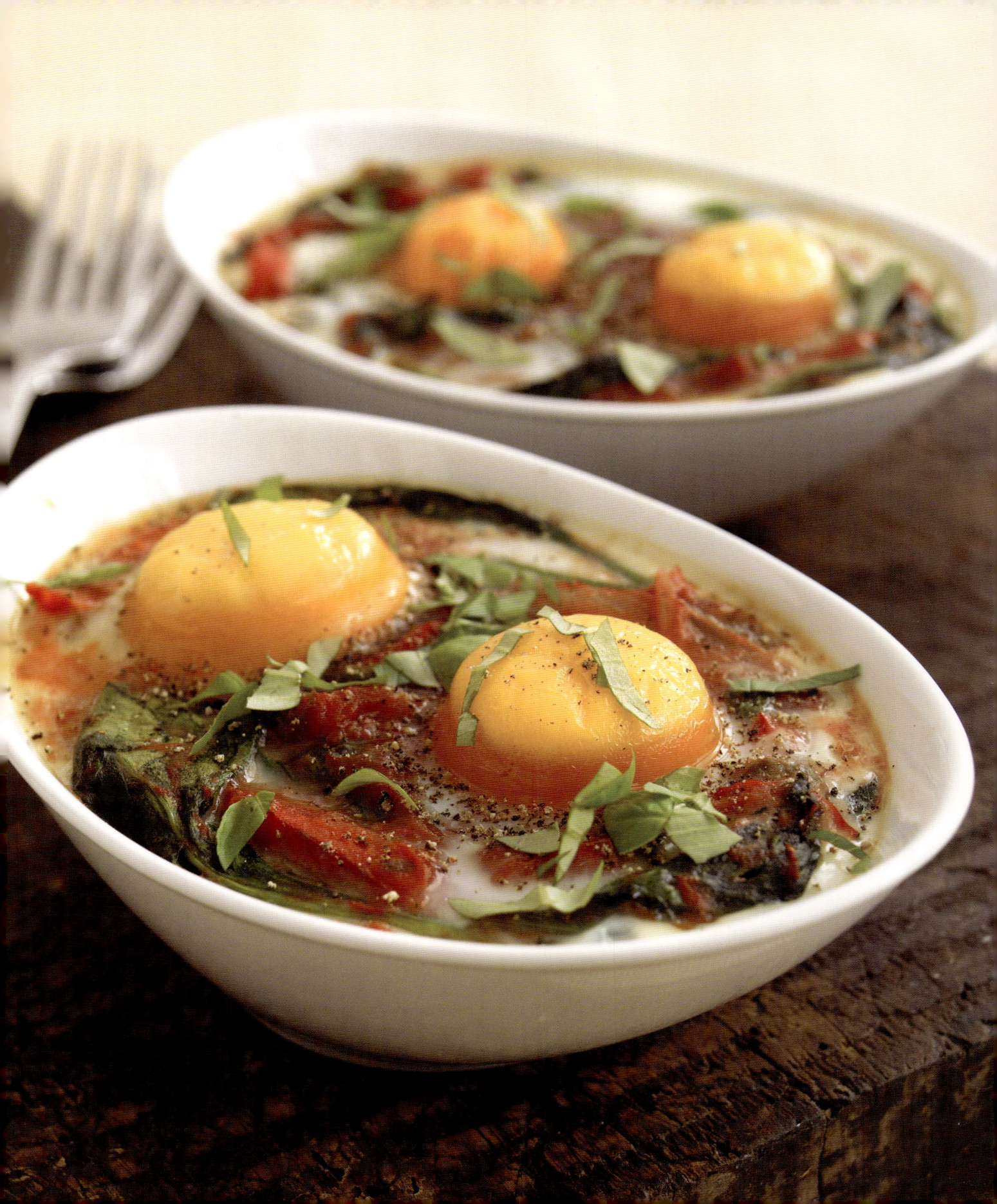

Soups, Salads and Light Meals

Vegetable stock

Home-made vegetable stock adds so much flavour to vegetable-based soups and rice dishes. It's suitable for freezing so you can always have some on hand.

3 onions, quartered
½ bunch celery, trimmed and
   cut into 5 cm lengths
2 carrots, peeled and cut into
   5 cm pieces
1 head garlic, cut in half widthwise
5 black peppercorns
2 fresh or dried bay leaves
4 litres water

Place all ingredients in a large saucepan or stockpot and bring to the boil. Reduce heat and simmer for 1½ hours. Strain the vegetables and reserve liquid in containers ready to freeze once cooled.

Makes 3 litres

Chicken stock

Nothing beats the flavour of home-made stock. Chicken carcasses are available at most butchers.

4 chicken carcasses, washed
5 litres water
2 sticks celery, cut into 5 cm lengths
2 onions, quartered
5 cloves garlic, crushed
10 black peppercorns
3 fresh or dried bay leaves

Place the carcasses in a large saucepan or stockpot and fill with water until just covered. Bring to the boil and skim off any scum that rises to the surface. Add the remaining ingredients, reduce heat and gently simmer for 3 hours. Remove from the heat and skim again. Allow to cool then strain into containers and store in the fridge or freezer.

Makes 3 litres

Bacon, lentil and tomato soup

A lovely, hearty soup for winter, and suitable for freezing.

olive oil spray
2 onions, diced
2 cloves garlic, crushed
1 stick celery, diced
4 rashers rindless bacon, trimmed and chopped
4 sprigs thyme
½ cup brown lentils, rinsed
1 x 400 g can salt-reduced diced tomatoes
1 litre water
2 fresh or dried bay leaves
4 tablespoons chopped coriander leaves

* Note: a 400 g can of lentils may be used instead of dried lentils. If using canned, reduce the cooking time to 20 minutes.

Heat a large saucepan over a low heat and spray lightly with oil. Add onions, garlic and celery and cook gently for a few minutes until soft. Add bacon and thyme and cook for a further 2 minutes. Add lentils, tomatoes, water and bay leaves, increase heat and bring to the boil. Reduce the heat, cover and simmer for 1 hour, stirring occasionally, until lentils are tender.

Remove bay leaves and thyme and serve topped with coriander leaves.

Serves 4

NUTRITION ANALYSIS
PER SERVE
Total kJ: 773 kJ
Carbohydrates: 14.9 g
Fat: 6.2 g
Saturated fat: 2.2 g
Protein: 14.8 g
Fibre: 5.4 g

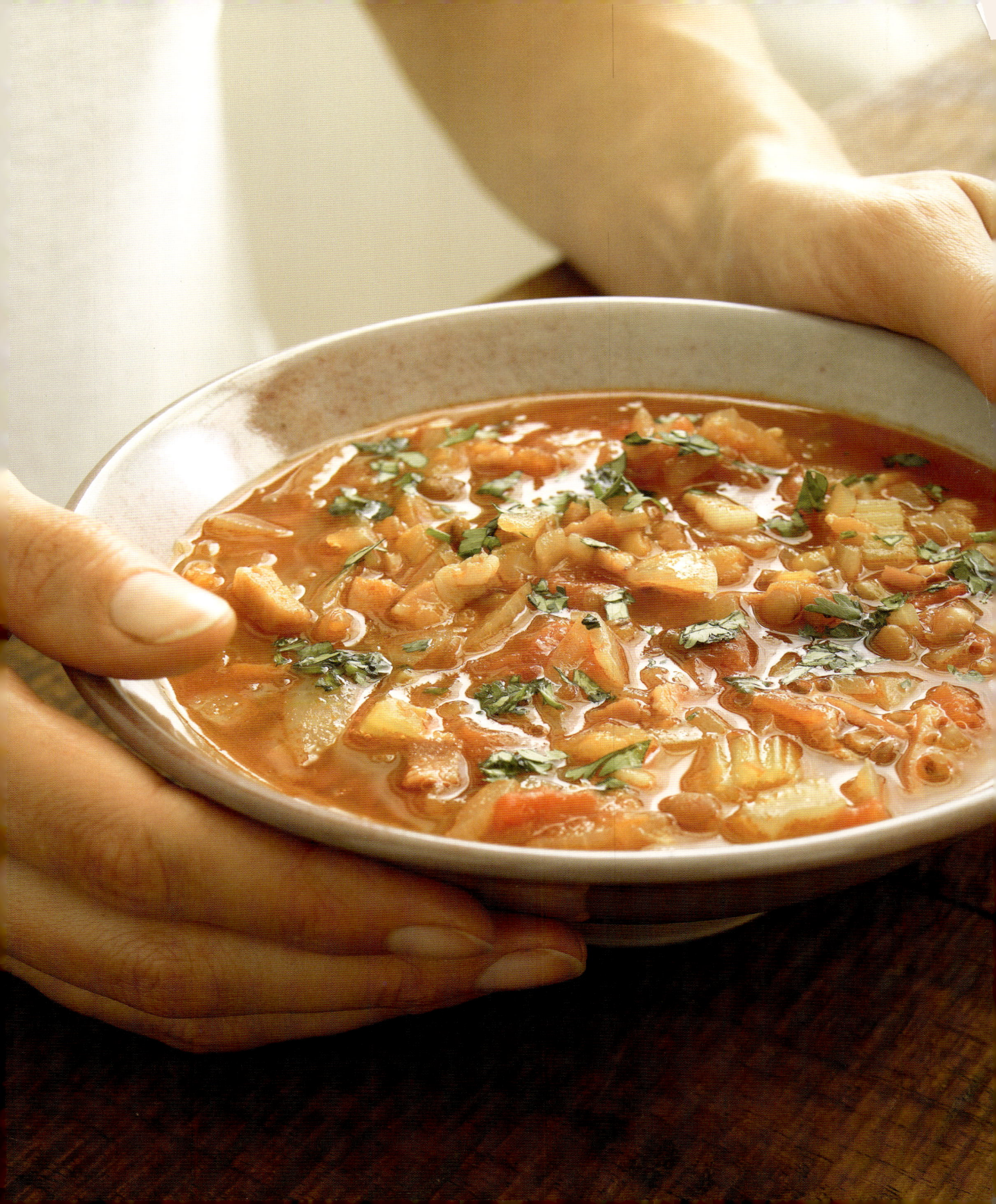

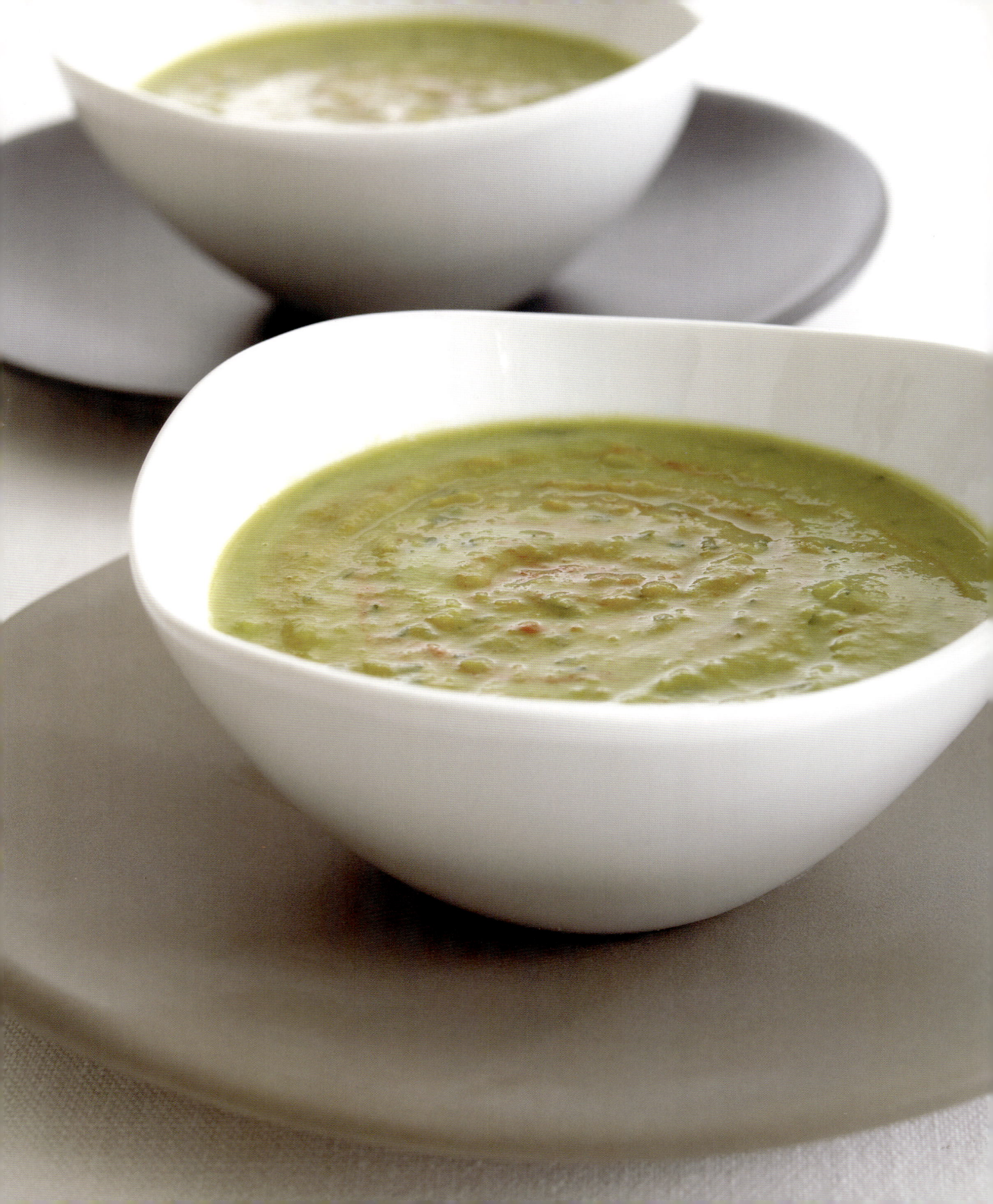

Minted pea soup

This soup is delicious in summer, topped with harissa sauce for a spicy twist.

olive oil spray
2 onions, finely diced
2 cloves garlic, crushed
700 ml chicken stock (see recipe on page 167)
500 g frozen peas
1 cup roughly chopped mint leaves
2 tablespoons harissa* or Harissa Dressing (see page 180)

* Harissa paste is available from delicatessens.

Heat a large saucepan over a low heat and spray lightly with oil. Cook the onions and garlic gently for a few minutes until soft. Add chicken stock and bring to the boil. Add peas and bring back to the boil for 5–7 minutes.

Remove from the heat and allow to cool slightly. Add mint leaves and purée using a blender or hand-held processor. Serve topped with a swirl of harissa if desired. The soup will keep in the fridge for up to 4 days, but is best served immediately as its vibrant green colour will fade.

Serves 4

NUTRITION ANALYSIS

PER SERVE
Total kJ: 504 kJ
Carbohydrates: 13.8 g
Fat: 1.2 g
Saturated fat: 0.3 g
Protein: 9.7 g
Fibre: 8.1 g

Lamb and barley hotpot

Barley is related to wheat and has a nutty flavour. This is a wonderfully hearty soup for winter.

olive oil spray
1 onion, diced
3 cloves garlic, crushed
2 sticks celery, diced
2 carrots, diced
300 g lamb chuck fillets, trimmed and cut into cubes
3 sprigs rosemary
2 tablespoons tomato paste or ¼ cup Napoli Sauce (see page 182)
1½ litres chicken stock (recipe on page 167)
2 fresh or dried bay leaves
1 cup pearl barley
125 g green beans, cut into 4 cm lengths
2 tablespoons chopped flat-leaf parsley

Heat a large saucepan over a low heat and spray lightly with oil. Add onion, garlic, celery and carrots and cook gently for a few minutes until soft. Add lamb and rosemary and cook until the meat is browned on all sides. Cover with napoli sauce and cook for a further 2 minutes. Add the chicken stock and bay leaves and bring to the boil.

Add the barley and reduce heat. Cover and simmer gently for 1½ hours until the barley is tender. Add beans and simmer for another 30 minutes until tender.

Remove the bay leaves and rosemary sprigs and serve sprinkled with parsley.

Serves 4

NUTRITION ANALYSIS

PER SERVE
Total kJ: 1085 kJ
Carbohydrates: 17.1g
Fat: 8.2 g
Saturated fat: 4.0 g
Protein: 26 g
Fibre: 6.4 g

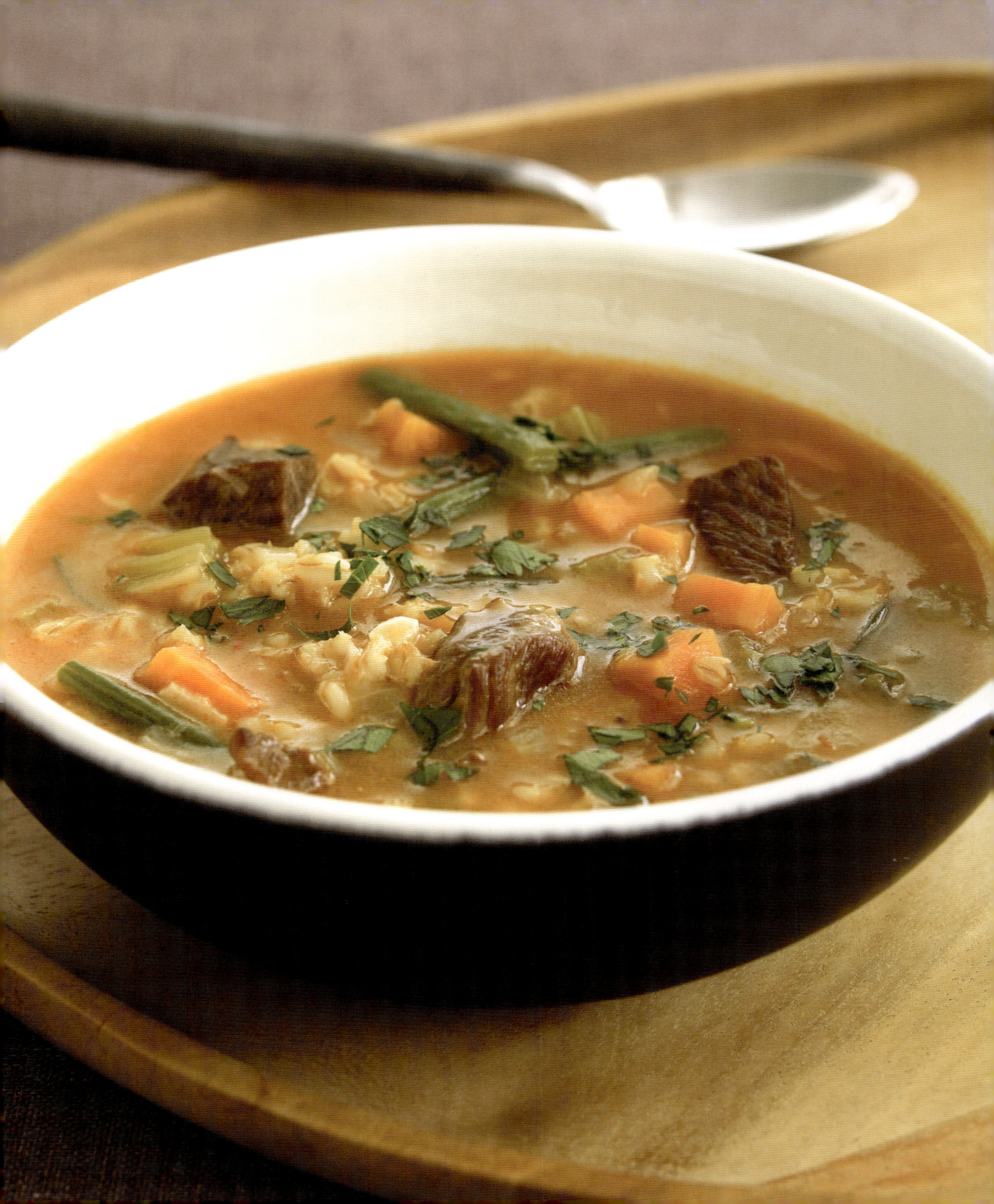

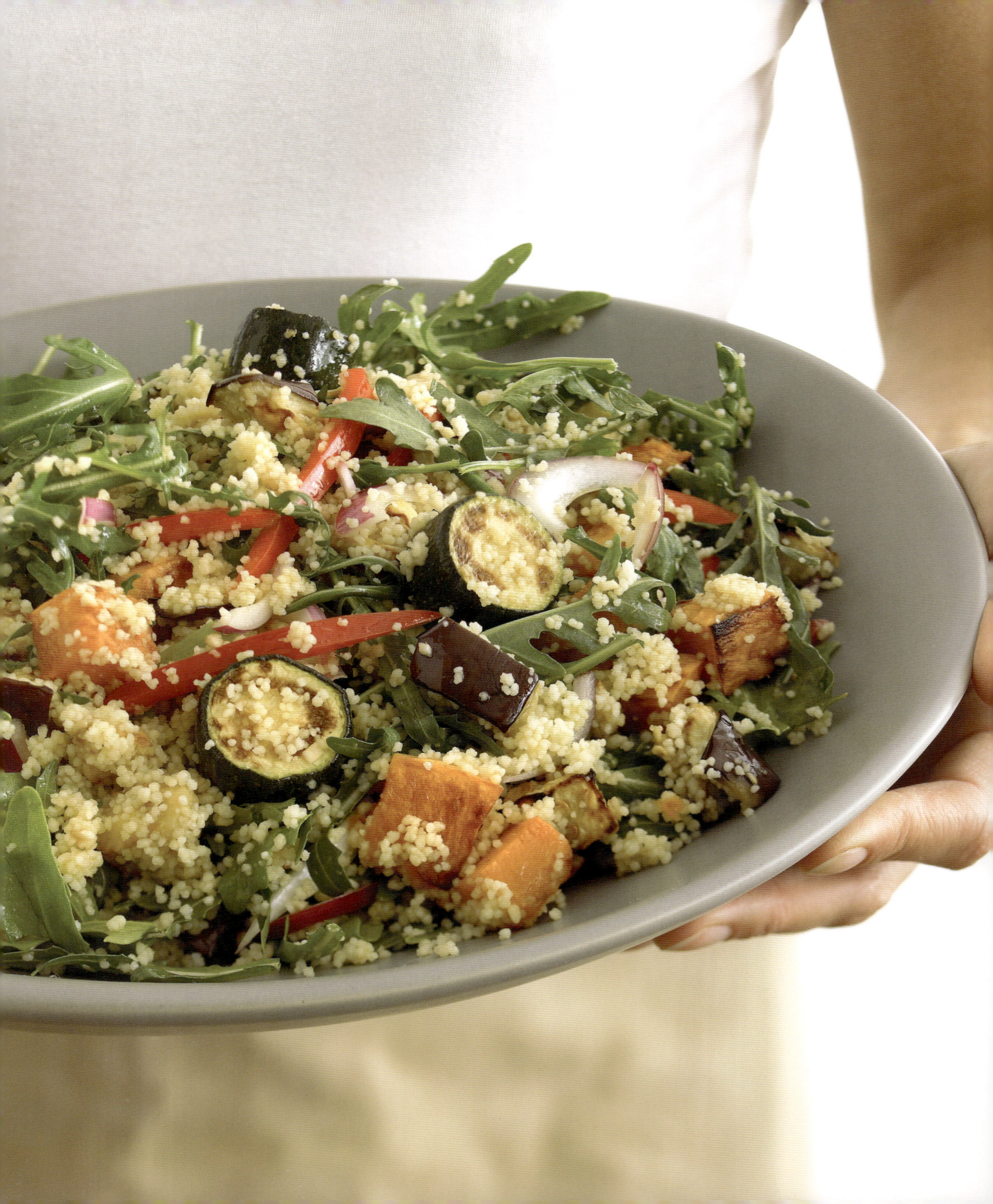

Roasted vegetable and couscous salad

This salad is a satisfying meal. The vegetables can be pre-roasted and combined with the other ingredients when ready to serve.

¼ butternut pumpkin, peeled, seeded and cut into 2 cm pieces
olive oil spray
½ eggplant, cut into 2 cm cubes
1 zucchini, cut into 2 cm pieces
¾ cup couscous
¾ cup boiling water
½ red onion, finely sliced
½ red capsicum, finely sliced
150 g baby rocket leaves

DRESSING
1 clove garlic, crushed
2 teaspoons red wine vinegar
1 teaspoon balsamic vinegar
⅓ cup extra-virgin olive oil
¼ teaspoon honey

Preheat oven to 250°C (480°F).

Place pumpkin pieces in a deep baking tray and spray lightly with oil to coat. Bake for 10 minutes then add the eggplant and zucchini (also sprayed lightly with oil). Roast for a further 20 minutes or until cooked. Remove from oven and set aside.

Combine the couscous and boiling water in a bowl, mix with a fork, cover with plastic wrap and let stand for 7 minutes.

To make the dressing place all ingredients in an airtight jar and shake until combined.

Loosen the couscous with a fork until light and fluffy. Add the roast vegetables, onion, capsicum and rocket leaves. Mix the dressing through the salad until coated.

Serves 4

NUTRITION ANALYSIS
PER SERVE
Total kJ: 801 kJ
Carbohydrates: 11.7 g
Fat: 13.0 g
Saturated fat: 1.5 g
Protein: 4.2 g
Fibre: 5.6 g

Chicken, beetroot and walnut salad

A sweet and colourful summer salad with a nutty crunch.

4 large beetroot, washed and trimmed
2 medium skinless chicken breasts
150 g baby spinach leaves
2 tablespoons roughly chopped walnuts
½ red onion, thinly sliced

DRESSING

1 clove garlic, crushed
2 teaspoons red wine vinegar
1 teaspoon balsamic vinegar
⅓ cup extra-virgin olive oil
¼ teaspoon honey

Preheat oven to 150°C (300°F).

Wrap each beetroot in foil and roast on an oven rack for 1½–2 hours until soft. Allow to cool then peel and slice into 8 wedges.

Grill or chargrill the chicken breasts for 5 minutes on each side until cooked through. Allow to cool slightly and cut into 2½ cm slices.

To make the dressing place all ingredients in an airtight jar and shake to combine.

Combine the spinach leaves, walnuts and onion in a bowl then add the chicken and beetroot. Toss the dressing through the salad and serve warm.

Serves 4

NUTRITION ANALYSIS
PER SERVE
Total kJ: 1336 kJ
Carbohydrates: 5.5 g
Fat: 16.9 g
Saturated fat: 3.9 g
Protein: 35.1 g
Fibre: 3.0 g

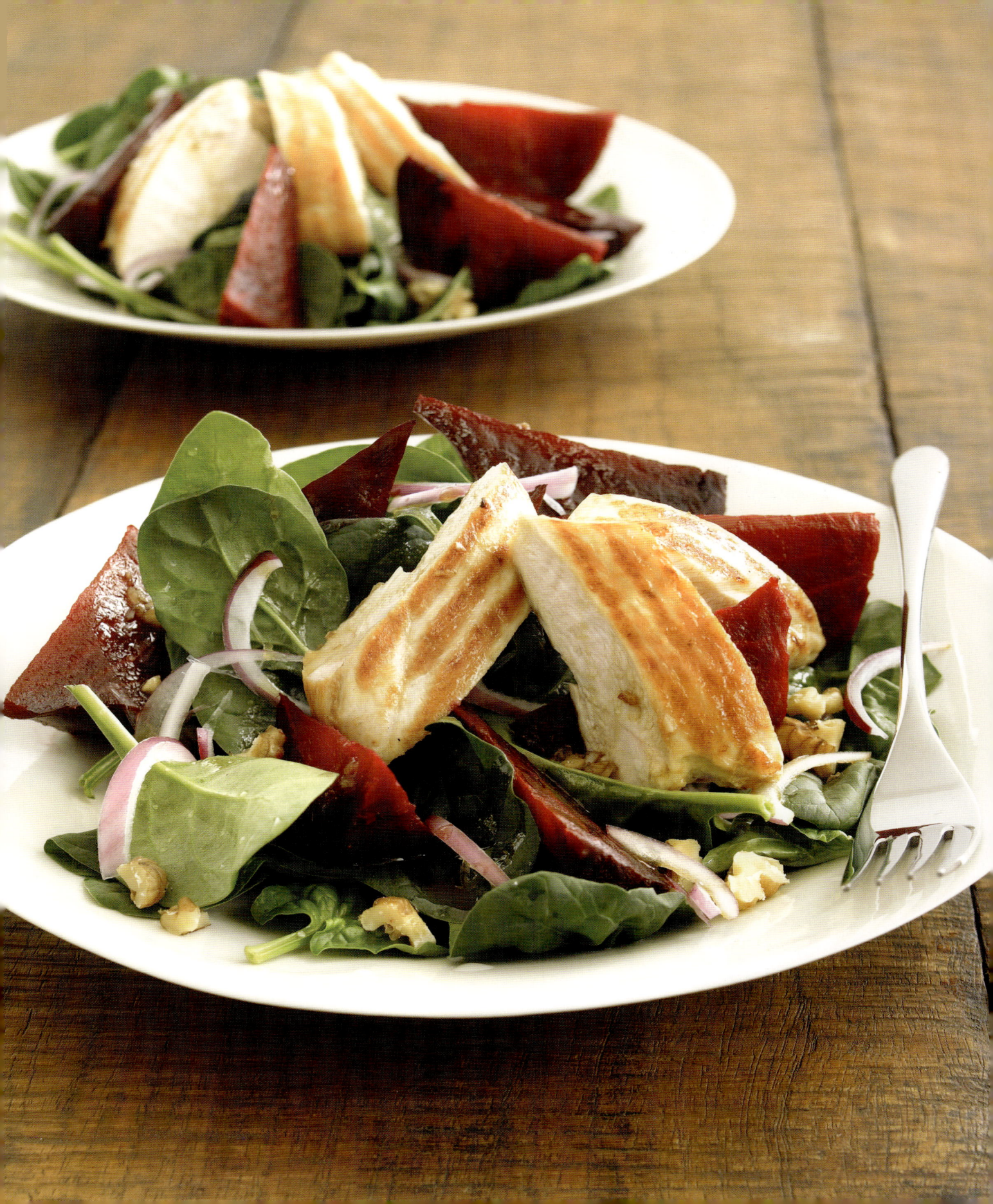

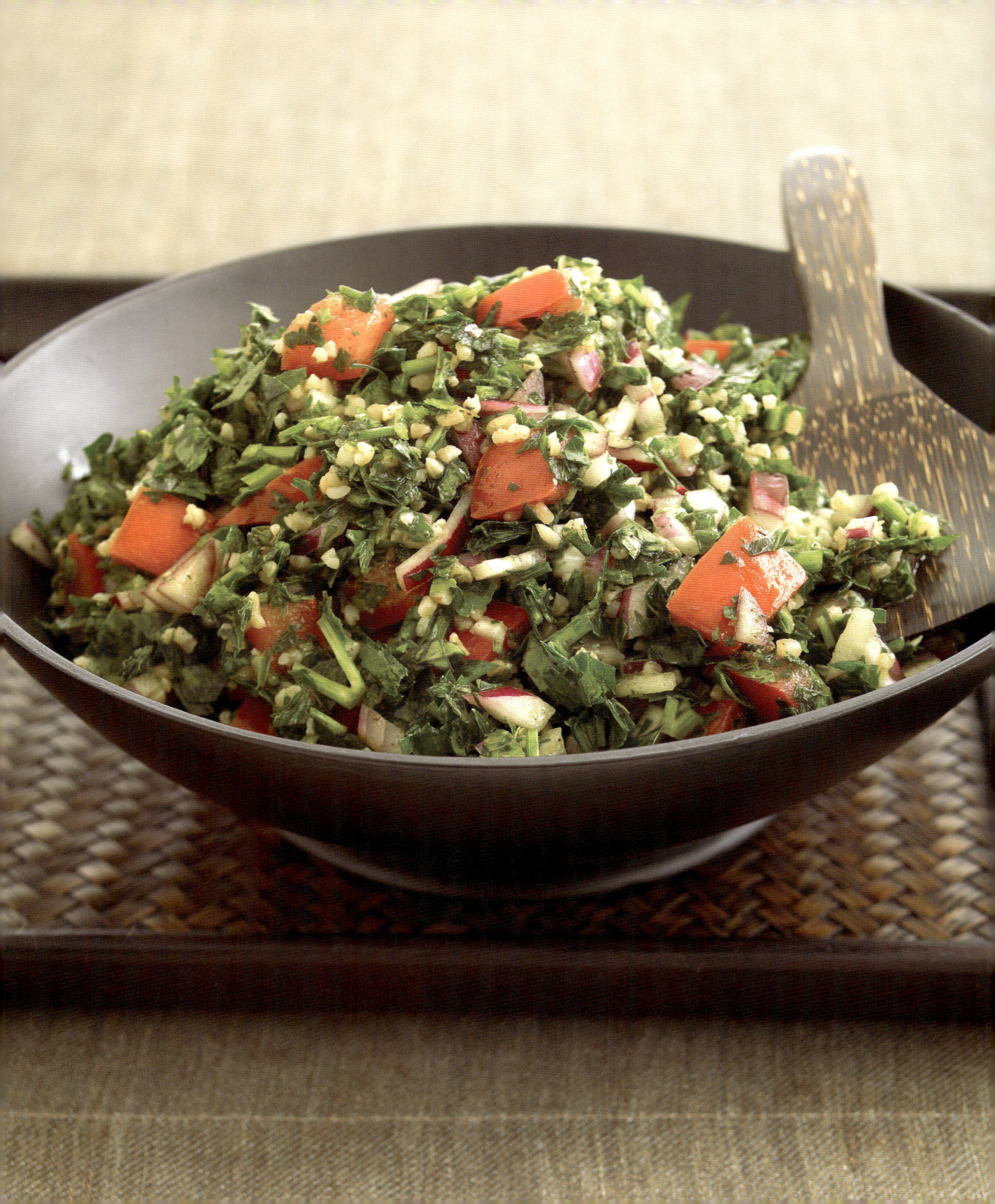

Tabouleh

This salad is a wonderful accompaniment for lamb cutlets. It can be made in advance and the dressing added when ready to serve.

2 tablespoons coarse burghul (cracked wheat)
2 tablespoons boiling water
1½ cups (roughly 1 bunch) finely chopped flat-leaf parsley
¼ cup finely chopped mint leaves
1 tomato, seeds removed, diced
1 red onion, finely diced
1 teaspoon ground cinnamon
½ teaspoon ground allspice

DRESSING
juice of 2 lemons
1 clove garlic, crushed
½ cup extra-virgin olive oil
¼ cup flaxseed oil

Place burghul and water in a bowl and set aside for 10 minutes.

To make the dressing place all ingredients in an airtight jar and shake until combined.

Combine parsley, mint, tomato and onion in a mixing bowl. Loosen the burghul with your fingertips to separate the grains. Add to the other ingredients along with the cinnamon and allspice. Toss the dressing through and serve.

Serves 4

NUTRITION ANALYSIS

PER SERVE
Total kJ: 642 kJ
Carbohydrates: 6.4 g
Fat: 12.5 g
Saturated fat: 1.5 g
Protein: 2.0 g
Fibre: 2.8 g

Harissa dressing

A great spicy accompaniment for salads or fritters. It can also be added to soups. The dressing will keep for up to 2 weeks in an airtight container in the fridge.

20 small red (birdseye) chillies, seeded and roughly chopped
5 cloves garlic, roughly chopped
1 teaspoon dried mint
1 teaspoon ground coriander
2 tablespoons extra-virgin olive oil

Place all ingredients in a food processor and process to a smooth paste.

Serves 4

> **NUTRITION ANALYSIS**
> PER SERVE
> Total kJ: 394 kJ
> Carbohydrates: 1.3 g
> Fat: 9.3 g
> Saturated fat: 1.3 g
> Protein: 0.8 g
> Fibre: 1.4 g

Fennel and orange salad

Fennel has a lovely aniseed flavour and is a good palate cleanser. This salad goes well with fish, chicken or pork dishes.

2 medium fennel bulbs, trimmed and finely sliced lengthwise
2 oranges, peeled and cut into segments
½ red onion, finely sliced
¼ cup flat-leaf parsley
1 radicchio lettuce, shredded

DRESSING
juice of 2 lemons
1 clove garlic, crushed
½ cup extra-virgin olive oil
¼ cup flaxseed oil

Place the fennel in a bowl of iced water for 5 minutes (this will make it crisper and sweeter).

To make the dressing place all ingredients in an airtight jar and shake until combined.

Drain the fennel and combine all salad ingredients. Toss the dressing through until well coated.

Serves 4

> **NUTRITION ANALYSIS**
> PER SERVE
> Total kJ: 706 kJ
> Carbohydrates: 9.7 g
> Fat: 12.5 g
> Saturated fat: 1.5 g
> Protein: 2.1 g
> Fibre: 4.9 g

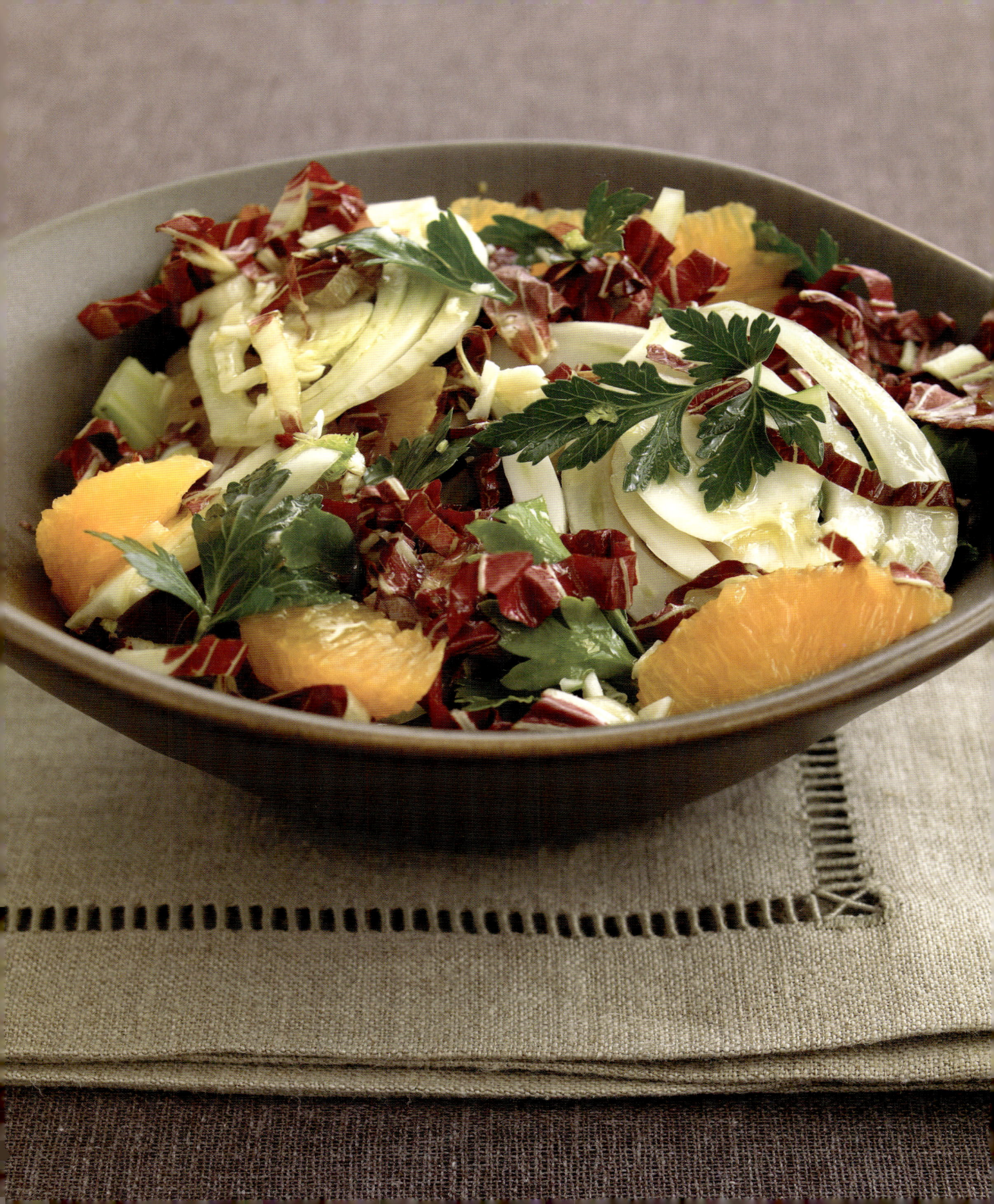

Napoli sauce

A zesty tomato sauce to use on pizzas and in all sorts of other dishes.

olive oil spray
2 onions, finely diced
4 cloves garlic, crushed
3 x 400 g cans salt-reduced crushed tomatoes
2 fresh or dried bay leaves

Heat a large saucepan over a low heat and spray lightly with oil. Cook the onions and garlic gently for a few minutes until soft. Add the tomatoes and bay leaves and simmer for 1 hour. Remove the bay leaves, allow to cool slightly, then purée using a blender or hand-held processor if desired.

Makes 1 litre

NUTRITION ANALYSIS
PER SERVE
Total kJ: 178 kJ
Carbohydrates: 5.4 g
Fat: 1.2 g
Saturated fat: 0.1 g
Protein: 1.5 g
Fibre: 2.0 g

Tuna and asparagus salad

You can assemble this salad so quickly – it's perfect to take to work.

1 x 425 g can tuna in springwater
2 bunches asparagus, sliced into 7 cm lengths
½ cup corn kernels
½ red capsicum, finely sliced
4 spring onions, finely sliced
50 g mixed lettuce leaves
½ cup coriander leaves

DRESSING
1 tablespoon Dijon mustard
1½ teaspoons seeded mustard
1 tablespoon low-fat natural yoghurt
1½ teaspoons white wine vinegar
juice of 1 lemon

Drain the tuna. Steam the asparagus for 3–5 minutes until tender then allow to cool. To make the dressing place all ingredients in an airtight jar and shake until combined. Combine all salad ingredients and drizzle with dressing.

Serves 4

NUTRITION ANALYSIS
PER SERVE
Total kJ: 825 kJ
Carbohydrates: 9.6 g
Fat: 3.2 g
Saturated fat: 1.1 g
Protein: 30.0 g
Fibre: 3.7 g

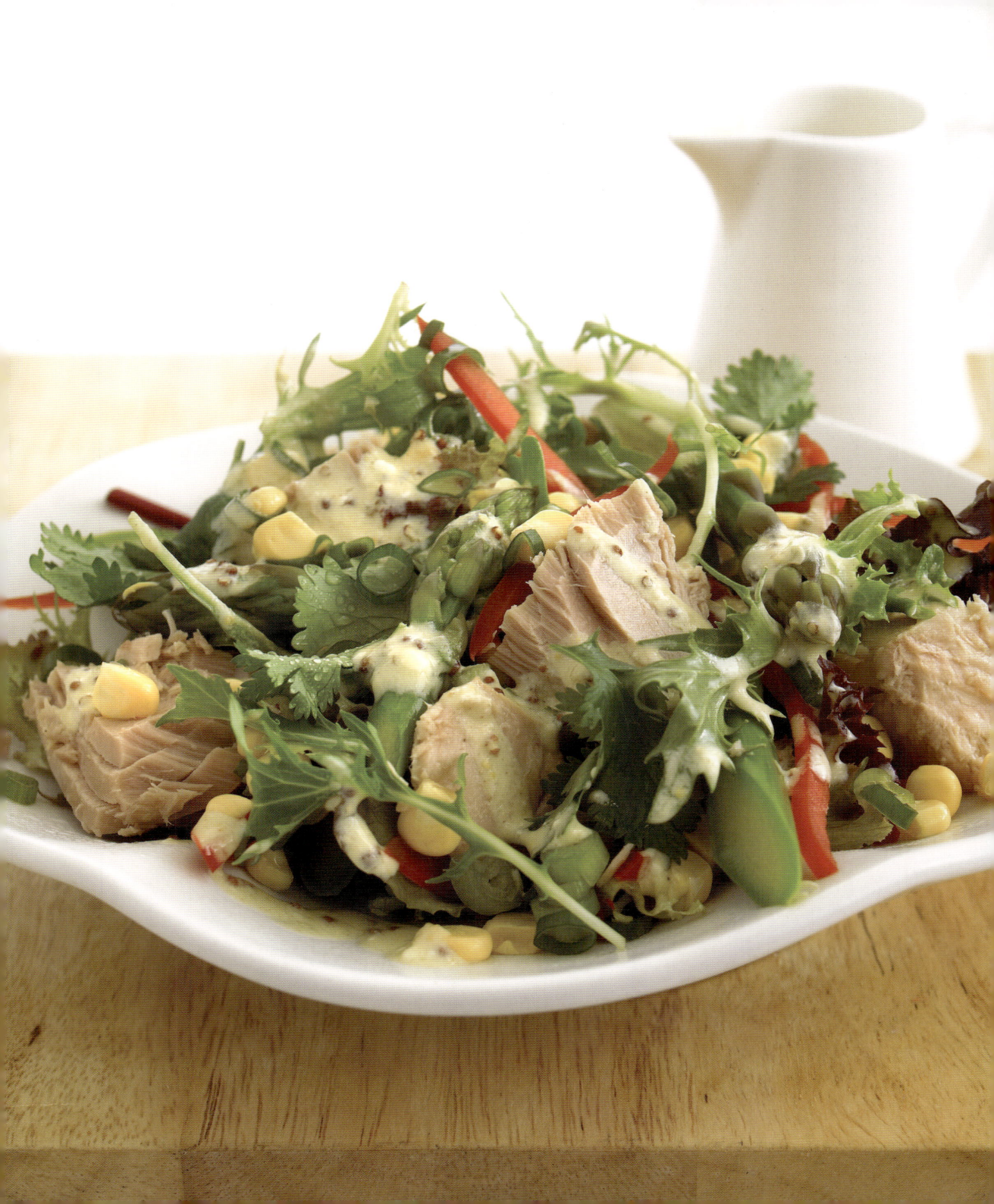

Chickpea, fetta and coriander tarts

These savoury tarts are easy to make and are great for picnics.

1 x 400 g can chickpeas, rinsed and drained
1 cup tomato passata or Napoli Sauce
    (see page 182)
100 g reduced-fat fetta, crumbled
½ cup chopped coriander leaves
freshly ground black pepper
1 egg
4 sheets filo pastry
olive oil spray

Preheat oven to 220°C (430°F).

Place the chickpeas in a mixing bowl and mash with a fork. Add the passata, fetta and coriander and mix together well. Season with pepper to taste then stir in egg.

Lay a sheet of filo on the bench, keeping the remainder covered to prevent them from drying out. Spray the sheet lightly with oil and fold in half. Repeat this once then cut in half, giving you 2 rectangles of pastry.

Spray a muffin tin lightly with oil and line each mould with a filo piece, pressing it down around the base and edges. Fill the moulds evenly with the chickpea mixture and bake for 20 minutes or until the pastry is golden brown.

Makes 8 tarts (2 per serve)

NUTRITION ANALYSIS

PER SERVE
Total kJ: 995 kJ
Carbohydrates: 23.0 g
Fat: 7.6 g
Saturated fat: 3.1 g
Protein: 16.6 g
Fibre: 6.1 g

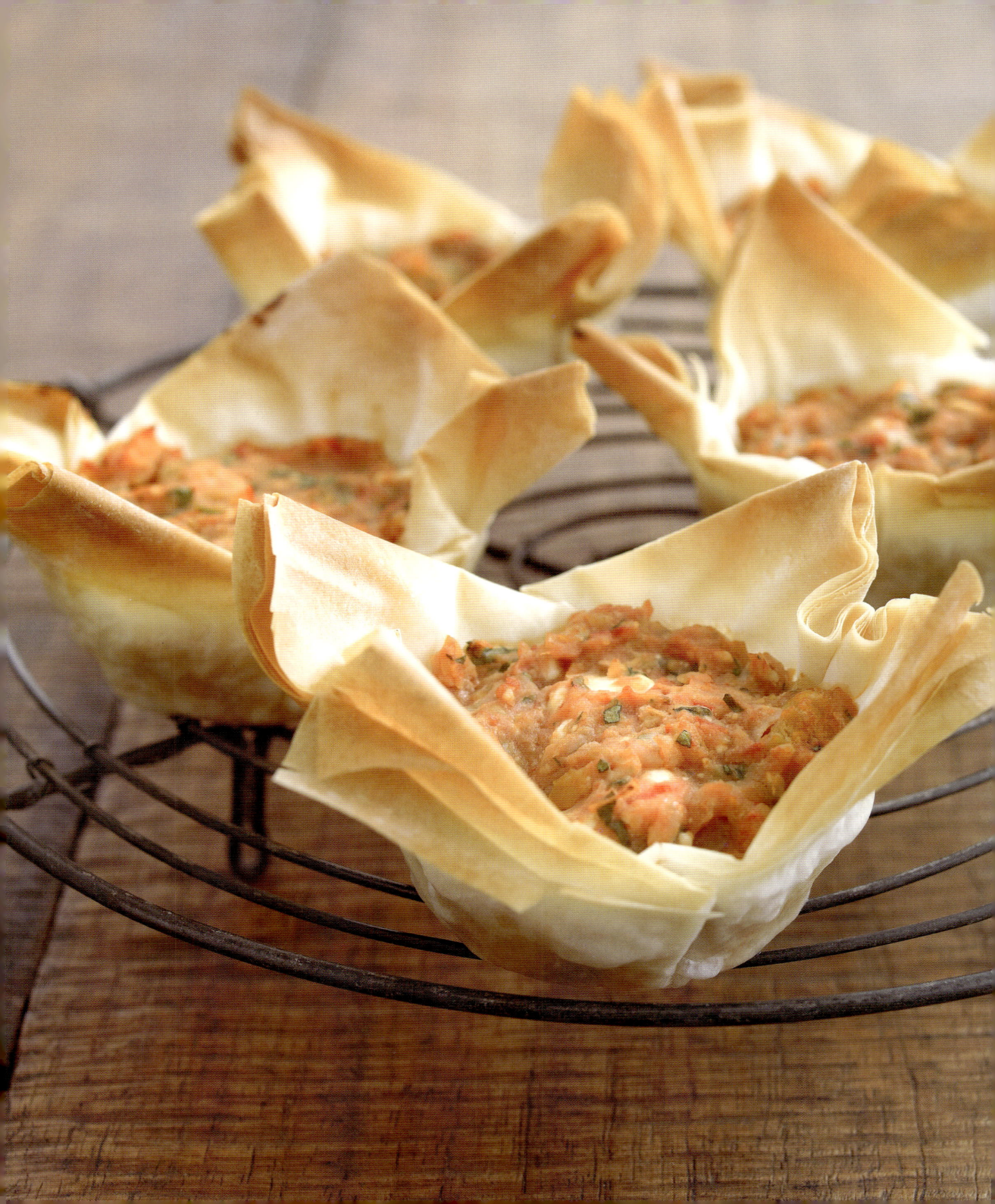

Zucchini, tomato and basil frittata

This is very simple to make and lovely served warm or cold with a simple green salad and Harissa Dressing (see page 180).

olive oil spray
2 red onions, finely sliced
2 cloves garlic, crushed
3 zucchini, grated
3 ripe roma tomatoes, diced
6 eggs
½ cup grated reduced-fat cheddar cheese
4 tablespoons finely shredded basil

Preheat oven to 150°C (300°F).

Heat a large, ovenproof pan over a low heat. Spray lightly with oil and gently cook the onions and garlic for a few minutes until soft. Add zucchini and tomatoes and warm through.

Whisk eggs, cheese and basil in a mixing bowl and pour into the hot pan, mixing thoroughly. Increase the heat slightly and cook without stirring for 5 minutes. Transfer to the oven for a further 25–30 minutes or until golden and set in the middle.

Remove from oven and let stand for a further 5 minutes before loosening the edges with a knife. Turn out onto a plate and serve.

Serves 4

NUTRITION ANALYSIS

PER SERVE
Total kJ: 952 kJ
Carbohydrates: 9.0 g
Fat: 11.7 g
Saturated fat: 4.5 g
Protein: 19.4 g
Fibre: 4.5 g

Spiced lamb pockets

These pockets make a tasty lunch or a quick dinner the whole family will love. To reduce the carbohydrate content serve patties with salad and dressing only.

500 g lean lamb mince
1½ teaspoons ground cumin
2 tablespoons finely chopped flat-leaf parsley
1 egg
1 tablespoon harissa* or Harissa Dressing (see page 180)
olive oil spray
1 onion, finely diced
1 clove garlic, crushed

DRESSING

4 tablespoons low-fat natural yoghurt
1 teaspoon harissa*
juice of 1 lemon

*Harissa paste is available from delicatessens.

TO SERVE

4 small wholemeal pita bread pockets
1 roma tomato, finely sliced
½ cup shredded iceberg lettuce
½ red onion, finely sliced

Combine lamb, cumin, parsley, egg and harissa in a large mixing bowl.

Heat a large frying pan over a low heat and spray lightly with oil. Add onion and garlic and cook gently for a few minutes until soft. Add to the lamb mixture and combine. Shape mixture into 12 patties, roughly 7 cm in diameter.

Spray a little more oil in the pan and cook patties for 6–8 minutes on each side.

To serve, gently open pita bread pockets and divide tomato, lettuce and onion evenly among them. Place lamb patties in pockets and drizzle with dressing.

Serves 4

NUTRITION ANALYSIS

PER SERVE
Total kJ: 1770 kJ
Carbohydrates: 25.5 g
Fat: 18.1 g
Saturated fat: 8.9 g
Protein: 37.1 g
Fibre: 4.4 g

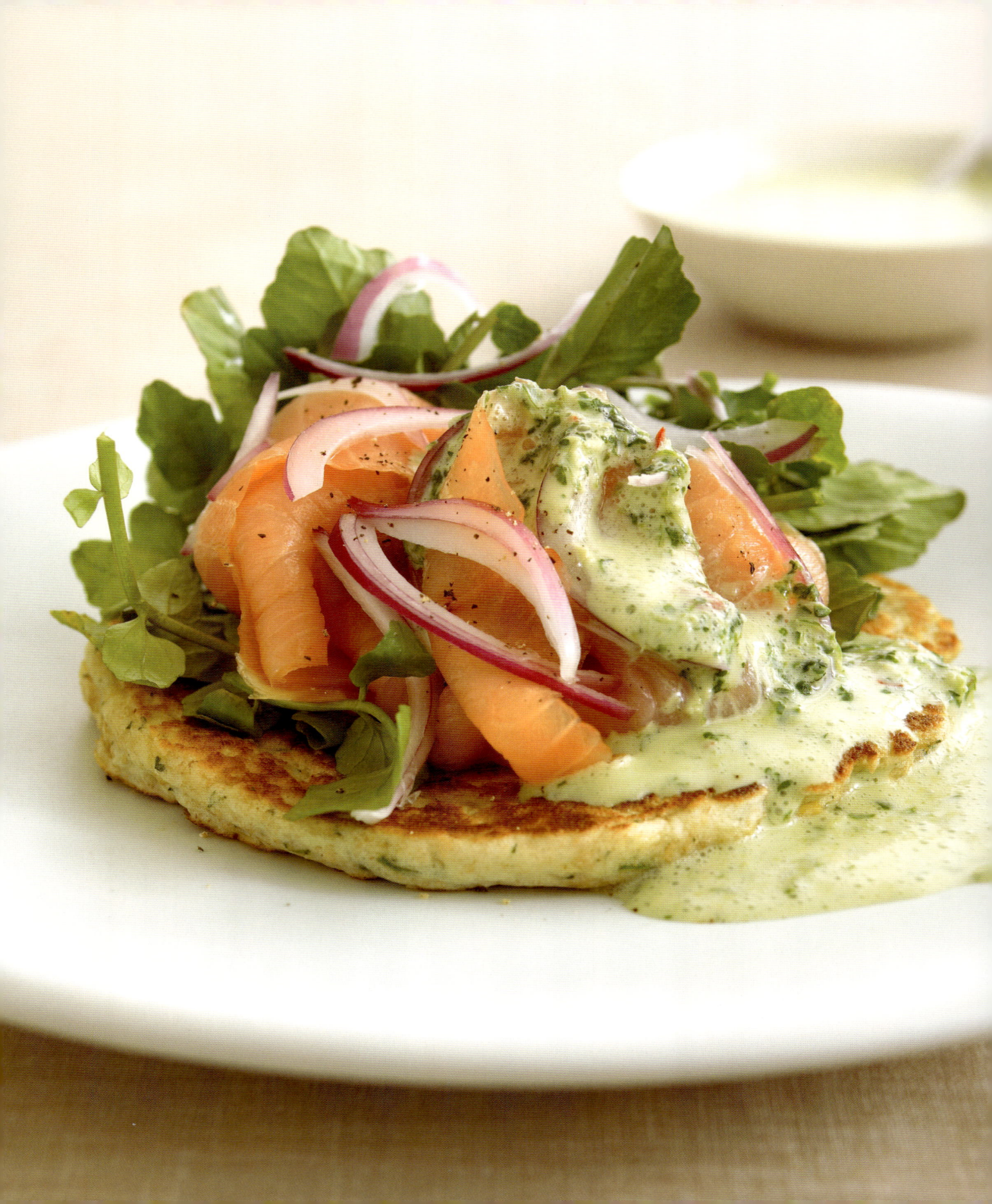

Corn fritters with smoked salmon and coriander dressing

A light and satisfying meal, perfect for weekend lunches.

DRESSING
1 cup chopped coriander leaves
juice ½ lemon
2 cloves garlic, roughly chopped
2 small red (birdseye) chillies, seeded and finely sliced
5 tablespoons low-fat natural yoghurt

½ cup wholemeal self-raising flour
¼ teaspoon baking powder
2 spring onions, finely sliced
1 tablespoon chopped dill
1 x 200 g cooked corn cob, kernels removed, or 200 g can corn kernels
4 tablespoons low-fat milk
2 egg whites
olive oil spray
freshly ground black pepper
8 slices smoked salmon, cut into 5 cm pieces
125 g watercress
¼ red onion, finely sliced

To make the dressing place coriander, lemon juice, garlic and chillies in a food processor and process to a smooth paste. Add the yoghurt and set aside.

Combine flour, baking powder, spring onions, dill and corn in a mixing bowl. Add milk and stir thoroughly.

In another bowl whisk egg whites until fluffy then gently fold through the flour mixture.

Heat a large frying pan over a medium heat and spray lightly with oil. Spoon the mixture into the pan and cook until small bubbles form on the surface.

Turn the fritters over and cook for a further 5 minutes or until golden.

Combine the salmon, watercress and onion and arrange on top of the fritters. Drizzle with coriander dressing. The dressing will keep for up to 3 days stored in an airtight container in the fridge.

Serves 4

NUTRITION ANALYSIS
PER SERVE
Total kJ: 1095 kJ
Carbohydrates: 29.0 g
Fat: 5.0 g
Saturated fat: 1.1 g
Protein: 21.0 g
Fibre: 5.6 g

Spicy beef and mushroom kebabs

These are fantastic done on the barbecue. Use any combination of vegetables.

MARINADE
2 tablespoons grated ginger
2 cloves garlic, crushed
juice of 2 limes
2 small red (birdseye) chillies, seeded and finely sliced
½ cup oyster sauce
1 teaspoon sesame oil
2 tablespoons vegetable oil

500 g lean beef, cut into cubes
2 corn cobs, husks removed and cut into 2½ cm rounds
1 red capsicum, cored, seeded and cut into squares
1 zucchini, cut into 2½ cm rounds
1 red onion, cut into wedges
8 flat mushrooms, wiped, stalks removed, and cut in half

Combine marinade ingredients and pour over beef pieces, tossing to coat. Marinate overnight or for a minimum of 2 hours.

If using bamboo skewers, soak in water for 30 minutes.

Steam corn for 5–7 minutes or until tender.

Thread alternating pieces of beef and vegetables onto skewers. Use any leftover marinade to baste during cooking.

Place skewers under a hot grill and cook for for 8–10 minutes, turning once. Serve with a salad of mixed green leaves.

Serves 4

NUTRITION ANALYSIS
PER SERVE
Total kJ: 1230 kJ
Carbohydrates: 11.4 g
Fat: 10.2 g
Saturated fat: 4.3 g
Protein: 37.0 g
Fibre: 3.3 g

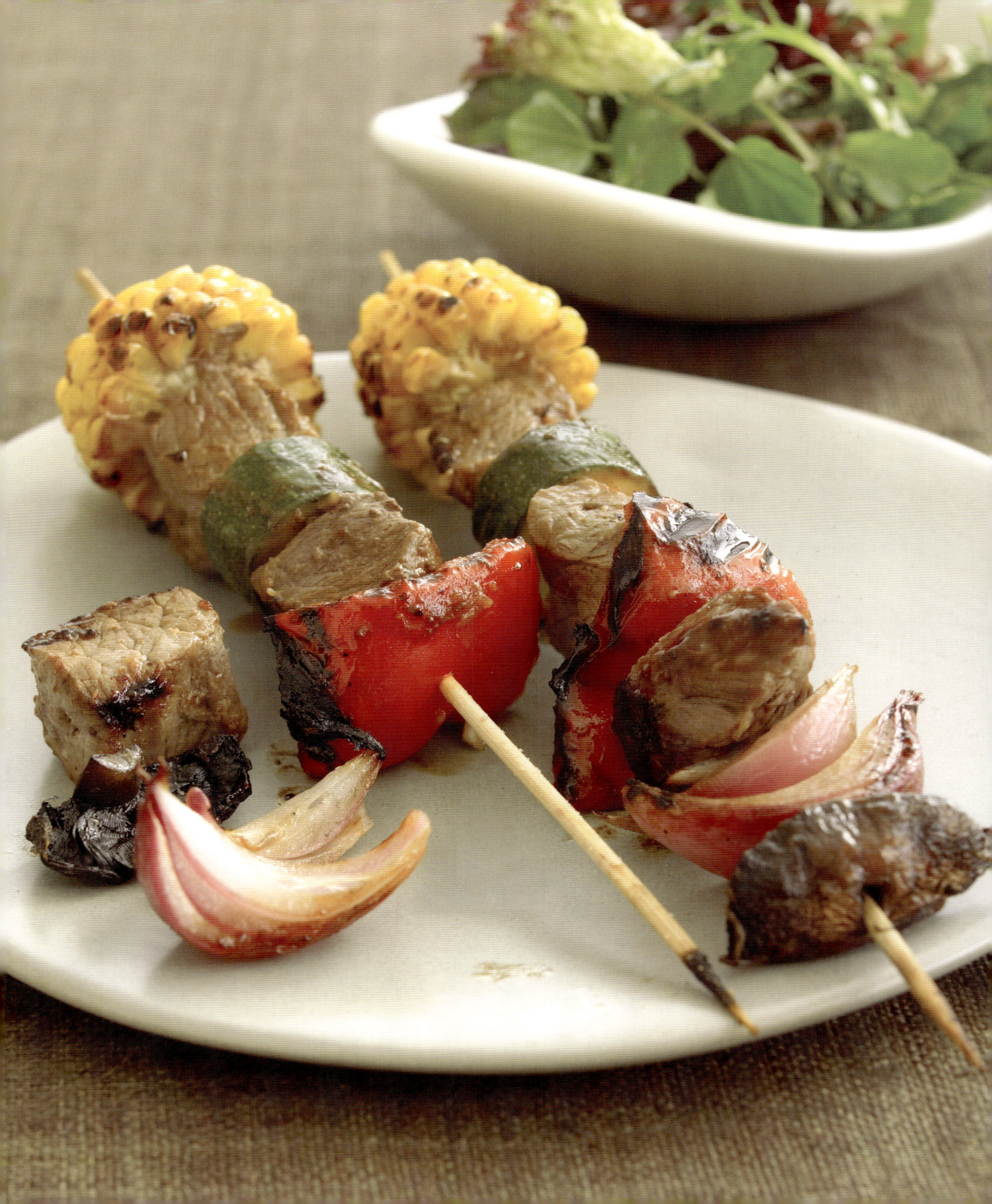

Lamb and pine nut pizza

This pizza base is easy to make and is enough for a 12-inch pizza base. Alternatively you could use a piece of pita bread.

BASE
2½ cups wholemeal self-raising flour
3 heaped tablespoons low-fat natural yoghurt

olive oil spray
250 g lamb fillets, trimmed
3 tablespoons tomato paste, or 5 tablespoons Napoli Sauce (see page 182)
½ red onion, finely sliced
1 tablespoon pine nuts
50 g baby rocket leaves
2 tablespoons low-fat natural yoghurt

Preheat oven to 220°C (430°F).

Sift the flour into a mixing bowl, make a well in the centre and add the yoghurt. Mix well to form a smooth dough. Press dough into a lightly greased pizza tray so that it covers the base evenly (about 1 cm thick).

Heat a large frying pan over a medium heat and spray lightly with oil. Add the lamb and brown on all sides. Transfer to an ovenproof dish and cook for a further 5 minutes in the oven. Remove, allow to cool slightly and cut into 1 cm slices. Keep warm.

Bake pizza base for 7 minutes until golden around the edges. Remove base from oven, top with napoli sauce and arrange onion and lamb slices. Bake for a further 10 minutes.

Toast the pine nuts in a dry pan over a low heat until golden.

Serve pizza topped with rocket leaves, pine nuts and yoghurt.

Serves 4

NUTRITION ANALYSIS
PER SERVE
Total kJ: 1884 kJ
Carbohydrates: 61.0 g
Fat: 8.2 g
Saturated fat: 1.3 g
Protein: 25.0 g
Fibre: 11.3 g

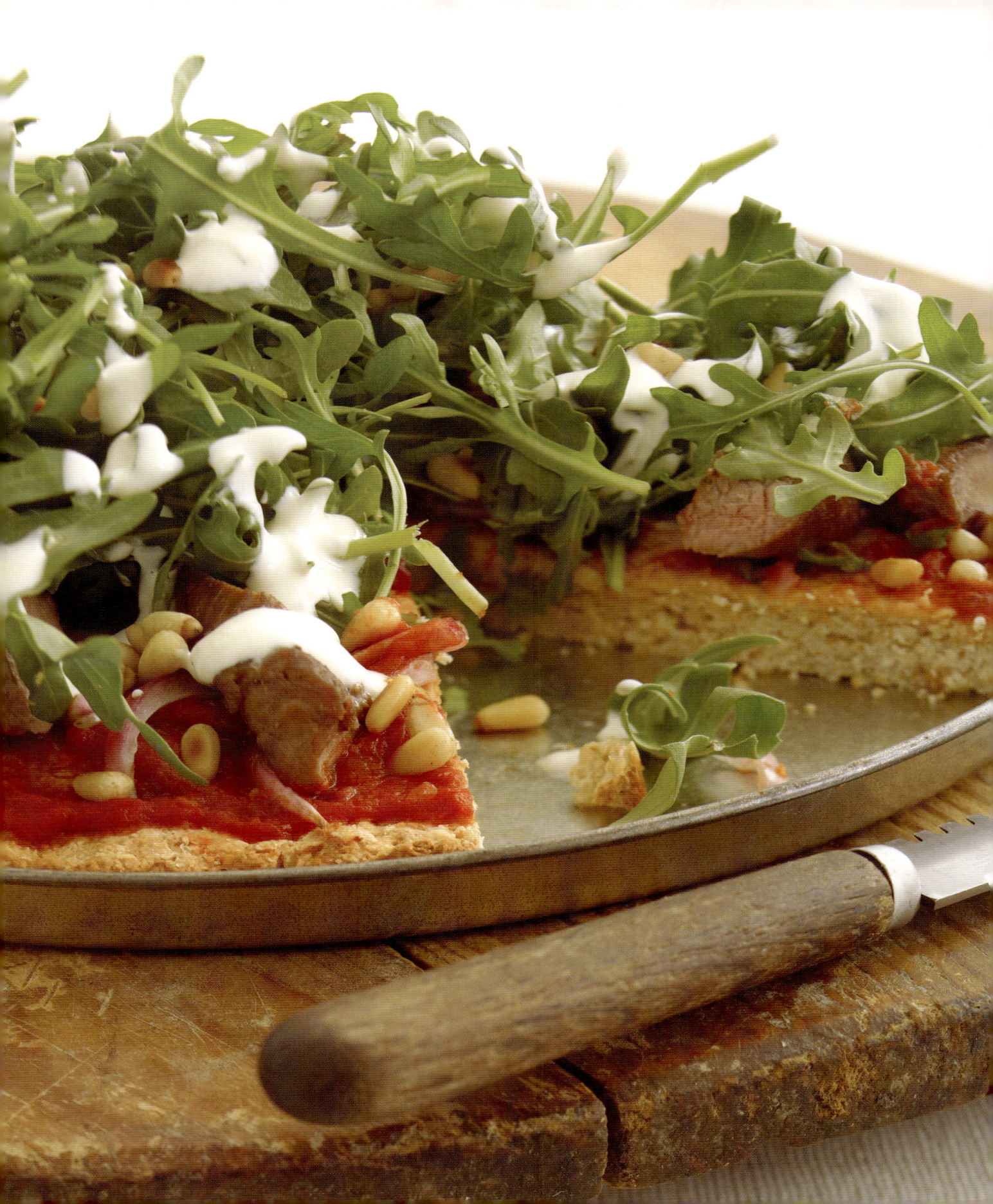

Dinners

Chicken cacciatore

A delicious winter warmer that requires little preparation – just pop it into the oven and relax.

olive oil spray
1 leek, trimmed, finely sliced and washed
3 sticks celery, finely diced
2 carrots, peeled and finely diced
2 cloves garlic, crushed
3 chicken thigh fillets, trimmed and each cut into 4 pieces
2 tablespoons tomato paste
4 tablespoons red wine
2 sprigs thyme
200 g mushrooms, finely sliced
2 x 400 g cans salt-reduced crushed tomatoes
½ cup chicken stock (recipe on page 167)
50 g roughly chopped pitted black olives
2 bay leaves
2 tablespoons balsamic vinegar

Preheat the oven to 200°C (400°F).

Heat a large, ovenproof pan over a low heat and spray lightly with oil. Cook the leek, celery, carrots and garlic gently for a few minutes until soft. Increase the heat, add chicken pieces and brown for 4–5 minutes. Add the tomato paste and cook for a further 3 minutes, stirring. Add the red wine to the pan and cook for a further 2 minutes. Add the thyme and mushrooms and cover with the tomatoes and chicken stock. Bring to the boil then remove from heat. Add the olives, bay leaves and balsamic vinegar and transfer the dish to the oven. Cook for 45 minutes, turning chicken pieces two or three times, until tender. Remove bay leaves and serve with brown rice.

Serves 4

NUTRITION ANALYSIS
PER SERVE
Total kJ: 541 kJ
Carbohydrates: 41.5 g
Fat: 9.4 g
Saturated fat: 2.5 g
Protein: 23.3 g
Fibre: 8.7 g

Chicken san choy bau

A quick and easy dish to prepare that is great for entertaining. Fried noodles are 5 cm lengths of precooked thin noodles, found in the Asian section of the supermarket.

olive oil spray
2 teaspoons grated ginger
2 onions, finely diced
4 cloves garlic, crushed
1 small red (birdseye) chilli, seeded and finely sliced
350 g chicken mince
1 teaspoon cornflour
1 egg yolk
4 iceberg lettuce leaf cups, washed
1 teaspoon sesame oil
1 teaspoon fish sauce
2 tablespoons lime juice
2 tablespoons light soy sauce
2 teaspoons kecap manis (sweet soy sauce)
¼ cup fried shallots
¼ cup fried noodles
¼ cup coriander leaves
¼ cup Vietnamese mint leaves

Heat a large frying pan or wok over a low heat, spray lightly with oil and cook ginger, onions, garlic and chilli gently until soft. Increase the heat, add chicken mince and cook for a few minutes, breaking up with a wooden spoon.

Combine cornflour and egg yolk to form a smooth paste.

Drain off any excess liquid from the mince before adding the sesame oil, fish sauce, lime juice, soy sauce, kecap manis and egg mixture. Cook for 5 minutes over a medium heat, stirring occasionally, then remove from heat and mix through the fried shallots and noodles.

Divide mixture evenly between the lettuce cups and top with coriander and mint leaves.

Serves 4

NUTRITION ANALYSIS
PER SERVE
Total kJ: 1107 kJ
Carbohydrates: 9 g
Fat: 11.9 g
Saturated fat: 3.3 g
Protein: 27.9 g
Fibre: 3.5 g

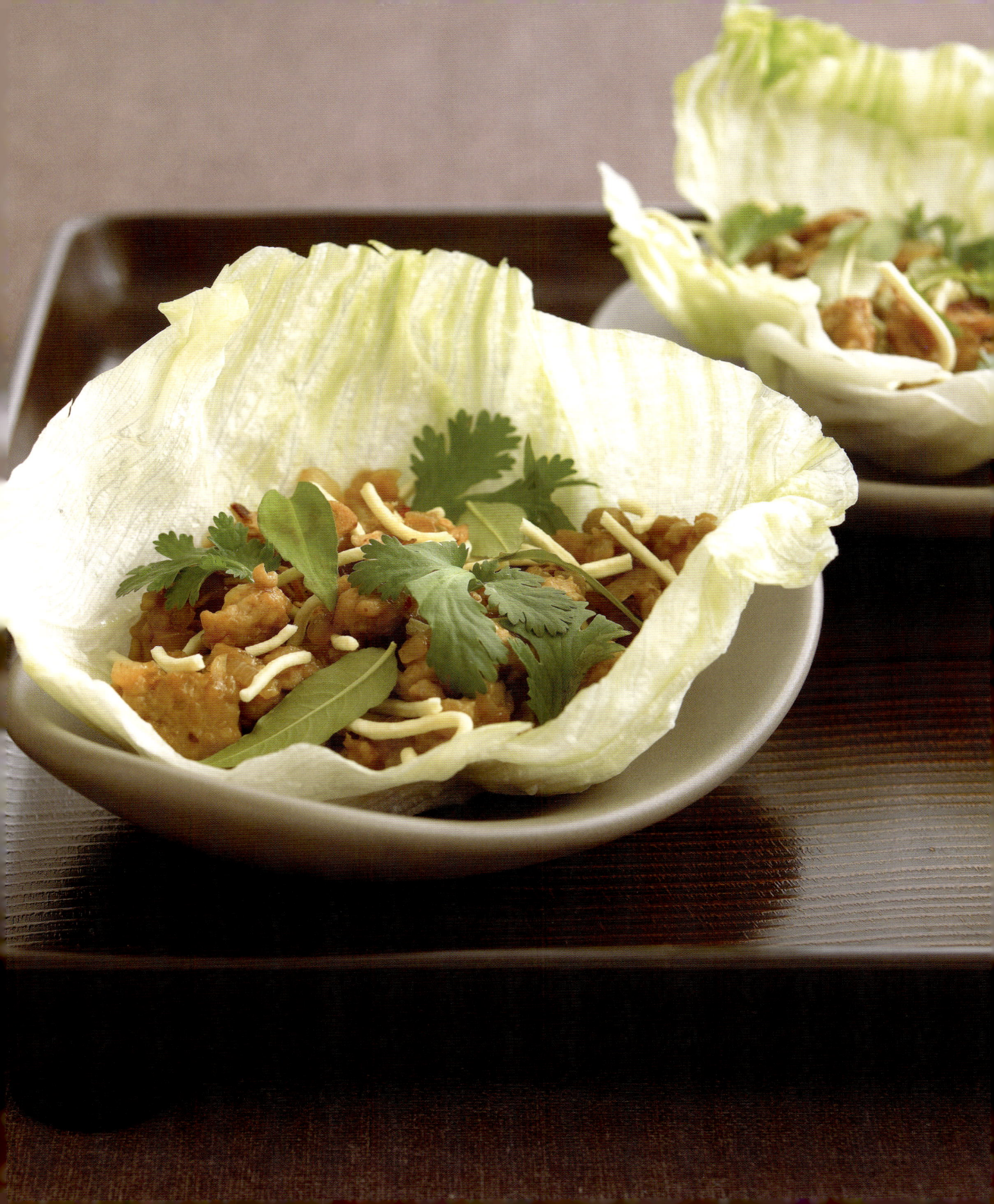

Chicken and cashew stir-fry

The combination of tender chicken pieces and crunchy vegetables and cashews make this stir-fry a winner.

MARINADE
- 1 tablespoon grated ginger
- ½ small red chilli (birdseye), seeded and finely sliced
- 2 cloves garlic, crushed
- 1 tablespoon soy sauce
- 1 teaspoon kecap manis (sweet soy sauce)
- ½ teaspoon fish sauce
- 1 tablespoon lime juice
- ½ teaspoon oyster sauce
- ½ teaspoon mirin (Japanese rice wine)

- 2 medium skinless chicken breasts, cut into 1 cm strips
- olive oil spray
- 2 onions, finely sliced
- 1 tablespoon grated ginger
- 4 cloves garlic, crushed
- 120 g baby corn spears, cut into thirds
- 1 large head broccoli, cut into small florets
- ½ red capsicum, finely sliced
- ¼ cup water
- 100 g rice vermicelli noodles
- 1 teaspoon cornflour
- 7 water chestnuts, sliced
- ¼ cup raw cashew nuts, roughly chopped
- ¼ cup chopped coriander leaves

Combine marinade ingredients and pour half over the chicken pieces, tossing to coat. Leave to marinate for 2 hours.

Heat a wok or large frying pan over a low heat, spray lightly with oil, add the onions and cook gently for a few minutes until soft. Add the ginger, garlic and corn and cook lightly for a couple of minutes. Remove chicken pieces from the marinade, reserving any remaining liquid, and add to the wok. Increase heat and toss for 3 minutes until browned. Add the broccoli, capsicum and water. Reduce to a simmer and cook for 7 minutes, stirring occasionally, until tender. Stir the remaining marinade through and heat.

Cover the vermicelli noodles with boiling water and let stand for 2 minutes, then drain. Mix the cornflour with a teaspoon of water. Move all ingredients to one side of the wok and add the cornflour mixture, stirring until it thickens to a sauce. Add the noodles, water chestnuts, cashew nuts and coriander leaves, mix everything together thoroughly and serve.

Serves 4

NUTRITION ANALYSIS
PER SERVE
Total kJ: 1816 kJ
Carbohydrates: 17.6 g
Fat: 18.3 g
Saturated fat: 4.4 g
Protein: 46.9 g
Fibre: 4.6 g

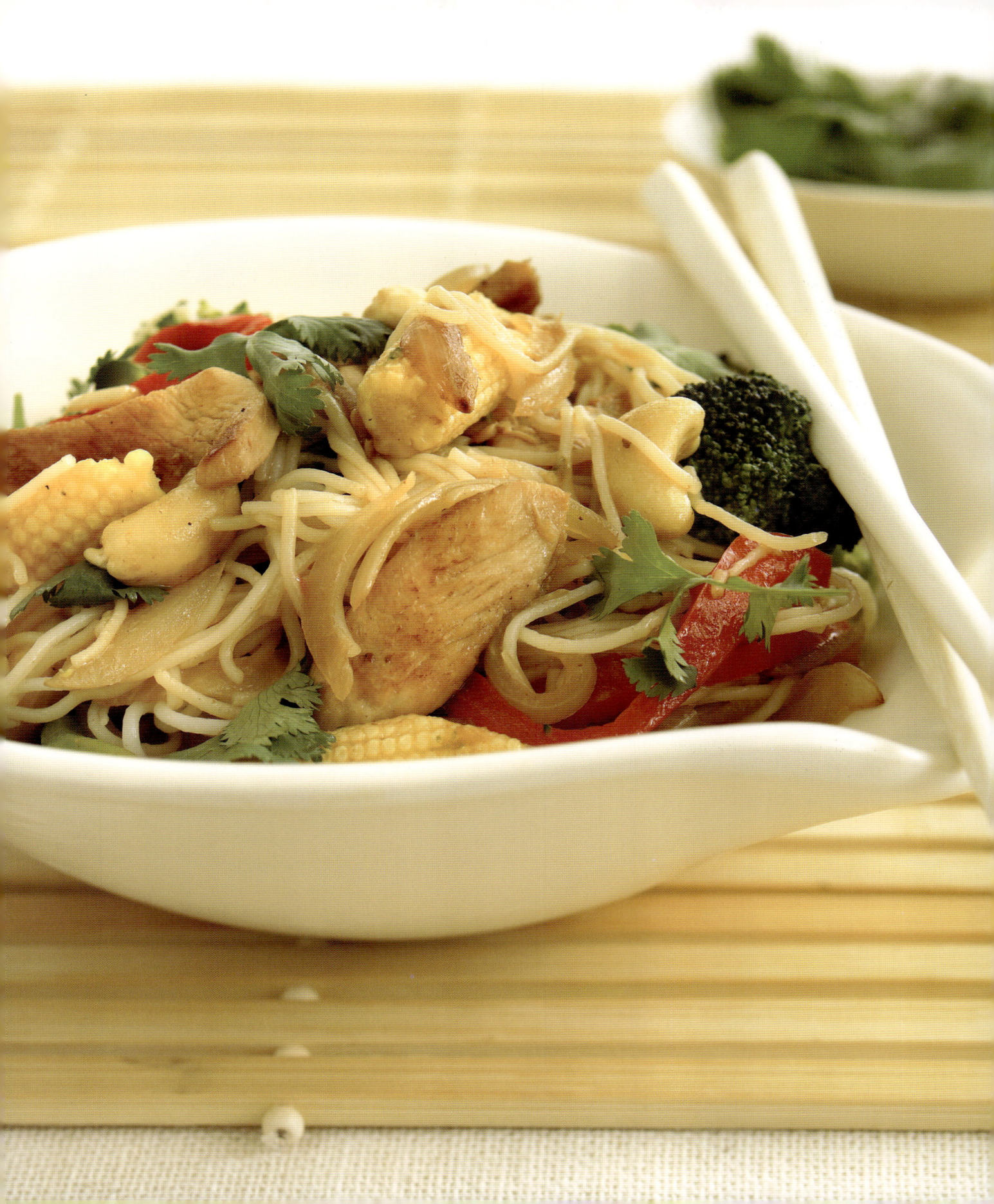

Chicken and spinach lasagne

This delicious lasagne comes with a with a twist: no pasta.

olive oil spray
1 onion, finely diced
4 cloves garlic, crushed
½ bunch spinach, stemmed, washed and roughly chopped
3 chicken thigh fillets, trimmed, cut into 1 cm strips
3 cups tomato passata or Napoli Sauce (see page 182)
200 g low-fat ricotta, crumbled
½ cup grated reduced-fat cheddar cheese
350 g sweet potato, peeled and cut into wafer-thin slices

Preheat oven to 200°C (400°F).

Heat a large frying pan over a medium heat, spray lightly with oil and cook the onion and garlic gently until soft. Add half the spinach, and cook gently until wilted then tip mixture into a bowl. Add the remaining spinach to the pan and cook until wilted, then add to the bowl and allow to cool.

Add more oil and cook the chicken until lightly browned. Add the tomato passata or napoli sauce and stir to combine. Remove from heat.

Squeeze any excess water from the spinach and chop roughly. Combine with the ricotta and cheddar cheese.

Spray the base and sides of an ovenproof dish lightly with oil and cover the base with sweet potato slices. Spoon a third of the chicken and tomato sauce mixture onto it, and then a layer of the chopped spinach and ricotta mixture. Repeat this process twice, finishing with a layer of cheese. Cover the dish with a lid or tightly with foil and place in the oven. After 30 minutes remove the lid or foil and bake for a further 20 minutes until golden.

Remove from oven and let stand for 10 minutes before serving with a simple green salad.

Serves 4

NUTRITION ANALYSIS
PER SERVE
Total kJ: 1440 kJ
Carbohydrates: 13.1 g
Fat: 16.3 g
Saturated fat: 7.8 g
Protein: 32.9 g
Fibre: 6.2 g

Beef stir-fry with hokkien noodles

Colourful, delicious and quick to prepare, this dish is also extremely versatile. Any combination of vegetables can be used.

MARINADE

- 2 tablespoons cornflour
- 1 teaspoon bicarbonate of soda
- 1 teaspoon sesame seeds
- 2 tablespoons lime juice
- 2 tablespoons kecap manis (sweet soy sauce)

- 400 g lean beef strips
- olive oil spray
- 2 onions, finely sliced
- 2 tablespoons grated ginger
- 4 cloves garlic, crushed
- 1 carrot, peeled and finely sliced
- 1 red capsicum, finely sliced
- 100g snow peas, trimmed and cut in half
- ¼ cup water
- 200 g hokkien noodles

Combine marinade ingredients and pour over the beef strips, tossing to coat. Leave to marinate for 5–10 minutes.

Heat a wok or large frying pan over a medium heat and spray lightly with oil. Add onions and cook gently until soft, then add ginger, garlic and carrot and cook lightly for a few minutes until they begin to soften. Move vegetables to one side of the wok, increase heat and add the beef, reserving any remaining marinade. Cook over a high heat, stirring vigorously, until beef is browned on all sides, then mix everything thoroughly. Add the capsicum, snow peas, water and noodles and cook for 3–5 minutes until vegetables are tender.

Add any remaining marinade, stir through to heat and serve.

Serves 4

NUTRITION ANALYSIS

PER SERVE

Total kJ: 1435 kJ
Carbohydrates: 20.6 g
Fat: 10.8 g
Saturated fat: 4.4 g
Protein: 38.7 g
Fibre: 3.1 g

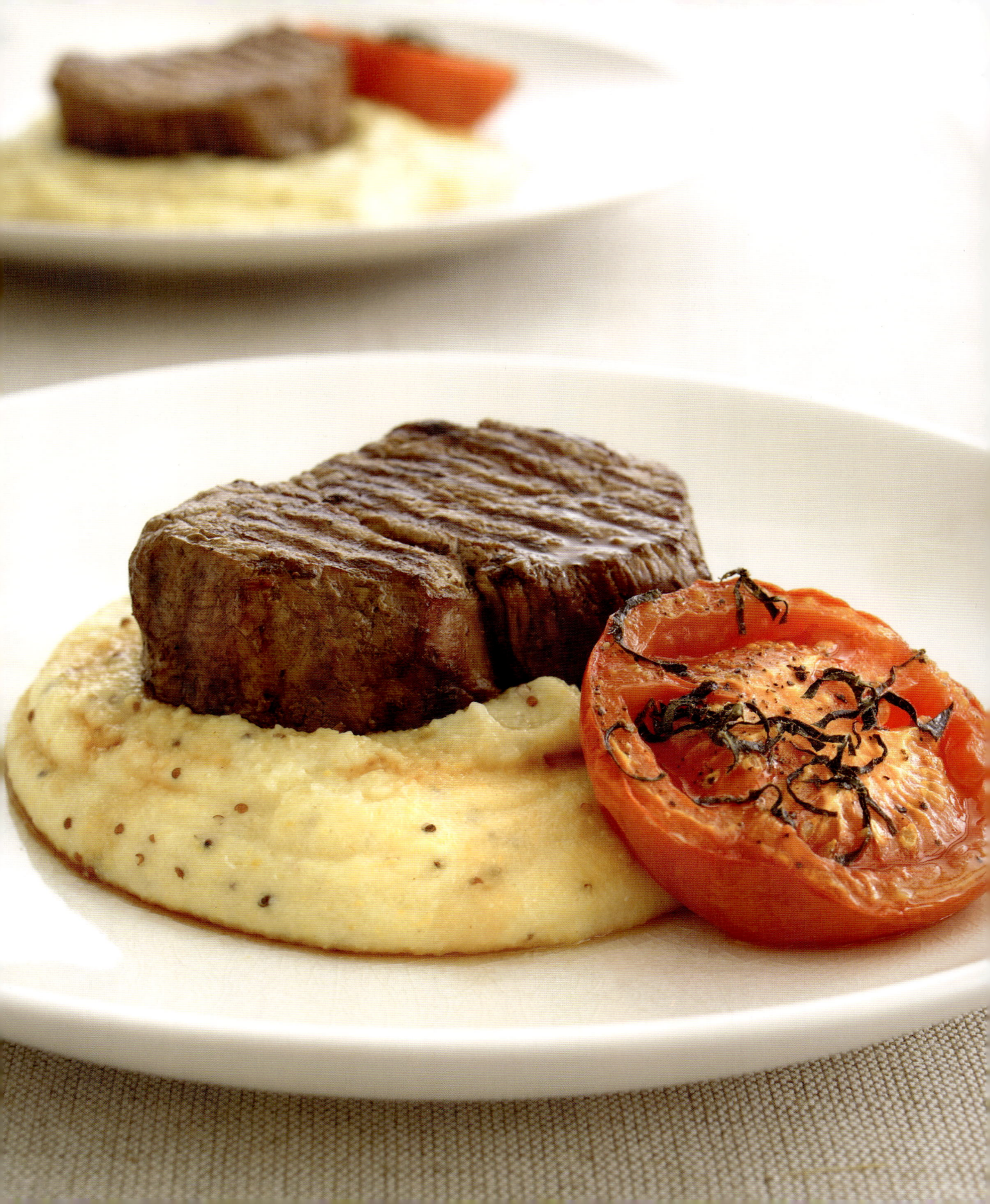

Grilled eye fillet with mustard polenta

Polenta is derived from corn so is great for those on a gluten-free diet.

2 tomatoes, cut in half widthwise
olive oil spray
2 teaspoons chopped oregano leaves
freshly ground black pepper
4 x 200 g eye fillet steaks

POLENTA

2 cups water
1½ cups low-fat milk
⅔ cup polenta
1½ teaspoons hot English mustard
1½ tablespoons seeded mustard

Preheat oven to 150°C (300°F).

Place tomatoes on a baking tray and spray lightly with oil. Top with oregano leaves and pepper. Bake in the oven for 30–40 minutes until tender.

Bring water and milk to the boil in a saucepan over a medium heat. Whisk in the polenta, ensuring it is well combined. Reduce heat and simmer for 40 minutes, whisking occasionally, until smooth and thick.

Halfway through the polenta cooking time, cook steaks under a hot grill for 5–7 minutes on each side. Alternatively, heat a large frying pan over a high heat and spray lightly with oil. Cook the steaks for 5–7 minutes on each side or as desired.

Set steaks aside to rest for 5 minutes in a warm place, loosely covered with foil. Add the mustards to the polenta and mix well. Spoon polenta onto each plate and place steak on top. Drizzle over any juices from the pan and serve with the roasted tomatoes.

Serves 4

NUTRITION ANALYSIS
PER SERVE
Total kJ: 1158 kJ
Carbohydrates: 3.9 g
Fat: 11.3 g
Saturated fat: 5.2 g
Protein: 39.0 g
Fibre: 0.8 g

Thai beef salad

A light and satisfying meal with lots of flavour.

MARINADE

2½ teaspoons oyster sauce
½ teaspoon sesame oil
4 tablespoons mirin (Japanese rice wine)
½ small red (birdseye) chilli, seeded and finely sliced
1 tablespoon grated ginger
2 cloves garlic, crushed

500 g rump steak, trimmed
olive oil spray
1 cup torn Vietnamese mint leaves
1 cup torn basil leaves
½ cup chopped coriander leaves
1½ teaspoons sesame seeds
4 spring onions, finely sliced
1 cup fried noodles
8 mango cheeks (roughly half a 425 g can), drained and cut into 1 cm slices, reserving 3 tablespoons juice/syrup for the dressing
2 small red (birdseye) chillies, seeded and finely sliced
2 tablespoons fried shallots
10 cherry tomatoes, halved

DRESSING

1½ tablespoons soy sauce
3 tablespoons lime juice
2 cloves garlic, crushed
1½ teaspoons grated ginger
2 teaspoons mirin (Japanese rice wine)
3 tablespoons reserved mango juice
½ teaspoon sesame oil
1 tablespoon oyster sauce

Combine marinade ingredients and pour over beef, tossing to coat. Leave to marinate overnight (or for a minimum of 4 hours).

Heat a frying pan over a high heat and spray lightly with oil. Cook the steaks for 3–5 minutes on each side, then remove from the pan and allow to cool slightly.

Combine the remaining salad ingredients. To make dressing place all ingredients in an airtight jar and shake until combined. Slice the beef diagonally into 1 cm strips, add to the salad and drizzle with dressing.

Serves 4

NUTRITION ANALYSIS

PER SERVE
Total kJ: 1397 kJ
Carbohydrates: 15.2 g
Fat: 13.6 g
Saturated fat: 5.4 g
Protein: 30.4 g
Fibre: 4.1 g

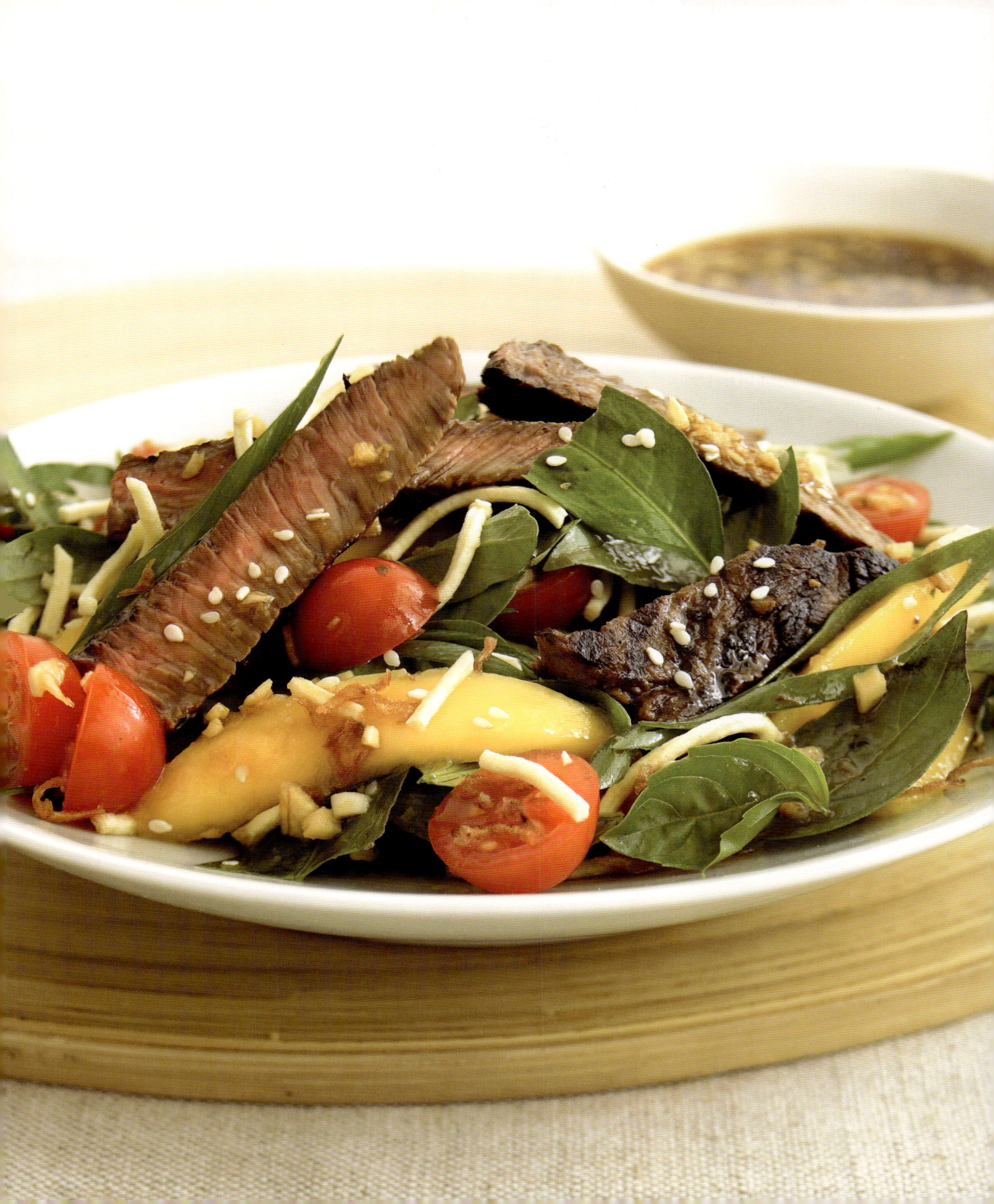

Steak sandwich

If you can't find minute steaks use tenderised rump steaks instead.

olive oil spray
150 g cherry tomatoes, halved
100 g mushrooms, wiped and chopped
4 x 150 g minute steaks
125 g lettuce leaves
1 red onion, finely sliced
4 slices sourdough bread
2 tablespoons horseradish cream
freshly ground black pepper

Heat a large frying pan over a medium heat and spray lightly with oil. Place the tomatoes and mushrooms in the pan and cook gently for a couple of minutes. Remove the tomatoes and put them in a warm place. Move mushrooms to one side of the frying pan and add the steaks. Cook for 2–4 minutes on each side.

Arrange the lettuce, onion, tomatoes and mushrooms on unbuttered slices of toasted sourdough finish with a dollop of horseradish cream and pepper to taste. Serve immediately.

Serves 4

NUTRITION ANALYSIS

PER SERVE
Total kJ: 1032 kJ
Carbohydrates: 16.6 g
Fat: 8.9 g
Saturated fat: 3.6 g
Protein: 23.2 g
Fibre: 3.5 g

Nachos

The delicious sauce here is suitable for freezing and can be used in other dishes such as tacos or enchiladas. Vegetarians can adapt the recipe, substituting beef with additional beans and adding carrots or celery.

SAUCE

olive oil spray
1 onion, diced
2 cloves garlic, crushed
250 g lean beef mince
1 red capsicum, cut into 1 cm dice
1 tablespoon sweet paprika
2 teaspoons ground cumin
1 teaspoon cayenne pepper
freshly ground black pepper
200 g canned red kidney beans, rinsed and drained
1 x 400 g can salt-reduced crushed tomatoes

4 pieces wholemeal mountain bread, cut into small triangles
½ cup grated reduced-fat cheddar cheese
½ ripe avocado, cut into 2 cm pieces
juice of ½ lemon
freshly ground black pepper

Preheat oven to 150°C (300°F).

Heat a large saucepan over a medium heat and spray lightly with oil. Add the onion and garlic and cook gently for a few minutes until soft. Add the mince, breaking it up with a wooden spoon, and cook until brown. Add the capsicum and spices and cook for a further 2 minutes. Add the beans and tomatoes and bring to the boil, then lower heat and simmer for 1 hour stirring occasionally.

Arrange the mountain bread pieces on a baking tray and bake in the oven for 15 minutes until crisp. Cover with the tomato–bean mixture and sprinkle cheese over the top. Return to the oven for 5 minutes until golden.

Place the avocado in a bowl and mix through the lemon juice and a little pepper using a fork.

Serve nachos topped with avocado.

Serves 4

NUTRITION ANALYSIS
PER SERVE
Total kJ: 1625 kJ
Carbohydrates: 26.1 g
Fat: 14.3 g
Saturated fat: 6.1 g
Protein: 33.7 g
Fibre: 6.4 g

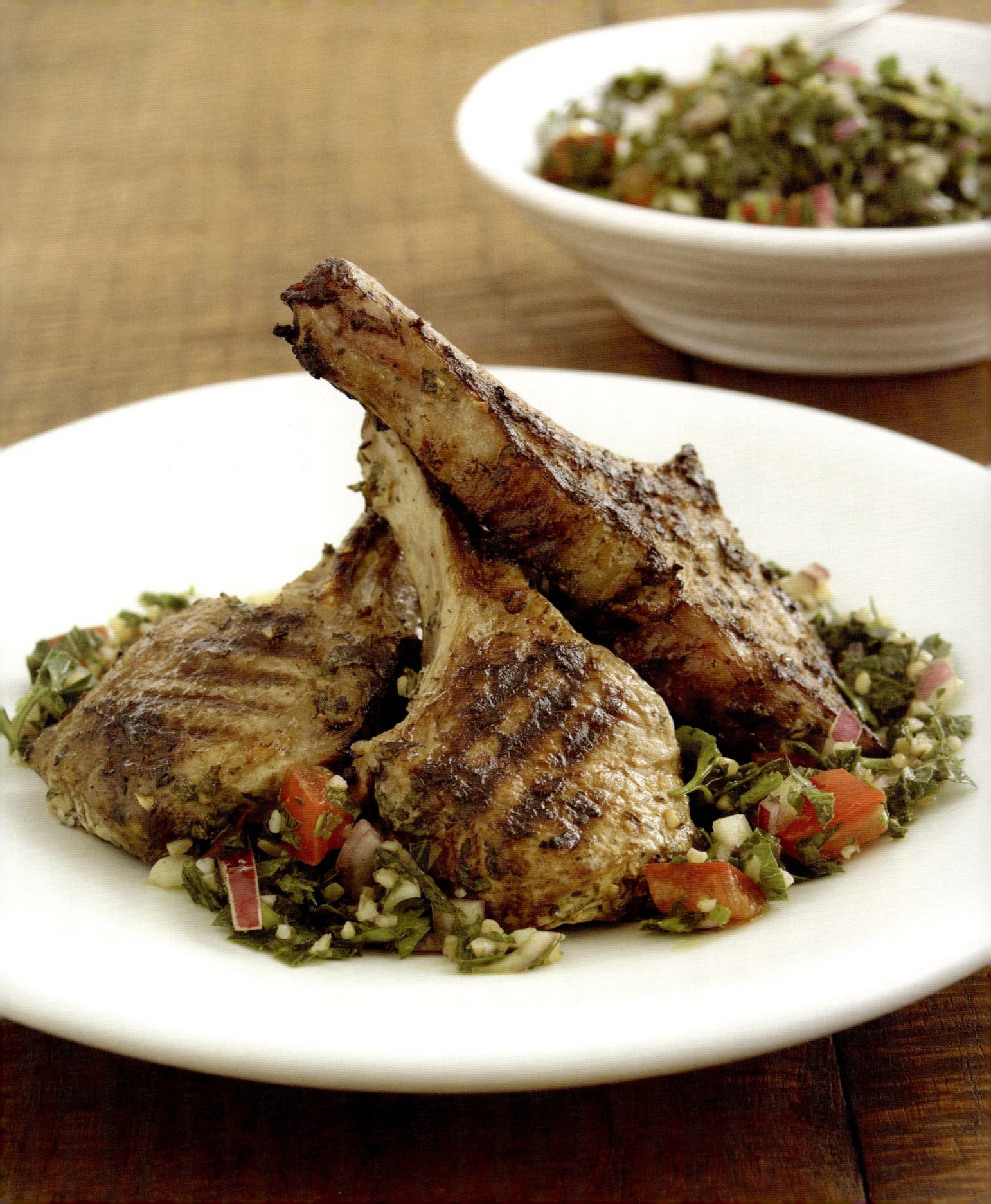

Yoghurt-marinated lamb cutlets

These cutlets, done on the barbecue and served with Tabouleh (see page 179), are the perfect summer meal.

¼ cup low-fat natural yoghurt
4 tablespoons finely shredded mint leaves
1 teaspoon dried mint
2 cloves garlic, crushed
½ teaspoon ground cumin
¼ teaspoon freshly ground black pepper
olive oil spray
12 lamb cutlets, trimmed

Mix the yoghurt, mint, garlic, cumin and pepper together. Toss the cutlets through the mix until evenly coated. Marinate overnight or for a minimum of 5 hours.

Heat a large frying pan over a medium heat and spray lightly with oil. (The cutlets can also be cooked under a hot grill or on the barbecue.) Cook for 5–8 minutes on each side. Cooking time will vary depending upon the thickness of the cutlets. Rest for 5 minutes, loosely covered with foil, before serving.

Serves 4

NUTRITION ANALYSIS

PER SERVE
Total kJ: 1152 kJ
Carbohydrates: 3.8 g
Fat: 12.9 g
Saturated fat: 6.8 g
Protein: 36.9 g
Fibre: 0.4 g

Braised lamb shanks with lentil and onion stew

When buying shanks, ask your butcher to cut the tendon. This helps the meat to fall off the bone while cooking, making it more flavoursome and tender.

4 lamb shanks
2 tablespoons plain flour
olive oil spray
2 onions, finely diced
3 sticks celery, finely diced
2 carrots, scraped and finely diced
4 sprigs thyme
3 tablespoons tomato paste
½ cup red wine
3 cups chicken stock (recipe on page 167)
½ cup brown lentils, rinsed
1 head garlic, cut in half widthwise
8 shallots, peeled
freshly ground black pepper

Preheat oven to 180°C (350°F).

Coat the shanks with flour. Heat a large frying pan over a high heat and spray lightly with oil. Brown shanks on all sides then remove. Add more oil if necessary, lower heat and cook the onions, celery, carrots and thyme gently for a few minutes until soft. Add tomato paste and cook for 2 minutes. Add the red wine and reduce for a further 2 minutes, then add the chicken stock and the shanks. Increase heat and bring to the boil.

Transfer the contents of the pan to a deep baking dish. Add lentils, garlic and shallots, cover with a lid or foil and cook for 2 hours in the oven. Turn the shanks every 30 minutes to ensure even cooking.

Remove the foil and cook for a further 30 minutes until meat is falling off the bone. Remove the shanks and keep in a warm place. Skim any fat from the surface of the liquid, remove the thyme and pour into a saucepan. Bring to the boil then turn down the heat and cook for 7–10 minutes. The sauce should reduce to a thick, stew-like consistency. Return the lamb shanks to the pan, stir gently to combine, season with pepper to taste and serve.

Serves 4

NUTRITION ANALYSIS
PER SERVE
Total kJ: 1284 kJ
Carbohydrates: 11.8 g
Fat: 11 g
Saturated fat: 5.5 g
Protein: 36.0 g
Fibre: 4.2 g

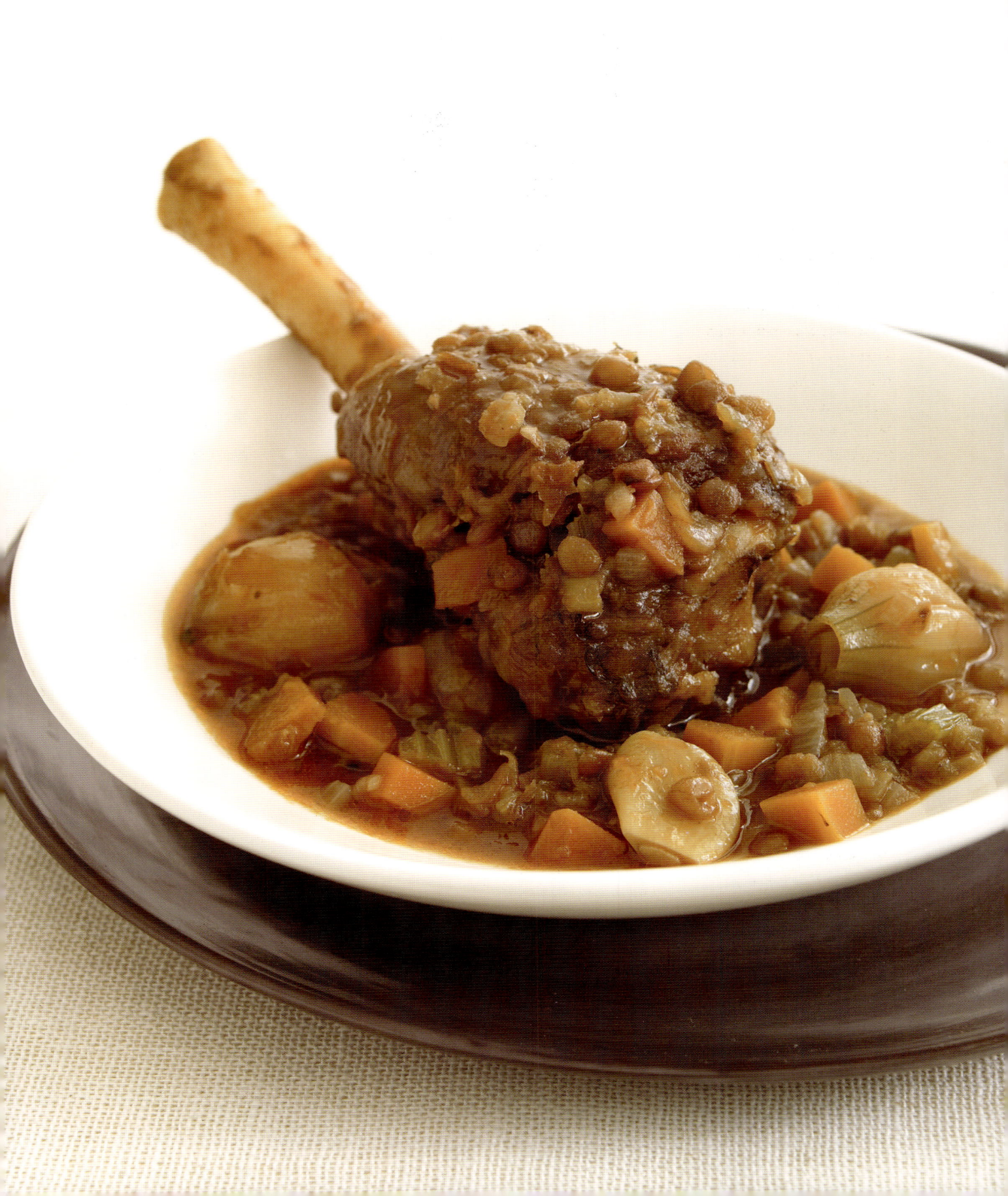

Herb-crusted grilled pork

This dish is perfect for barbecues and goes well with Fennel and Orange Salad (see page 180).

1 teaspoon coriander seeds
2 teaspoons fennel seeds
1 teaspoon cumin seeds
freshly ground black pepper
rind of 2 oranges, grated
4 x 200 g pork mid-loin chops, trimmed

Using a mortar and pestle crush the coriander, fennel and cumin seeds. If you prefer, use the same quantities of ground seeds.

Mix the spices and orange rind. Roll the edges of the pork chops in the spice mix to coat evenly. Cook under a hot grill for 5–7 minutes on either side until golden brown.

Rest in a warm place for 5 minutes, loosely covered with foil, before serving.

Serves 4

NUTRITION ANALYSIS
PER SERVE
Total kJ: 1300 kJ
Carbohydrates: 0.0 g
Fat: 20.0 g
Saturated fat: 7.9 g
Protein: 32.8 g
Fibre: 0.0 g

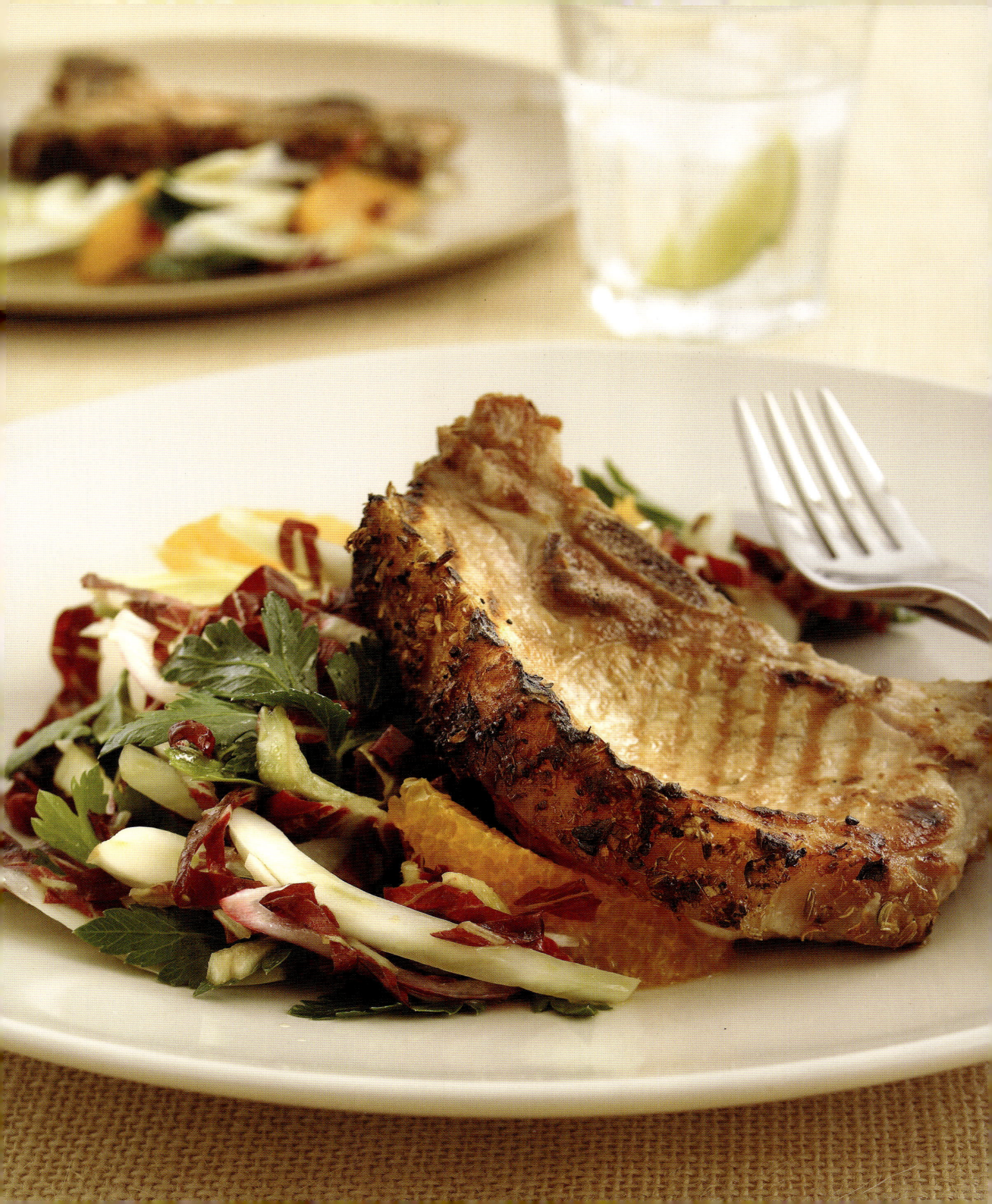

Prawns with avocado and mango salsa

A dish that's perfect when entertaining in summer.

600 g green (raw) peeled prawns
1 ripe avocado, cut into 2 cm pieces
1 small red chilli (birdseye), seeded and finely diced
1 large mango, peeled and diced (or 1 x 425 g can mango cheeks, drained and diced)
½ red onion, finely diced
juice of 2 limes
¼ cup chopped coriander leaves
¼ cup reduced-fat mayonnaise

Bring a saucepan of water to the boil, add the prawns and cook for 5 minutes until pink. Drain and allow to cool.

Mix the avocado, chilli, mango, onion, lime juice and coriander leaves together. Add the mayonnaise and stir until all the ingredients are coated. To serve, spread the salsa on a plate and top with prawns.

Serves 4

NUTRITION ANALYSIS

PER SERVE
Total kJ: 1389 kJ
Carbohydrates: 12.3 g
Fat: 12.6 g
Saturated fat: 2.7 g
Protein: 40.1 g
Fibre: 2.4 g

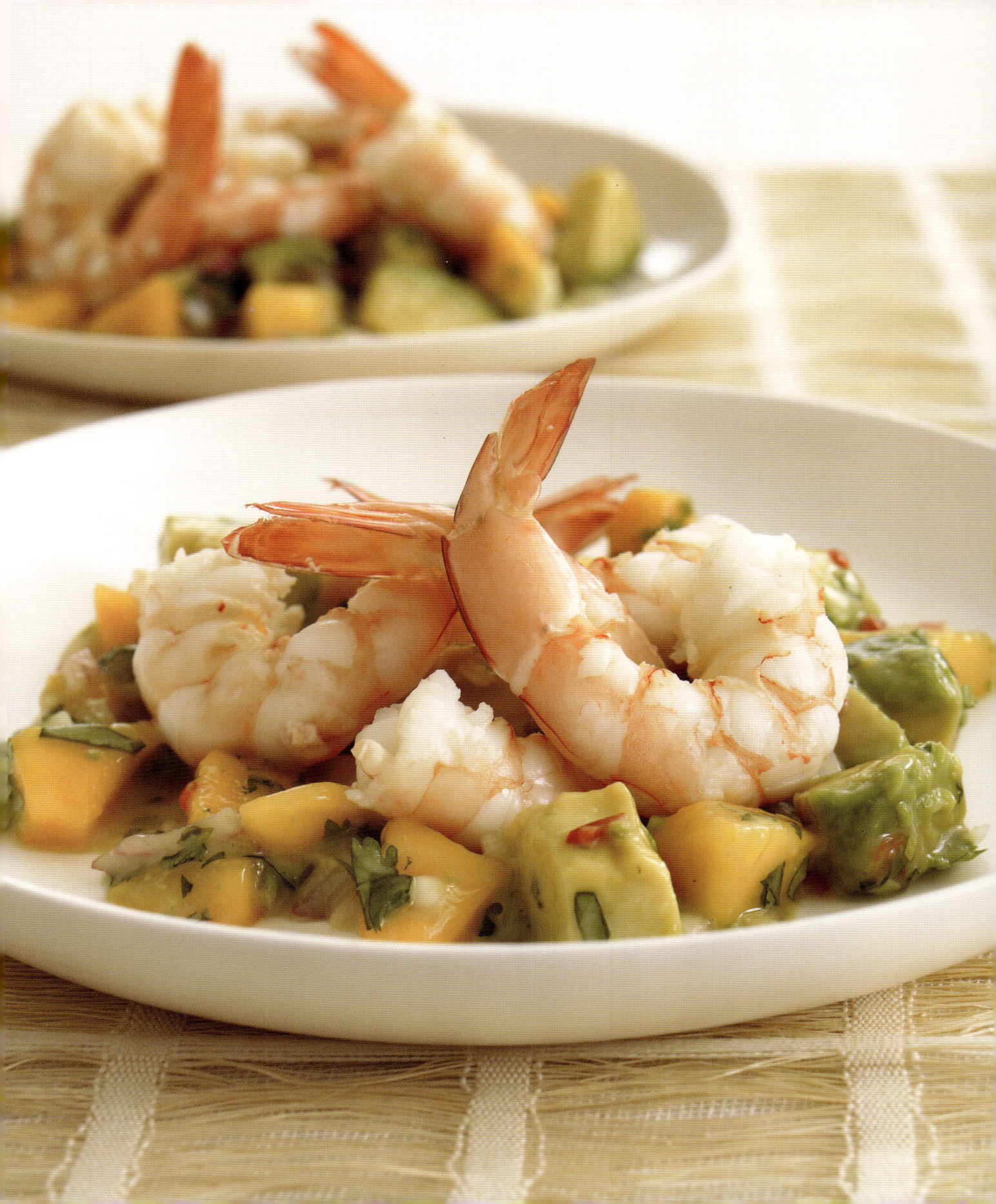

Ocean trout panzanella salad

This salad is perfect for entertaining: not only is it extremely colourful and attractive on the plate, it is also very easy to make.

4 x 300 g ocean trout fillets
1½ pieces mountain bread, cut into 5 cm squares
1 red capsicum
olive oil spray
1 tomato, diced
3 tablespoons roughly chopped pitted olives
1 Lebanese cucumber, halved lengthwise, seeded and roughly chopped
½ red onion, finely sliced
2 tablespoons roughly chopped capers
3 tablespoons torn basil leaves
2 tablespoons chopped flat-leaf parsley
4 tablespoons red wine vinegar
4 tablespoons extra-virgin olive oil

Preheat oven to 150°C (300°F).

Place ocean trout fillets on a lined baking tray and roast in the oven for 10 minutes. When cooked the flesh should separate but remain firm when pressed lightly.

Arrange the mountain bread squares on a baking tray and place in the oven for about 20 minutes to crispen.

Spray the capsicum lightly with oil and hold over a flame or under a grill until the skin blackens. Allow to cool, then peel, seed and cut into 2 cm strips.

Combine the bread, capsicum, tomato, olives, cucumber, onion and capers. Using your fingers, gently flake the ocean trout into the salad. Add the basil and parsley leaves, drizzle vinegar and oil over and mix thoroughly.

Serves 4

NUTRITION ANALYSIS
PER SERVE
Total kJ: 1310 kJ
Carbohydrates: 7.4 g
Fat: 22.0 g
Saturated fat: 3.5 g
Protein: 19.8 g
Fibre: 1.3 g

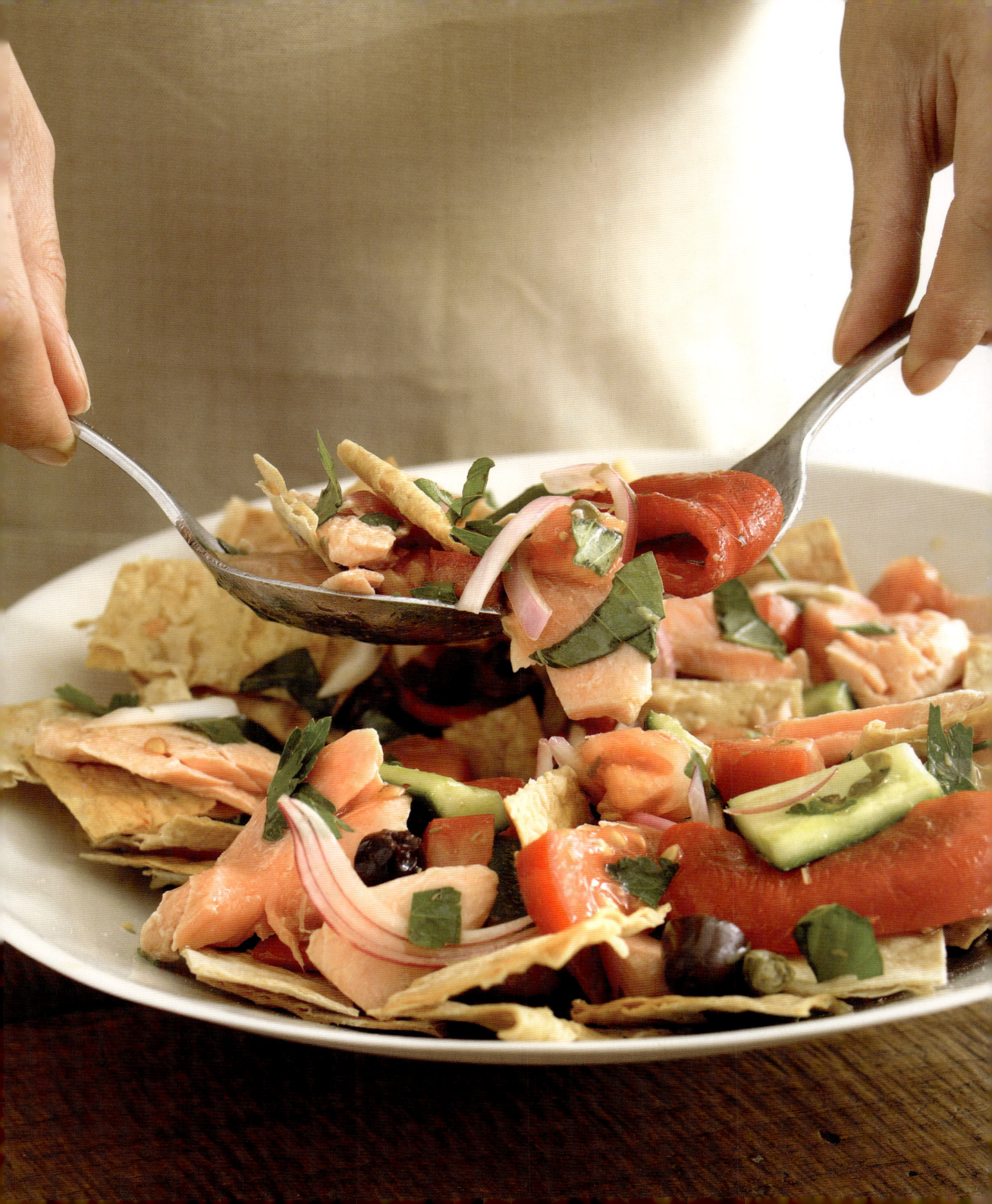

Sardines Provençale

This recipe uses canned sardines, but for an interesting variation cook fresh sardines separately first. Sardine bones are soft and edible, and a great source of calcium.

olive oil spray
2 onions, diced
4 cloves garlic, crushed
2 tomatoes, diced
¼ cup white wine
2 tablespoons chopped oregano leaves
1 cup chicken stock (recipe on page 167)
400 g canned sardines in springwater, drained
2 tablespoons roughly chopped black olives
2 tablespoons basil leaves
freshly ground black pepper

Heat a large frying pan over a medium heat and spray lightly with oil. Cook the onions and garlic gently until soft. Add the tomatoes and white wine and cook until the wine has reduced by half. Add the oregano and chicken stock, increase heat and bring to the boil. Cook until the sauce begins to thicken. Add the sardines to the pan and allow to warm through. Add the olives, basil leaves and pepper to taste, and serve immediately.

Serves 4

NUTRITION ANALYSIS
PER SERVE
Total kJ: 907 kJ
Carbohydrates: 9.0 g
Fat: 9.8 g
Saturated fat: 2.5 g
Protein: 21.0 g
Fibre: 2.3 g

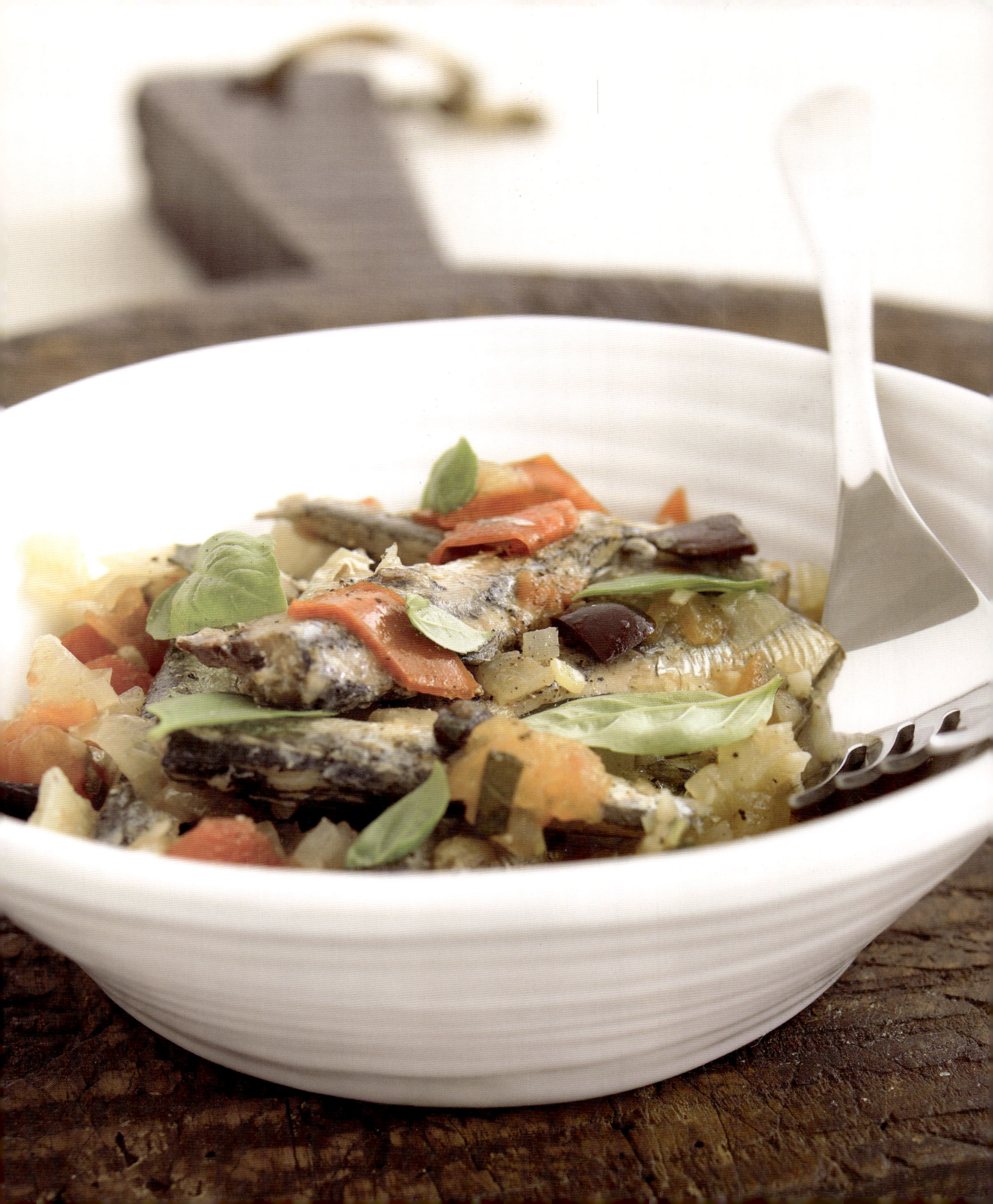

Crisp-skinned salmon with lemon and Asian greens

This dish is simple and tasty. The salt causes the salmon skin to crispen, and also adds wonderful flavour, so use the best-quality salt you can find.

4 x 180–200 g Atlantic salmon fillets, skin on
rind (julienned) and juice of 1 lemon
1 teaspoon sea salt flakes
olive oil spray
2 bunches baby bok choy, outer leaves removed, and cut into strips

Pat the salmon skin dry using a paper towel. Drizzle about a tablespoon of the lemon juice over the skin then coat evenly with salt flakes.

Heat a large frying pan over a medium–high heat and spray lightly with oil. Cook the salmon skin-side down in the hot pan for 3–5 minutes, gently shaking the pan occasionally to ensure the skin doesn't stick, then carefully flip over and cook for another 3–5 minutes. The salmon should be golden brown and crisp.

Meanwhile, steam the bok choy for 5 minutes then mix through the lemon rind and remaining lemon juice. Serve salmon fillets with bok choy.

Serves 4

NUTRITION ANALYSIS
PER SERVE
Total kJ: 1245 kJ
Carbohydrates: 1.1 g
Fat: 15.7 g
Saturated fat: 3.7 g
Protein: 37.2 g
Fibre: 1.0 g

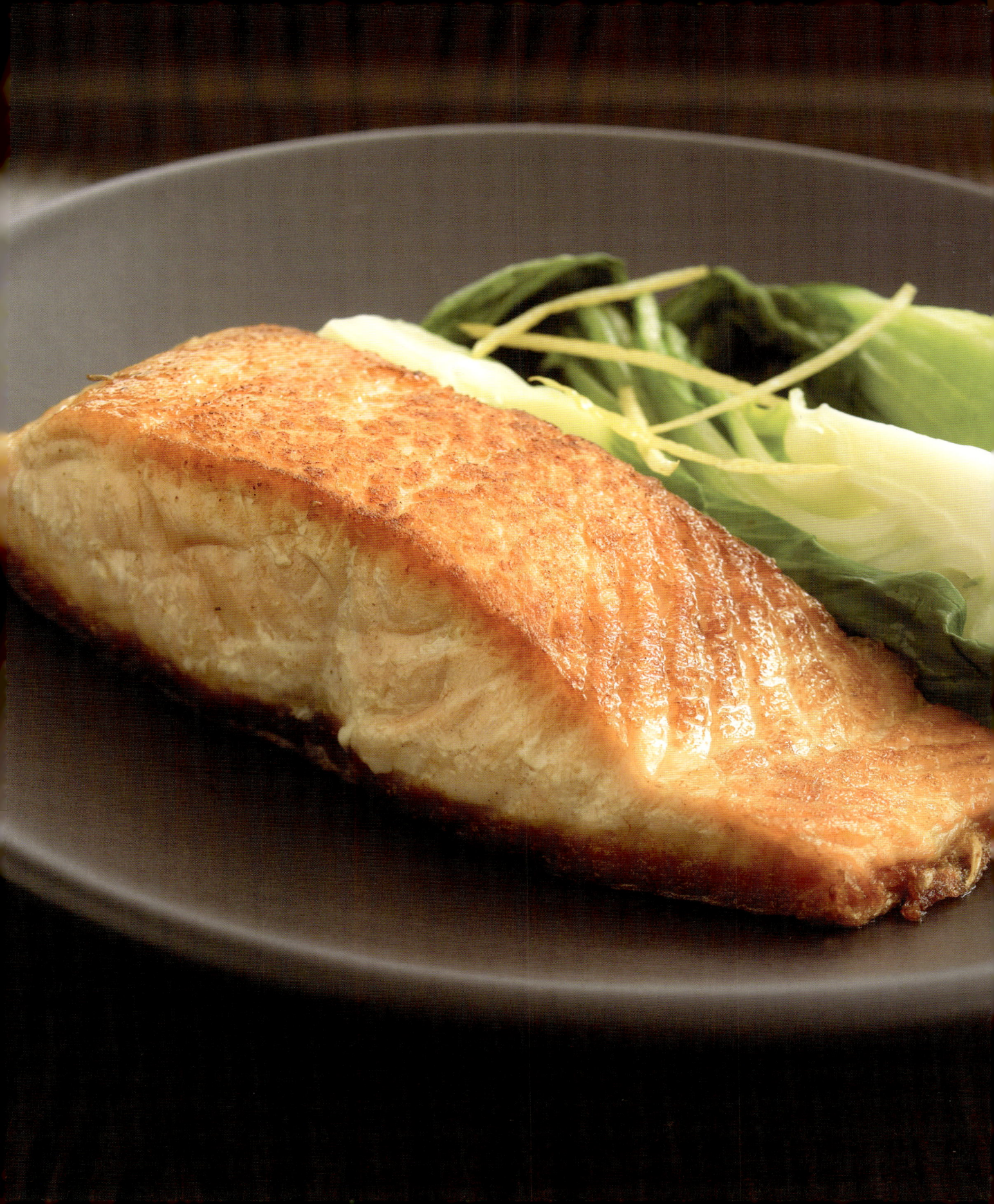

Snapper with Greek salad

Snapper is a firm white fish with a mild flavour, very low in fat and high in protein.

olive oil spray
4 x 180–200 g snapper fillets, skin on

SALAD
2 tomatoes, diced
1 Lebanese cucumber, sliced lengthwise, seeded and diced
1 red onion, finely sliced
½ teaspoon dried oregano
4 tablespoons roughly chopped black olives
4 tablespoons roughly chopped flat-leaf parsley
2 tablespoons reduced-fat fetta, crumbled

DRESSING
1 clove garlic, crushed
2 teaspoons red wine vinegar
1 teaspoon balsamic vinegar
⅓ cup extra-virgin olive oil
½ teaspoon honey

Heat a large frying pan over a high heat and spray lightly with oil. Cook the snapper fillets skin-side down for 3–5 minutes, then carefully flip over and cook for 3–5 minutes on the other side, gently moving the pan occasionally to ensure the skin doesn't stick to the pan.

Combine the tomatoes, cucumber, onion, oregano, olives and parsley in a mixing bowl.

To make the dressing place all ingredients in an airtight jar and shake until combined. Add the fetta to the salad. Mix the dressing through the salad and serve with snapper fillets on top.

Serves 4

NUTRITION ANALYSIS
PER SERVE
Total kJ: 1436 kJ
Carbohydrates: 5.8 g
Fat: 12 g
Saturated fat: 3.2 g
Protein: 51.5 g
Fibre: 2 g

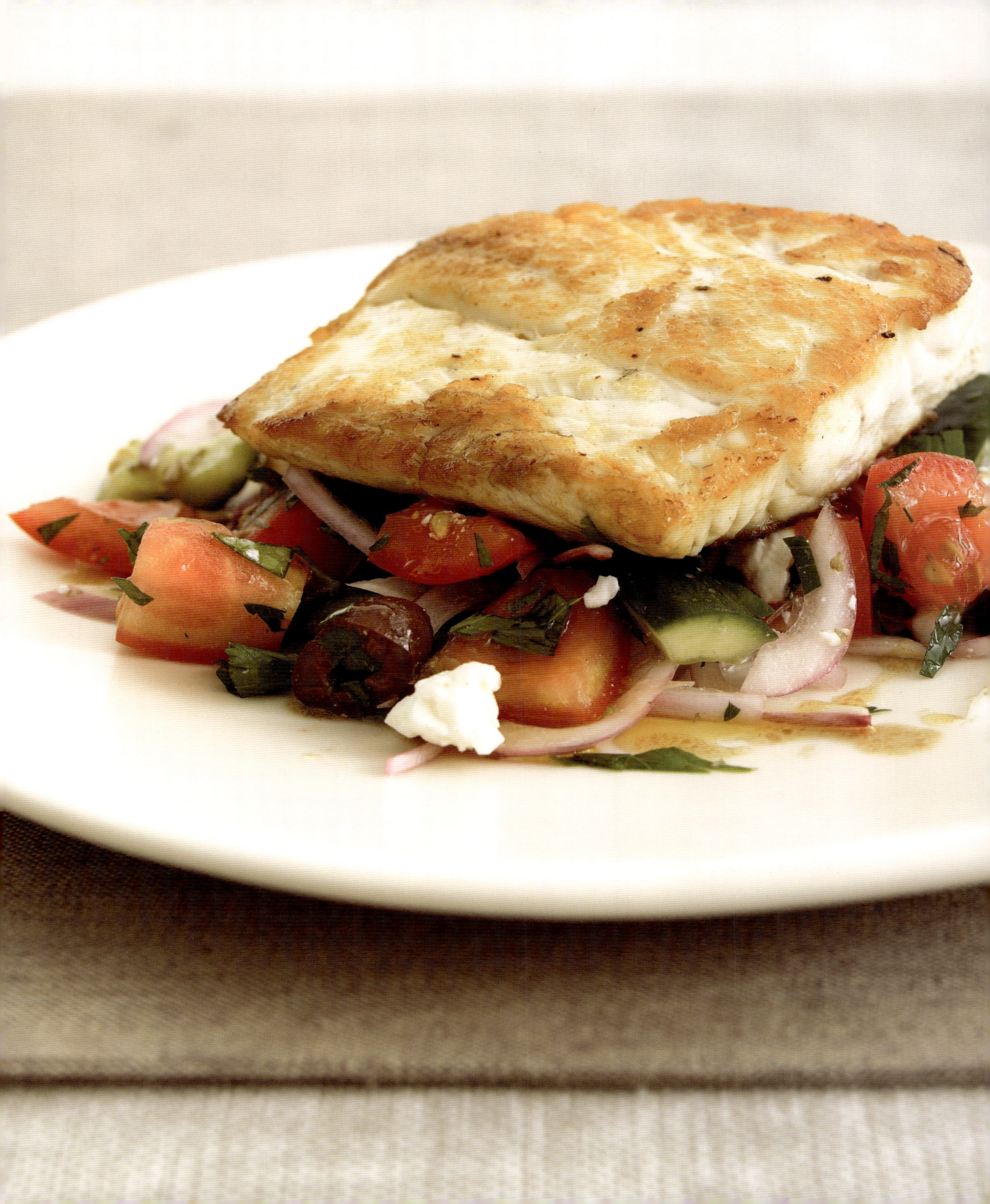

Swordfish with roast tomato and rocket salad

A very simple dish with a lovely herb flavour.

3 tomatoes, cut in half widthwise
olive oil spray
1 teaspoon chopped oregano leaves
4 x 180 g swordfish steaks
120 g rocket leaves
¼ cup balsamic vinegar

Preheat oven to 150°C (300°F).

Place tomatoes on a baking tray, spray lightly with oil and sprinkle with oregano leaves. Roast in the oven for 1 hour until soft.

Heat a large frying pan over a medium–high heat and spray lightly with oil. Cook the swordfish for 5 minutes on each side until cooked through. Remove from the pan and set aside in a warm place.

Spray the frying pan again lightly with oil and heat. Chop the tomato halves and place in the heated frying pan. Cook for 1–2 minutes over a high heat then add the rocket. Toss through the tomatoes and allow to wilt slightly. Add the balsamic vinegar and mix through. Remove from the pan and serve immediately with the swordfish.

Serves 4

NUTRITION ANALYSIS
PER SERVE
Total kJ: 1043 kJ
Carbohydrates: 2.4 g
Fat: 5.3 g
Saturated fat: 1.6 g
Protein: 45.8 g
Fibre: 1.6 g

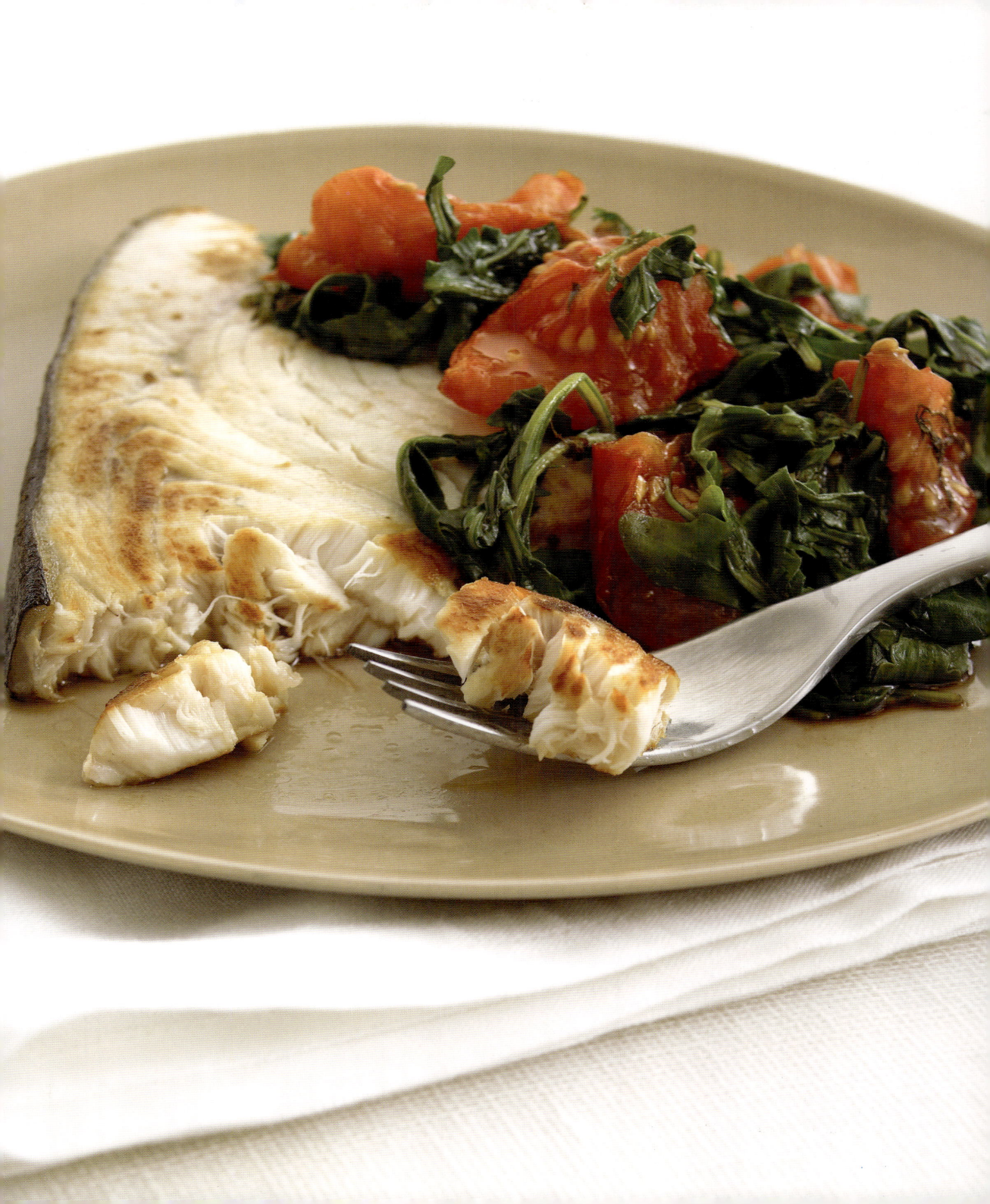

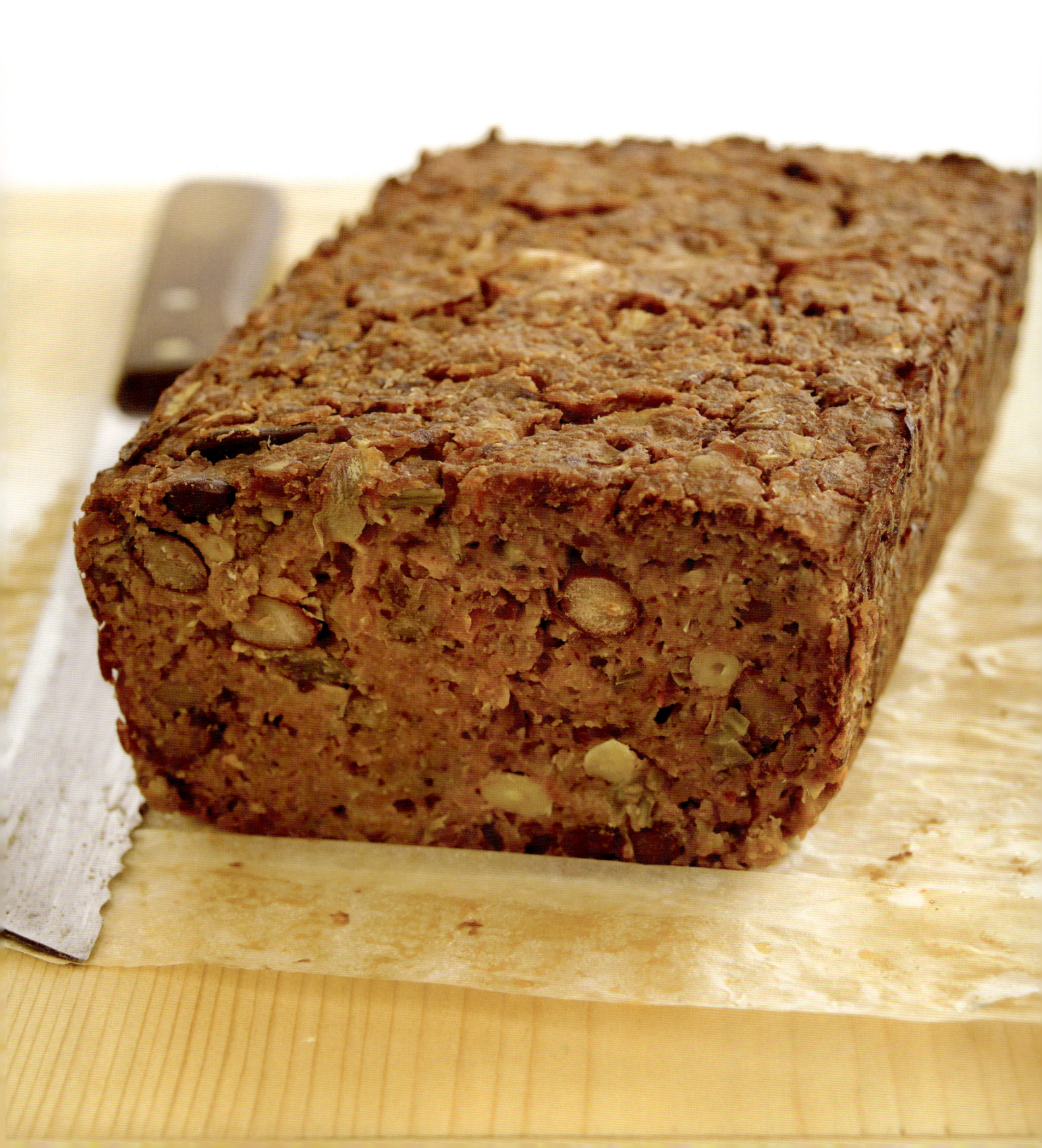

Spiced bean loaf

This is a great high-fibre alternative to meatloaf. Serve with a green salad.

olive oil spray
1 onion, finely diced
2 cloves garlic, crushed
2 sticks celery, finely diced
1 x 400 g can lentils, rinsed and drained
1 x 420 g can red kidney beans, rinsed and drained
½ zucchini, grated
½ carrot, grated
2 eggs
½ cup tomato passsata or Napoli Sauce (see page 182)
1½ tablespoons pine nuts
½ teaspoon ground cumin
½ teaspoon cayenne pepper
1 teaspoon sweet paprika
¾ cup wheatgerm

Preheat oven to 200°C (400°F).

Line a loaf tin (5-cup capacity) with greaseproof paper. Heat a large frying pan over a medium heat, spray lightly with oil and cook the onion, garlic and celery until soft. Remove from heat and allow to cool. Combine the lentils and beans and purée two-thirds of the mix. Stir through remaining beans, onion mixture and the remaining ingredients. Tip into the loaf tin and press firmly into shape.

Bake in the oven for 50 minutes until the centre of the loaf is firm to the touch. Serve hot or cold.

Serves 4

NUTRITION ANALYSIS

PER SERVE
Total kJ: 1361 kJ
Carbohydrates: 30.4 g
Fat: 10.3 g
Saturated fat: 1.5 g
Protein: 20.3 g
Fibre: 14.0 g

Vegetables stuffed with spiced rice

These can be served as either a vegetarian main meal or in smaller portions as an entrée or side dish.

- 2 small eggplants, cut in half lengthwise and skin pierced a couple of times with a skewer
- 2 zucchini, cut in half lengthwise
- 2 red capsicums, cut in half lengthwise, cored and seeded
- 2 tomatoes, cut in half widthwise, seeds removed and saved

STUFFING
- olive oil spray
- 2 onions, finely diced
- 4 cloves garlic, crushed
- 3 cups cooked brown rice
- 1 x 400 g can salt-reduced crushed tomatoes
- ¼ cup finely shredded mint leaves
- juice of 1 lemon
- freshly ground black pepper
- 1½ teaspoons cinnamon
- ½ teaspoon allspice

Preheat oven to 200°C (400°F).

Steam eggplants, zucchini and capsicums for 8–10 minutes until tender. Allow to cool, then using a teaspoon gently scrape out the insides (leaving a 1–1½ cm wall) of the eggplant, zucchini and tomato. Dice the flesh and set aside.

Heat a large frying pan over a medium heat, spray lightly with oil and cook the onion and garlic gently until soft. Add the eggplant, zucchini and tomato flesh and cook for a further 3 minutes. Add the cooked rice, tomatoes, mint, lemon juice, pepper, cinnamon and allspice.

Pack the vegetable shells snugly into a baking dish and stuff. Cover the dish with foil and transfer to the oven for 40 minutes. Remove the foil and cook for a further 10 minutes.

Serves 4

NUTRITION ANALYSIS
PER SERVE
Total kJ: 593 kJ
Carbohydrates: 17.8 g
Fat: 1.4 g
Saturated fat: 0.1 g
Protein: 7.8 g
Fibre: 11.4 g

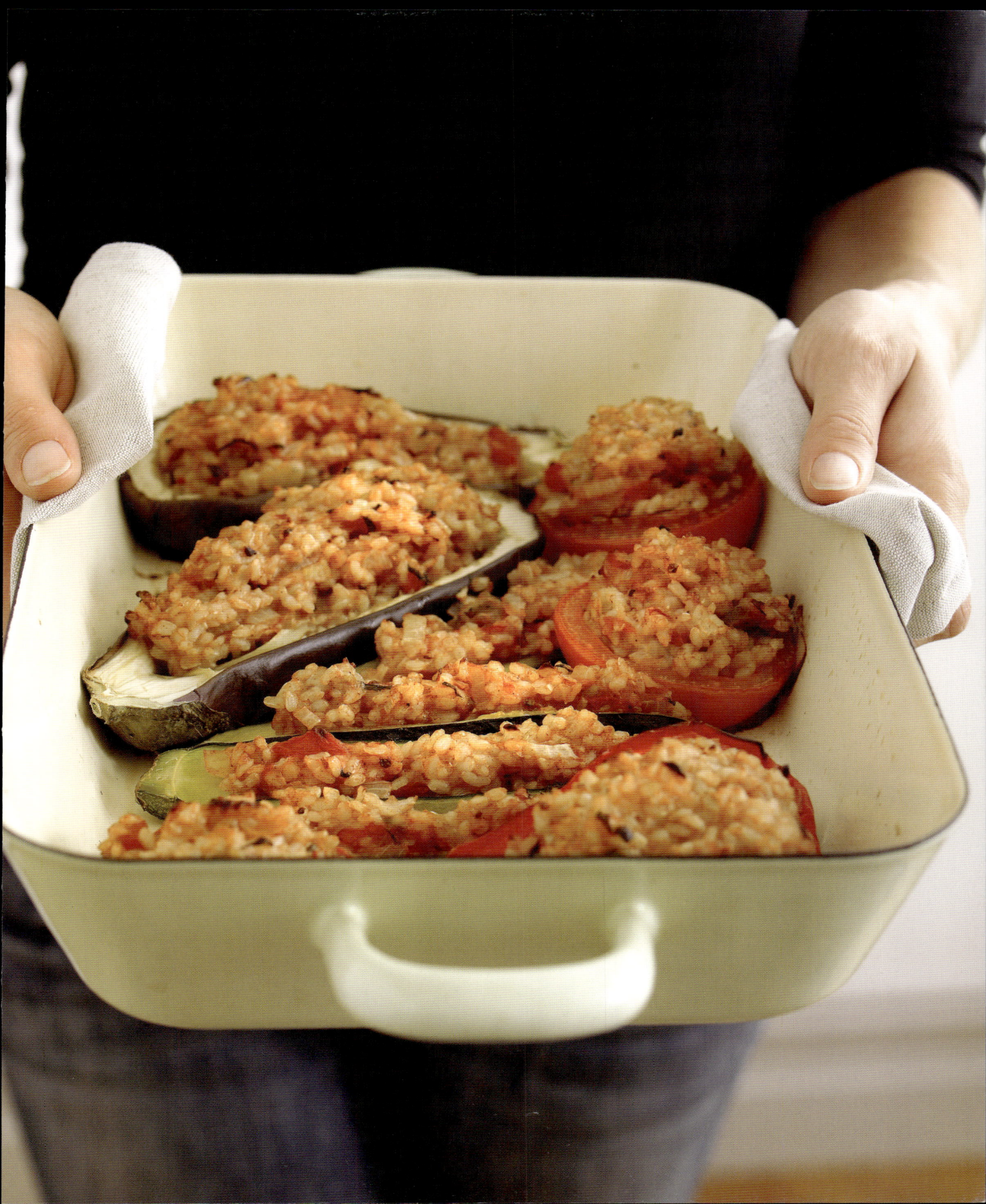

Spiced vegetable ratatouille with couscous

This is a great winter warmer. The spice mix may appear complicated but it is actually very easy to make. Keep the excess in the freezer and sprinkle onto roast vegetables for added flavour.

SPICE MIX

- 1 teaspoon cayenne pepper
- 1 teaspoon freshly ground black pepper
- 1½ teaspoons sweet paprika
- 1½ teaspoons ground ginger
- 1 tablespoon ground turmeric
- 2 teaspoons ground cinnamon
- 2 teaspoons ground cumin
- 1 teaspoon allspice
- ¼ teaspoon sea salt

- ¼ butternut pumpkin, peeled, seeded and cut into 2 cm pieces
- 1 carrot, scraped and diced
- ½ eggplant, diced
- olive oil spray
- 2 red onions, diced
- 2 sticks celery, diced
- 1 zucchini, diced
- 3 cloves garlic, crushed
- 2 cups tomato passsata or Napoli Sauce (see page 182)
- 2 cups water
- 1 x 400 g can chickpeas, rinsed and drained
- juice of ½ lemon
- 1 cup couscous
- 1 tablespoon unsalted butter
- 1 cup boiling water

Preheat oven to 220°C (430°F).

Combine all spice mix ingredients. Arrange pumpkin, carrot and eggplant pieces on a baking tray, spray lightly with oil and sprinkle 1 tablespoon of the spice mix over the top. Bake for 30 minutes until tender.

Heat a large saucepan over a low heat and spray lightly with oil. Cook the onion and celery until soft, add the zucchini, garlic and 1 teaspoon of spice mix, and cook for a further 2 minutes. Add the chickpeas, roasted vegetables, napoli sauce and water. Cover and simmer over a low heat for 40 minutes until all vegetables are soft. When cooked add lemon juice and more spice mix to taste.

Place couscous and butter in a bowl and pour over boiling water. Cover and let stand for 5 minutes, then stir gently with a fork to loosen the grains. To serve place the couscous in a large bowl and arrange the vegetables on top. The vegetables are delicious topped with low-fat yoghurt to temper the spice of the dish.

Serves 6

NUTRITION ANALYSIS

PER SERVE

Total kJ: 1028 kJ

Carbohydrates: 32.8 g

Fat: 6.0 g

Saturated fat: 2.8 g

Protein: 10.0 g

Fibre: 9.0 g

Desserts and Sweet Treats

Apple and mango frappé

½ cup mango pieces
2 tablespoons lime juice
½ cup apple juice
1 cup soda water

Purée the mango using a blender or hand-held processor. Combine with remaining ingredients and then pour into a plastic container, cover and freeze overnight. Use a fork to break into pieces when ready to serve.

Serves 4

NUTRITION ANALYSIS
PER SERVE
Total kJ: 140 kJ
Carbohydrates: 7.5 g
Fat: 0.0 g
Saturated fat: 0.0 g
Protein: 0.4 g
Fibre: 0.3 g

Apple and rhubarb crumble

4 cups Stewed Apple and Rhubarb (see page 155)
3 tablespoons butter
½ cup rolled oats
¼ cup shredded coconut
2 tablespoons almond meal
¼ teaspoon cinnamon

Preheat oven to 180°C (350°F).

Divide the stewed apple and rhubarb evenly between 4 individual (1-cup capacity) ramekins. Place the butter and half the oats in a food processor and process until the mixture is the consistency of breadcrumbs. Tip into a mixing bowl and add the rest of the oats, coconut, almond meal and cinnamon.

Spoon the crumble mix over the fruit and bake for 15–20 minutes until crisp and golden.

Remove from the oven and let stand for 5 minutes before serving. Delicious served with low-fat natural yoghurt.

Serves 4

NUTRITION ANALYSIS
PER SERVE
Total kJ: 1101 kJ
Carbohydrates: 11.3 g
Fat: 19.5 g
Saturated fat: 11.6 g
Protein: 5.4 g
Fibre: 8.1 g

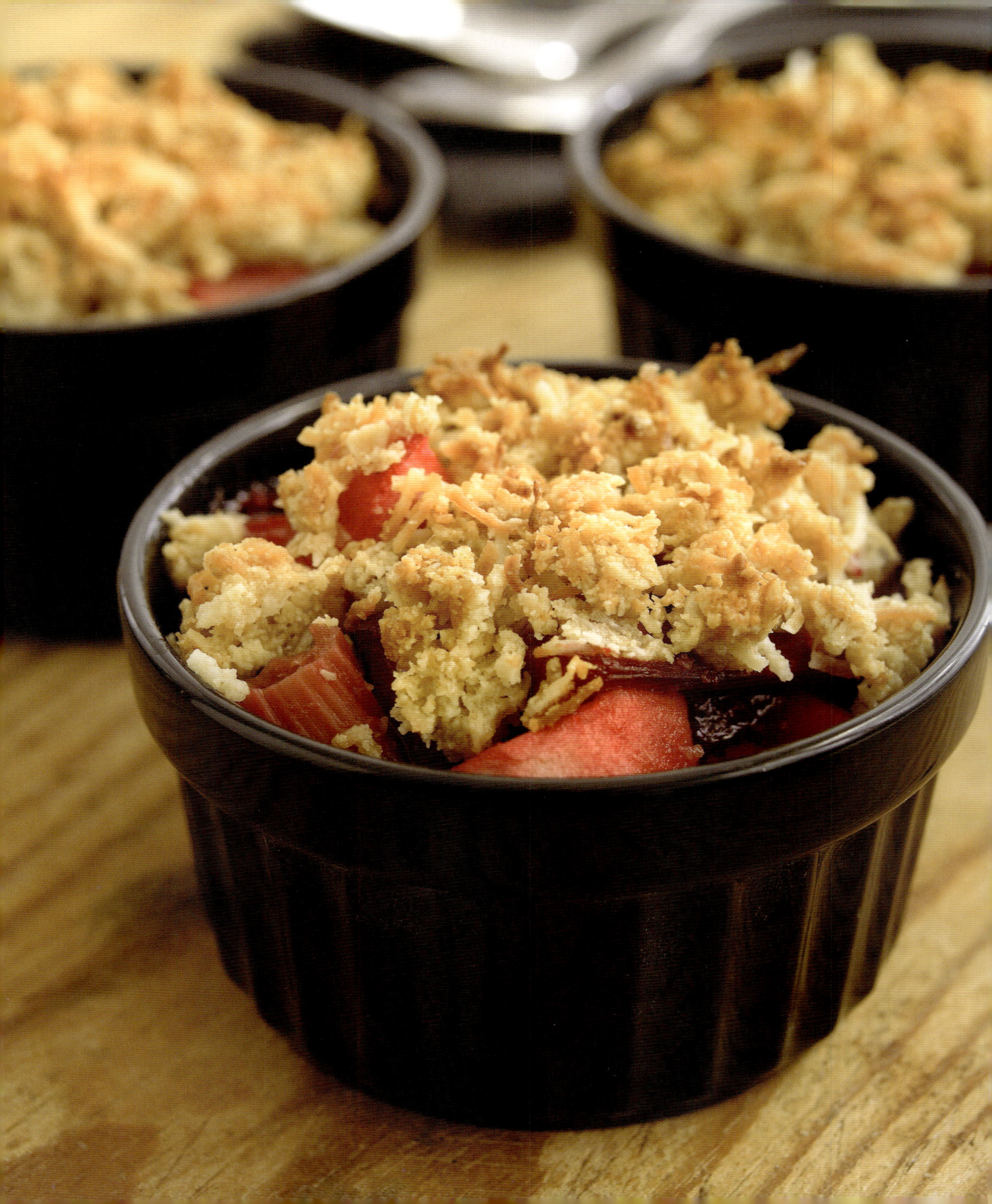

Passionfruit soufflés

10 passionfruit, or ½ cup canned pulp, strained to remove seeds
olive oil spray
¾ cup caster sugar
5 egg whites

Preheat oven to 200°C (400°F).

If using fresh passionfruit, remove seeds and pulp. Pass half the amount through a seive, reserving juice and discarding seeds.

Heat remaining seeds, juice and sugar in a saucepan over a low heat and cook, stirring, until thickened.

Spray 4 individual (1-cup capacity) ramekins lightly with oil, then sprinkle with a small amount of caster sugar, ensuring that the base and sides are lightly coated.

Whisk egg whites until they begin to thicken. Add the sugar slowly while whisking and continue until soft peaks form. Gently fold the passionfruit through, reserving a little of the syrup.

Spoon mixture into ramekins, leaving 1 cm at the top. Bake in the oven for 15–20 minutes until the soufflés have risen and are golden brown.

Drizzle with the reserved passionfruit syrup and serve.

Serves 4

NUTRITION ANALYSIS
PER SERVE
Total kJ: 853 kJ
Carbohydrates: 42.5 g
Fat: 0.1 g
Saturated fat: 0.0 g
Protein: 5.8 g
Fibre: 6.3 g

Pear and coconut spring rolls

3 cups (650 g) Spiced Poached Pears (see page 155), drained, patted dry and chopped, or use canned pears
½ cup shredded coconut
½ cup wheatgerm
6 sheets filo pastry
olive oil spray
2 tablespoons brown sugar

Place pears in a mixing bowl and combine with the coconut and wheatgerm.

Place 1 sheet of filo on a flat surface, covering the others to prevent them drying out. Spray the sheet lightly with oil and fold in half. Spray lightly again and sprinkle over a small amount of the brown sugar.

Spoon a sixth of the fruit mixture evenly along the bottom edge of the filo square and roll the square up tightly, spraying lightly with oil to finish and seal. Repeat for the remaining sheets.

Heat a large frying pan over a medium heat and spray lightly with oil. Cut the spring rolls in half and cook for 2 minutes on each side until golden brown. Serve hot.

Serves 4

NUTRITION ANALYSIS
PER SERVE
Total kJ: 1088 kJ
Carbohydrates: 40.0 g
Fat: 7.2 g
Saturated fat: 5.6 g
Protein: 6.0 g
Fibre: 6.9 g

Mango lassi

1 cup low-fat natural yoghurt
½ cup water
¼ teaspoon ground cardamom
½ cup canned mango cheeks in syrup (or fresh if in season)
½ teaspoon rosewater (optional)

Place all ingredients in a blender and mix until smooth. Drink immediately.

Serves 1

Berry and mint sorbet

½ cup caster sugar
1½ cups water
¾ cup mixed berries
½ cup roughly chopped mint leaves
extra mint leaves to garnish

Heat sugar and water in a saucepan, stirring occasionally until sugar dissolves. Bring to the boil over a medium heat, add berries and cook for a couple of minutes until soft. Remove from the heat, add the mint leaves and allow to cool completely.

Strain the mixture through a sieve to remove all the berry seeds and pour into a plastic container. Freeze overnight.

Serves 4

NUTRITION ANALYSIS
PER SERVE
Total kJ: 1040 kJ
Carbohydrates: 34.4 g
Fat: 4.5 g
Saturated fat: 2.9 g
Protein: 14.1 g
Fibre: 1.1 g

NUTRITION ANALYSIS
PER SERVE
Total kJ: 534 kJ
Carbohydrates: 32.0 g
Fat: 0.0 g
Saturated fat: 0.0 g
Protein: 0.6 g
Fibre: 1.0 g

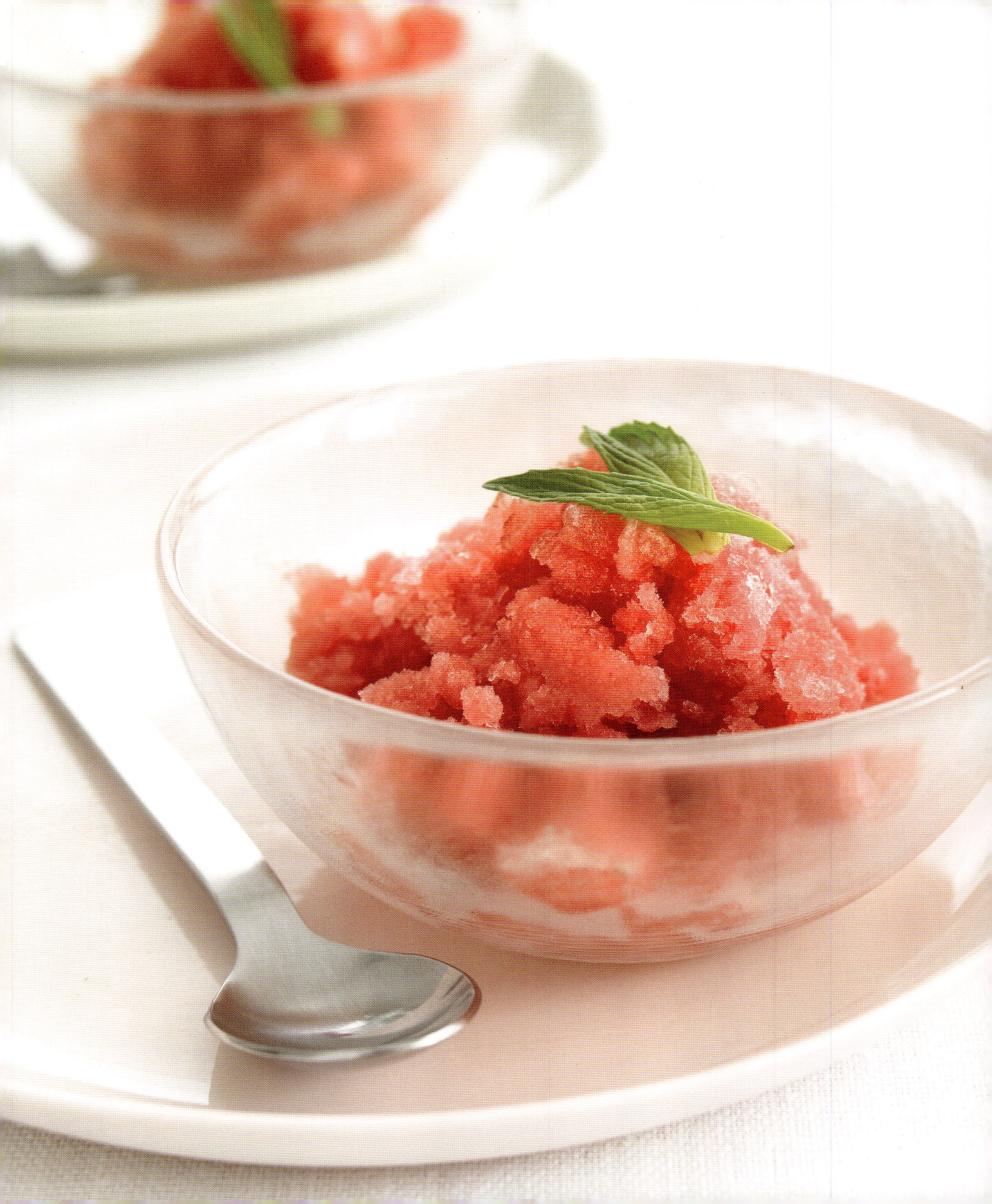

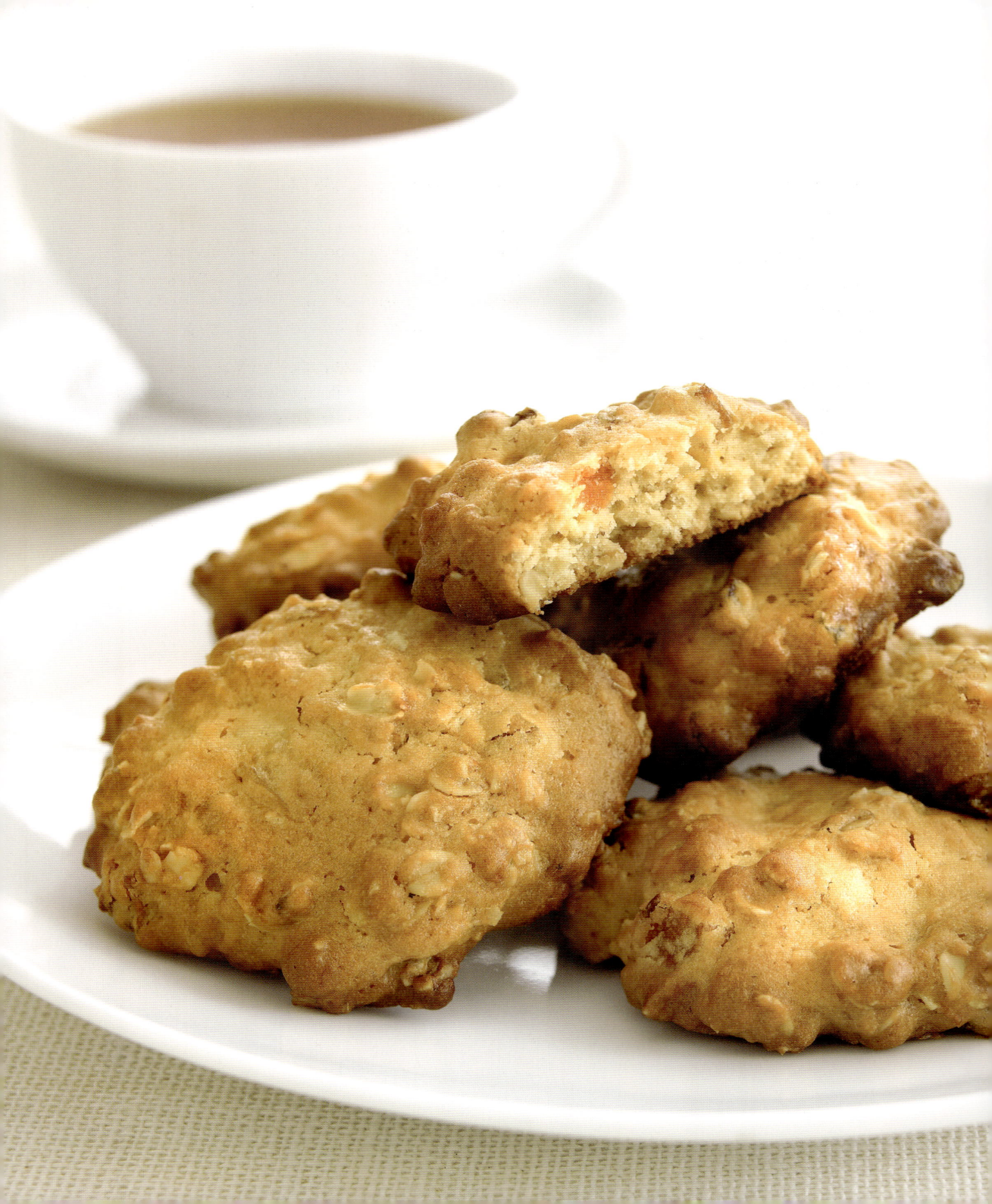

Apricot, ginger and honey cookies

1 cup plain flour
1 cup rolled oats
½ teaspoon baking powder
2 tablespoons brown sugar
100 g butter
¼ cup honey
rind of 1 orange, finely grated
1 egg
½ teaspoon vanilla essence
¼ cup finely diced dried apricots
2 tablespoons finely diced crystallised ginger

Preheat oven to 175°C (350°F).

Mix together the flour, oats, baking powder and sugar. In a small saucepan gently melt the butter and honey. Remove from heat and add the orange rind, egg and vanilla essence. Pour over the oat mixture and combine, adding the apricots and ginger.

Spoon onto a lined baking tray, leaving room between each. Press to flatten into 5 cm rounds, and bake in the oven for 20 minutes until golden brown.

Makes 18 cookies (3 per serve)

NUTRITION ANALYSIS
PER SERVE
Total kJ: 1494 kJ
Carbohydrates: 44.0 g
Fat: 17.0 g
Saturated fat: 9.6 g
Protein: 6.0 g
Fibre: 4.1 g

Carrot, sultana and walnut muffins

1 cup wholemeal self-raising flour
¾ cup self-raising flour
⅓ cup brown sugar
1½ teaspoons ground cinnamon
¾ cup orange juice
2 tablespoons light sour cream
1 egg
½ cup finely grated carrot
⅓ cup sultanas
2 tablespoons chopped walnuts

Preheat oven to 180°C (350°F).

Mix both types of flour, sugar and cinnamon in a large bowl. In a separate bowl combine orange juice, sour cream and egg.

Fold the mixture into the flour, add carrot, sultanas and walnuts and stir until well combined. Spoon into a greased muffin tin and bake for 20 minutes until golden and firm to the touch.

Makes 10 muffins

NUTRITION ANALYSIS
PER SERVE
Total kJ: 805 kJ
Carbohydrates: 33.2 g
Fat: 3.3 g
Saturated fat: 0.9 g
Protein: 5.4 g
Fibre: 3.8 g

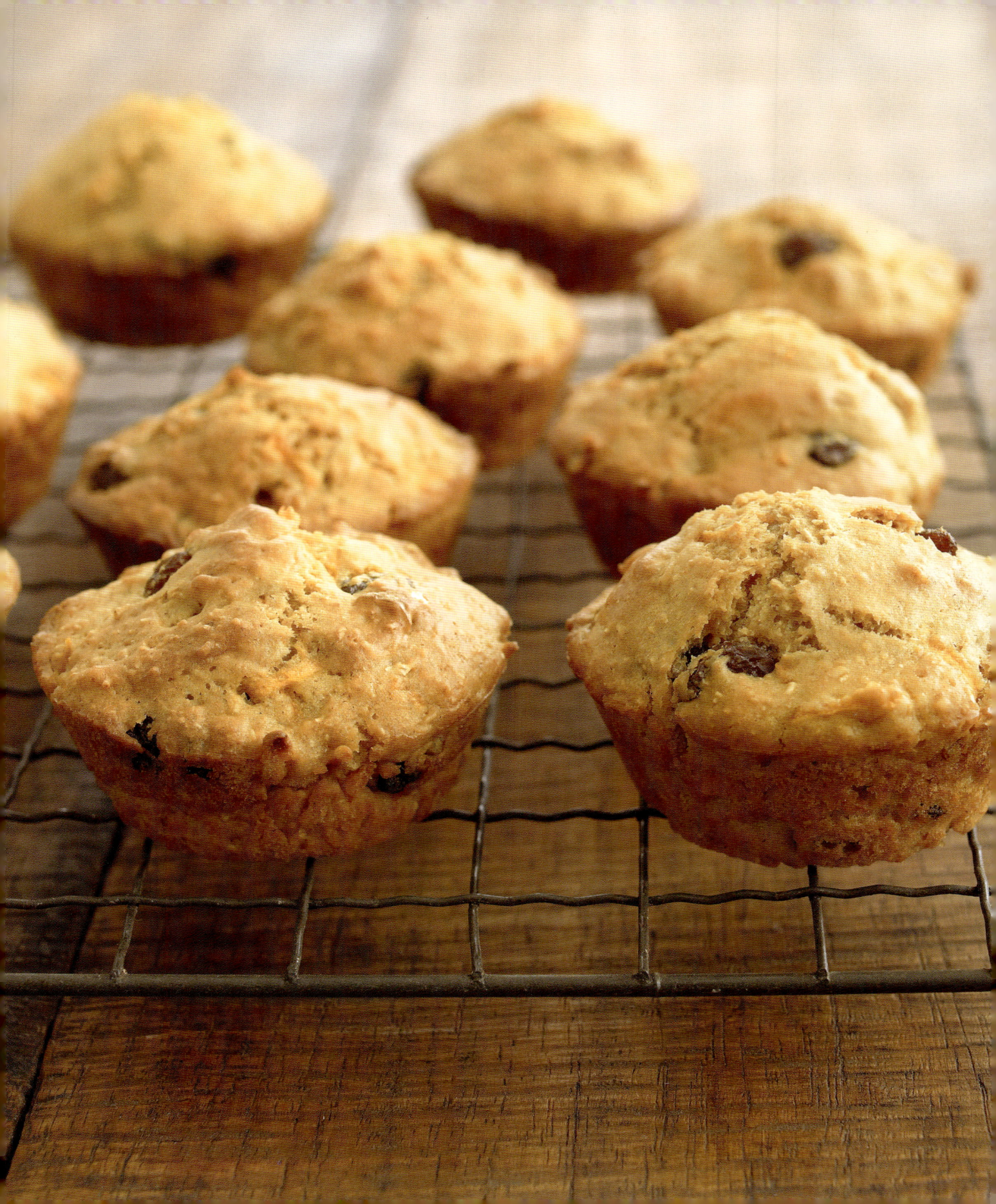

Date, almond and orange slice

250 g pitted dates
1 cup orange juice
rind of 1 orange
125 g butter
1 cup brown sugar
2 eggs
1 cup wholemeal self-raising flour
1 cup almond meal
olive oil spray
¼ cup flaked almonds

Preheat oven to 180°C (350°F).

Gently bring the dates, orange juice and rind to the boil in a small saucepan. Reduce heat to a simmer and cook for a further 8 minutes, stirring occasionally, until the mixture thickens. Take off the heat.

Beat the butter and sugar together until creamy. Mix in the eggs, flour and almond meal.

Spray an 18 x 28 cm cake tin lightly with oil. Pour half the batter into the tin and smooth to 1½ cm thickness.

Add the almonds to the date mixture, combine well and spread over the layer of batter. Top with the remaining batter and smooth the surface. Bake in the oven for 30 minutes until puffed and golden.

Leave in the tin to cool for 10 minutes before slicing.

Makes 16 pieces (2 per serve)

NUTRITION ANALYSIS
PER SERVE
Total kJ: 1967 kJ
Carbohydrates: 52.0 g
Fat: 24.0 g
Saturated fat: 9.6 g
Protein: 9.2 g
Fibre: 6.4 g

Index

accountability 38, 46, 72
aerobics 68
affirmations 5
alcohol 33, 34, 35
amino acids 56
animal protein 31
apples
　Apple and carrot buzz 150
　Apple and mango frappé 232
　Apple and rhubarb crumble 232
　Stewed apple and rhubarb 155
Apricot, ginger and honey cookies 239
Asian greens
　Crisp-skinned salmon with lemon and Asian greens 220
asparagus
　Tuna and asparagus salad 182
attitude
　and exercise 75
　and successful weight loss 12, 16–17, 47
avocado
　Avocado and fetta salsa 158
　Prawns with avocado and mango salsa 214

Bacon, lentil and tomato soup 168
bad days 23
Banana smoothie 149
basil
　Zucchini, tomato and basil frittata 186
beans, canned
　Spiced bean loaf 227

beef
　Beef stir-fry with hokkien noodles 201
　Grilled eye fillet with mustard polenta 203
　Spicy beef and mushroom kebabs 190
　Steak sandwich 206
　Thai beef salad 204
beetroot
　Chicken, beetroot and walnut salad 176
berries
　Berry and mint sorbet 236
　Berry compote 157
　Berry–mint smoothie 150
Biggest Loser, The
　7 Steps to fitness success 72–75
　10 Steps to weight-loss success 37–47
　eating plans 27–59, 65, 88–91, 97–127
　exercise plans 61–79, 92–95, 108–119, 119–126
　menu plans 88–89, 102–107
　recipes 165–217
　values 2
Bircher muesli 152
blood pressure 4
blood sugar levels 4, 42, 53, 54–55
BMI see Body Mass Index
body fat, distribution of 6
Body Mass Index (BMI) 7
Braised lamb shanks with lentil and onion stew 210
breakfast 42
Buckwheat pancakes 157

caffeinated drinks 35
cancer 4
carbohydrates 53–56
　complex (starches) 53
　dietary fibre 55
　GI and GL scales 54–55
　simple (sugars) 53
cardiovascular training 92, 108, 110–113, 122–123
carrot
　Apple and carrot buzz 150
　Carrot, sultana and walnut muffins 240
casseroles
　Braised lamb shanks with lentil and onion stew 210
　Chicken cacciatore 195
　Lamb and barley hotpot 172
cereals
　Bircher muesli 152
　Porridge 154
　Tropical muesli 149
cheese
　Avocado and fetta salsa 158
　Chickpea, fetta and coriander tarts 184
chicken
　Chicken and cashew stir-fry 198
　Chicken and spinach lasagne 200
　Chicken, beetroot and walnut salad 176
　Chicken cacciatore 195
　Chicken san choy bau 196
　Chicken stock 167
Chickpea, fetta and coriander tarts 184
children 51
chillies
　Harissa dressing 180

cholesterol 57
    HDL (high-density lipoprotein) cholesterol 57
    LDL (low-density lipoprotein) cholesterol 4, 56
coffee *see* caffeinated drinks
competition 47
cookies
    Apricot, ginger and honey cookies 239
cooking for health 98–100
coriander
    Chickpea, fetta and coriander tarts 184
    Corn fritters with smoked salmon and coriander dressing 189
couscous
    Roasted vegetable and couscous salad 175
    Spiced vegetable ratatouille with couscous 230
Crisp-skinned salmon with lemon and Asian greens 220
cycling 69

dairy protein (low fat) 32
dance 69
Date, almond and orange slice 242
desserts
    Apple and mango frappé 232
    Apple and rhubarb crumble 232
    Berry and mint sorbet 236
    Passionfruit soufflés 234
    Pear and coconut spring rolls 235
detox plans 48
diabetes (type 2) vii, 4, 54, 58
dietary fibre 55–56
dressings 175, 176, 179, 180, 182, 187, 204, 222

    Coriander dressing 189
    Harissa dressing 180
dried fruit
    Apricot, ginger and honey cookies 239
    Winter fruit compote 152
drinks 34–35
    Apple and carrot buzz 150
    Banana smoothie 149
    Berry–mint smoothie 150
    Mango lassi 236

eating
    Biggest Loser Eating Plan 27–59
    changing behaviour 12–17, 43, 45
    eating out 44
    healthy eating 3, 27, 53
    poor choices 12
    regular eating 42
    see also habits
eggs
    Italian omelette 160
    Passionfruit soufflés 234
    Scrambled eggs with smoked salmon 162
    Spanish-style baked eggs 164
    Zucchini, tomato and basil frittata 186
emotional eating 8, 38
    strategies for dealing with 9
    triggers for 8–9
energy 28
    and daily activity level 29
    and food 29, 53, 57
    and metabolism 28–29
    energy deficit 30, 59
exercise 45
    appropriate level 64, 108
    benefits of 63
    Biggest Loser Exercise Plans 61–79

    food 76
    KickStart Plan 92–95
    LifeStyle Plan 108–119, 119–126
    reasons for 62
    safe exercise 76
    types of exercise 68–69
    warm-ups and cool-downs 77, 92, 108, 110, 120
    where to start 66
    which is best 67
    see also habits, specific exercises

fad diets 13
fat 57
    cholesterol 57
    saturated fats 58
    trans fatty acids 58
    unsaturated fats 58
fat-soluble vitamins *see* vitamins
fatty acids 58
Fennel and orange salad 180
fertility problems 4
fish
    Ocean trout panzanella salad 216
    Sardines Provençale 218
    Snapper with Greek salad 222
    Swordfish with roast tomato and rocket salad 224
    Tuna and asparagus salad 182
    see also specific fish
fitness 67
    7 Steps to fitness success 72–75
food addiction 11
food, daily requirements *see* energy
food diary 9, 38

fruit 31, 53
    Lamb and pine nut pizza 192
    Passionfruit soufflés 234
    Winter fruit compote 152
    see also dried fruit; specific fruit

gallstones 4
GI see glycaemic index
GL see glycaemic load
glycaemic index 54
glycaemic load 54
goals 12, 18–19, 22, 38
    being realistic 18, 74
    exercise 74
    long-term 18, 22
    medium-term 22
    mini-goals 19
    'owning' 21
    short-term 4, 19, 22
    weight 4, 37
glucose see blood sugar
Grilled eye fillet with mustard polenta 203
guilt 23
gyms 70–71

habits, changing 3, 9, 12, 15–17, 37–47, 66, 73
Harissa dressing 180
HDL (high-density lipoprotein) cholesterol 57
healthy eating 3, 27, 53
    carbohydrates 53
    fats 57–58
    minerals 59
    proteins 56
    vitamins 59
    see also cooking for health
healthy 'extras' 33
healthy food 39
healthy weight range 6–7
heart disease vii, 4, 42, 56, 58

heart rate 79
heart-rate monitors 78
Herb-crusted grilled pork 212
herbs
    Herb-crusted grilled pork 212
    see also specific herbs
hydrogenated fats see trans fatty acids

insulin 54
Italian omelette 160

KickStart Plan 30, 48, 65, 83–95
    exercise program 92–95
    menu plans 88–91
    shopping lists 84–86
kilojoule counter book 30
kilojoules
    energy deficit 30, 59
    'extra' foods 11, 32
    food as source 28
    menu plans 88–91, 102–107
    overconsumption 28–30, 43, 50
    see also energy

lamb
    Braised lamb shanks with lentil and onion stew 210
    Lamb and barley hotpot 172
    Lamb and pine nut pizza 192
    Spiced lamb pockets 187
    Yoghurt-marinated lamb cutlets 209
LDL (low-density lipoprotein) cholesterol 56
lemon
    Crisp-skinned salmon with lemon and Asian greens 220
lentils
    Bacon, lentil and tomato soup 168
    Braised lamb shanks with lentil and onion stew 210

Spiced bean loaf 227
lifestyle habits 3
LifeStyle Plan 50, 65, 97–127
    cooking for health 98–100
    exercise programs 108–119, 119–126
    menu plans 102–107

mango
    Apple and mango frappé 232
    Mango lassi 236
    Prawns with avocado and mango salsa 214
marinades 190, 198, 201, 204
    Yoghurt marinade 209
meal planning 41
meal replacements 43
medications and weight gain 9
mental health 5
menu plans
    KickStart Plan 88–91
    LifeStyle Plan 102–107
metabolism 28, 42
Mifflin calculation 29
milk 53
minerals 59
mint
    Berry and mint sorbet 236
    Berry–mint smoothie 150
    Minted pea soup 171
    Yoghurt-marinated lamb cutlets 209
modifying recipes see cooking for health
monounsaturated fats see unsaturated fats
muffins
    Carrot, sultana and walnut muffins 240
mushrooms
    Slow-roasted garlic mushrooms 158

Spicy beef and mushroom
    kebabs 190

Nachos 207
Napoli sauce 182
noodles
    Beef stir-fry with hokkien
        noodles 201
nutrition labels 40
nutrition requirements 31, 42
nuts
    Carrot, sultana and walnut
        muffins 240
    Chicken and cashew stir-fry
        198
    Chicken, beetroot and walnut
        salad 176
    Date, almond and orange slice
        242

obesity 4, 42, 53, 58
    health risks 4
    incidence in Australia 6
    psychological problems 5
Ocean trout panzanella salad
    216
omega 3 fats see fatty acids
omega 6 fats see fatty acids
omega 9 fats see unsaturated fats
onions
    Braised lamb shanks with lentil
        and onion stew 210
oranges
    Date, almond and orange slice
        242
    Fennel and orange salad 180
organisation 40–41
osteoarthritis 4
overeating 8
    reasons for 8–10
    strategies for avoiding 11
    see also emotional eating
overweight

associated health risks 4
causes of 8–11
incidence in Australia 6
see also obesity

pancakes and fritters
    Buckwheat pancakes 157
    Corn fritters with smoked
        salmon and coriander
        dressing 189
Passionfruit soufflés 234
pastries, savoury
    Chickpea, fetta and coriander
        tarts 184
pastries, sweet
    Pear and coconut spring rolls
        235
pears
    Pear and coconut spring rolls
        235
    Spiced poached pears 155
peas
    Minted pea soup 171
personal trainer, finding 73
polenta 203
polycystic ovarian syndrome 4
polyunsaturated fats see
    unsaturated fats
pork
    Herb-crusted grilled pork 212
Porridge 154
portion size 28, 31–33, 43
positive thinking see attitude
Prawns with avocado and mango
    salsa 214
pregnancy 4, 49
prescription drugs (to aid weight
    loss) 52
professional support 47, 48
protein foods 31, 56–57
    complete 56
    incomplete 56

resistance band 114
resistance exercises, circuit
    134–142
resistance exercises, gym
    143–145
resistance training 92, 108,
    114–118, 123–126
resting metabolic rate (RMR)
    29, 50
rewards systems 10, 20
rhubarb
    Apple and rhubarb crumble
        232
    Stewed apple and rhubarb
        155
rice
    Vegetables stuffed with spiced
        rice 228
RMR see resting metabolic rate
Roasted vegetable and couscous
    salad 175
running 69

salads
    Chicken, beetroot and walnut
        salad 176
    Fennel and orange salad 180
    Greek salad 222
    Ocean trout panzanella salad
        216
    Roasted vegetable and
        couscous salad 175
    Swordfish with roast tomato
        and rocket salad 224
    Tabbouleh 179
    Thai beef salad 204
salmon
    Corn fritters with smoked salmon
        and coriander dressing 189
    Crisp-skinned salmon with
        lemon and Asian greens 220
    Scrambled eggs with smoked
        salmon 162

sandwiches and wraps
   Spiced lamb pockets 187
   Steak sandwich 206
Sardines Provençale 218
saturated fats 58
sauces
   Avocado and mango salsa 214
   for Nachos 207
   Napoli sauce 182
Scrambled eggs with smoked salmon 162
seafood
   Prawns with avocado and mango salsa 214
self-monitoring see accountability
shopping 41, 84–86
side-effects 48
skipping meals 42
sleep apnoea 4
Slow-roasted garlic mushrooms 158
Snapper with Greek salad 222
soft drinks 53
solution-focused approach 20
soups
   Bacon, lentil and tomato soup 168
   Lamb and barley hotpot 172
   Minted pea soup 171
Spanish-style baked eggs 164
Spiced bean loaf 227
Spiced lamb pockets 187
Spiced poached pears 155
Spiced vegetable ratatouille with couscous 230
Spice mix 230
Spicy beef and mushroom kebabs 190
spinach
   Chicken and spinach lasagne 200
sport 69

starches 53
Steak sandwich 206
Stewed apple and rhubarb 155
stir-fries
   Beef stir-fry with hokkien noodles 201
   Chicken and cashew stir-fry 198
stocks
   Chicken stock 167
   Vegetable stock 167
stress incontinence 4
stretch exercises 130–133
stroke, risks of 4
sugars 53
support systems 38, 46–47, 73
surgery 52
swimming 68
Swordfish with roast tomato and rocket salad 224

Tabbouleh 179
TEE see total energy expenditure
Thai beef salad 204
thermic effect of food 29
tomatoes
   Bacon, lentil and tomato soup 168
   Napoli sauce 182
   Swordfish with roast tomato and rocket salad 224
   Zucchini, tomato and basil frittata 186
total energy expenditure (TEE) 28, 29
training diary 72
trans fatty acids 58
treats 33
Tropical muesli 149
Tuna and asparagus salad 182

unsaturated fats 58

Vegetable stock 167
vegetables 31
   Chicken and spinach lasagne 200
   Roasted vegetable and couscous salad 175
   Spiced vegetable ratatouille with couscous 230
   Vegetable stock 167
   Vegetables stuffed with spiced rice 228
   see also specific vegetables
vegetarian protein 32, 56
very low energy diets 48
vitamins 59
VLED see very low energy diets

waist-to-hip ratio 7
walking 69
water 34, 48, 77
water-soluble vitamins see vitamins
weigh-ins 37, 47
weight circumference 6
weight loss
   10 Steps to Success 37–47
   benefits of 4
   children and 51
   eating to lose weight 30
   exercise and 12, 15
   how to achieve 12–17
   long-term 12
   maintaining 50–51
   mental attitude and 3, 12
   other weight-loss options 52
   reasons for 2
   safe rapid 48
   solution-focused approach 20
   see also The KickStart Plan
weight-loss groups see support systems
wholefoods see healthy food
wholegrains 32, 53

Winter fruit compote 152
wraps see sandwiches

yoga 69
yoghurt 53
    Banana smoothie 149
    Bircher muesli 152
    Mango lassi 236
    Yoghurt-marinated lamb
        cutlets 209

zucchini
    Zucchini, tomato and basil
        frittata 186